Cardiopulmonary Resuscitation: Clinical Updates and Perspectives

Cardiopulmonary Resuscitation: Clinical Updates and Perspectives

Editors

Timur Sellmann
Stephan Marsch

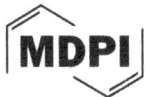

Basel • Beijing • Wuhan • Barcelona • Belgrade • Novi Sad • Cluj • Manchester

Editors
Timur Sellmann
Ev. Krankenhaus BETHESDA
zu Duisburg GmbH
Duisburg
Germany

Stephan Marsch
University Hospital Basel
Basel
Switzerland

Editorial Office
MDPI AG
Grosspeteranlage 5
4052 Basel, Switzerland

This is a reprint of articles from the Special Issue published online in the open access journal *Journal of Clinical Medicine* (ISSN 2077-0383) (available at: https://www.mdpi.com/journal/jcm/special_issues/cardiopulmonary_resuscitation).

For citation purposes, cite each article independently as indicated on the article page online and as indicated below:

Lastname, A.A.; Lastname, B.B. Article Title. *Journal Name* **Year**, *Volume Number*, Page Range.

ISBN 978-3-7258-1821-1 (Hbk)
ISBN 978-3-7258-1822-8 (PDF)
doi.org/10.3390/books978-3-7258-1822-8

© 2024 by the authors. Articles in this book are Open Access and distributed under the Creative Commons Attribution (CC BY) license. The book as a whole is distributed by MDPI under the terms and conditions of the Creative Commons Attribution-NonCommercial-NoDerivs (CC BY-NC-ND) license.

Contents

About the Editors vii

Stephan Marsch and Timur Sellmann
Cardiopulmonary Resuscitation: Clinical Updates and Perspectives
Reprinted from: *J. Clin. Med.* **2024**, *13*, 2717, doi:10.3390/jcm13092717 1

Jan Schmitz, Anton Ahlbäck, James DuCanto, Steffen Kerkhoff, Matthieu Komorowski, Vanessa Löw, et al.
Randomized Comparison of Two New Methods for Chest Compressions during CPR in Microgravity—A Manikin Study
Reprinted from: *J. Clin. Med.* **2022**, *11*, 646, doi:10.3390/jcm11030646 6

Jochen Hinkelbein, Lydia Kolaparambil Varghese Johnson, Nikolai Kiselev, Jan Schmitz, Martin Hellmich, Hendrik Drinhaus, et al.
Proteomics-Based Serum Alterations of the Human Protein Expression after Out-of-Hospital Cardiac Arrest: Pilot Study for Prognostication of Survivors vs. Non-Survivors at Day 1 after Return of Spontaneous Circulation (ROSC)
Reprinted from: *J. Clin. Med.* **2022**, *11*, 996, doi:10.3390/jcm11040996 17

Eujene Jung, Young Sun Ro, Jeong Ho Park, Hyun Ho Ryu and Sang Do Shin
Direct Transport to Cardiac Arrest Center and Survival Outcomes after Out-of-Hospital Cardiac Arrest by Urbanization Level
Reprinted from: *J. Clin. Med.* **2022**, *11*, 1033, doi:10.3390/jcm11041033 30

Cheng-Ying Chiang, Ket-Cheong Lim, Pei Chun Lai, Tou-Yuan Tsai, Yen Ta Huang and Ming-Jen Tsai
Comparison between Prehospital Mechanical Cardiopulmonary Resuscitation (CPR) Devices and Manual CPR for Out-of-Hospital Cardiac Arrest: A Systematic Review, Meta-Analysis, and Trial Sequential Analysis
Reprinted from: *J. Clin. Med.* **2022**, *11*, 1448, doi:10.3390/jcm11051448 41

Kevin Kunz, Sirak Petros, Sebastian Ewens, Maryam Yahiaoui-Doktor, Timm Denecke, Manuel Florian Struck and Sebastian Krämer
Chest Compression-Related Flail Chest Is Associated with Prolonged Ventilator Weaning in Cardiac Arrest Survivors
Reprinted from: *J. Clin. Med.* **2022**, *11*, 2071, doi:10.3390/jcm11082071 56

Sam Joé Brixius, Jan-Steffen Pooth, Jörg Haberstroh, Domagoj Damjanovic, Christian Scherer, Philipp Greiner, et al.
Beneficial Effects of Adjusted Perfusion and Defibrillation Strategies on Rhythm Control within Controlled Automated Reperfusion of the Whole Body (CARL) for Refractory Out-of-Hospital Cardiac Arrest
Reprinted from: *J. Clin. Med.* **2022**, *11*, 2111, doi:10.3390/jcm11082111 64

Timur Sellmann, Andrea Oendorf, Dietmar Wetzchewald, Heidrun Schwager, Serge Christian Thal and Stephan Marsch
The Impact of Withdrawn vs. Agitated Relatives during Resuscitation on Team Workload: A Single-Center Randomised Simulation-Based Study
Reprinted from: *J. Clin. Med.* **2022**, *11*, 3163, doi:10.3390/jcm11113163 78

Sangsoo Han, Hye Ji Park, Won Jung Jeong, Gi Woon Kim, Han Joo Choi, Hyung Jun Moon, et al.
Application of the Team Emergency Assessment Measure for Prehospital Cardiopulmonary Resuscitation
Reprinted from: *J. Clin. Med.* **2022**, *11*, 5390, doi:10.3390/jcm11185390 89

Timur Sellmann, Maria Nur, Dietmar Wetzchewald, Heidrun Schwager, Corvin Cleff, Serge C. Thal and Stephan Marsch
COVID-19 CPR—Impact of Personal Protective Equipment during a Simulated Cardiac Arrest in Times of the COVID-19 Pandemic: A Prospective Comparative Trial
Reprinted from: *J. Clin. Med.* **2022**, *11*, 5881, doi:10.3390/jcm11195881 97

Stephan Katzenschlager, Erik Popp, Jan Wnent, Markus A. Weigand and Jan-Thorsten Gräsner
Developments in Post-Resuscitation Care for Out-of-Hospital Cardiac Arrests in Adults—A Narrative Review
Reprinted from: *J. Clin. Med.* **2023**, *12*, 3009, doi:10.3390/jcm12083009 106

Sascha Macherey-Meyer, Sebastian Heyne, Max M. Meertens, Simon Braumann, Stephan F. Niessen, Stephan Baldus, et al.
Outcome of Out-of-Hospital Cardiac Arrest Patients Stratified by Pre-Clinical Loading with Aspirin and Heparin: A Retrospective Cohort Analysis
Reprinted from: *J. Clin. Med.* **2023**, *12*, 3817, doi:10.3390/jcm12113817 117

Anne-Kathrin Dathe, Anja Stein, Nora Bruns, Elena-Diana Craciun, Laura Tuda, Johanna Bialas, et al.
Early Prediction of Mortality after Birth Asphyxia with the nSOFA
Reprinted from: *J. Clin. Med.* **2023**, *12*, 4322, doi:10.3390/jcm12134322 128

Domagoj Damjanovic, Jan-Steffen Pooth, Yechi Liu, Fabienne Frensch, Martin Wolkewitz, Joerg Haberstroh, et al.
The Impact of Head Position on Neurological and Histopathological Outcome Following Controlled Automated Reperfusion of the Whole Body (CARL) in a Pig Model
Reprinted from: *J. Clin. Med.* **2023**, *12*, 7054, doi:10.3390/jcm12227054 142

About the Editors

Timur Sellmann

Timur Sellmann is a distinguished researcher currently serving as Head of Department at the Department of Anesthesiology and Intensive Care Medicine at Ev. Krankenhaus BETHESDA zu Duisburg. With a keen interest in cardiopulmonary resuscitation (CPR) and emergency care, Dr. Sellmann's work focuses on enhancing clinical outcomes through innovative research and advanced training methodologies. His current projects include the development of high-fidelity simulation models for CPR training, aimed at improving the skillset and decision-making abilities of healthcare providers in high-stress situations.

Dr. Sellmann's scientific interests encompass a broad range of topics within emergency medicine, particularly the optimization of pre-hospital care and post-resuscitation interventions. He is actively involved in research exploring the integration of artificial intelligence into emergency response systems and the utilization of telemedicine to improve early intervention strategies.

Throughout his career, Dr. Sellmann has been recognized for his contributions to the field with several awards. His dedication to advancing CPR practices and emergency care protocols has made him a prominent figure in his field, continually pushing the boundaries of medical research and practices.

Stephan Marsch

Until 2024, Stephan Marsch was the Professor of Intensive Care at the University of Basel and Chairman of the Intensive Care Unit at the University Hospital of Basel, Switzerland. Between 2010 and 2018, he served as Study Dean of the Medical Faculty of the University of Basel and was a member of the commission responsible for the Swiss Federal Licencing Exam in human medicine. His main scientific interest concerns human factors in medical emergencies, particularly in cardiopulmonary resuscitation. Together with his research group, he has conducted numerous simulation-based studies in this field, focusing predominantly on leadership, team-building, and gender.

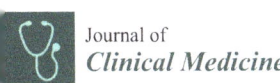

Editorial

Cardiopulmonary Resuscitation: Clinical Updates and Perspectives

Stephan Marsch [1] and Timur Sellmann [2,3,*]

[1] Department of Intensive Care, University Hospital, 4031 Basel, Switzerland; stephan.marsch@usb.ch
[2] Department of Anaesthesiology and Intensive Care Medicine, Bethesda Hospital, 47053 Duisburg, Germany
[3] Department of Anaesthesiology 1, Witten/Herdecke University, 58455 Witten, Germany
* Correspondence: timursellmann@yahoo.com

Cardiopulmonary resuscitation (CPR) stands as a cornerstone in emergency care, representing the crucial link between life and death for victims of cardiac arrest. Over the years, advancements in medical knowledge, technology, and training methodologies have propelled CPR into a dynamic field with continuous updates. In this closing editorial of the Special Issue "Cardiopulmonary Resuscitation: Clinical Updates and Perspectives", we sum up the major findings of the published articles. Nineteen manuscripts were submitted for consideration for the Special Issue, with thirteen papers finally accepted for publication and inclusion (eleven research articles and two reviews). The contributions as an overview of the published articles are listed below.

1. Simulation/Education

Effective CPR is an arduous task that requires skill, precision, and quick decision making—it is a stressful task per se. In view of the substantial evidence and the importance of simulation research, documented by high-ranking publications [1], innovative "high volume/high fidelity" simulation models are currently being developed. Models such as those enable us to measure the effectiveness of medical education and training methods in simulated CPR and to publish the results to increase the scope of available evidence and the visibility of scientific projects. Simulation models enable us to investigate relevant CPR questions using state-of-the-art methodology, avoiding methodological, logistical, and ethical challenges that would arise in studies with real patients. High-fidelity mannequins, virtual reality, and immersive scenarios nowadays enable healthcare providers to experience almost perfect realistic resuscitation situations. In this Special Issue, two papers on simulated cardiac circulation dealt with the effect of potential distractors on the overall performance of the teams during resuscitation. While both studies showed that randomly present relatives with different behavioral patterns (withdrawn or agitated) or carrying personal protective equipment (PPE) mentally stress the teams (measured by the NASA Task Load Index), no poorer performance during CPR could be demonstrated, at least for relatives' presence. For PPE, on the other hand, both the stress level and the significantly poorer performance are surprising, as the data were generated in 2021, i.e., after more than 2 years of pandemic experience. This made it possible to present results that might not have been intuitively expected. Simulation remains an ideal tool for analyzing special situations (e.g., rare, extremely time-consuming, and time-sensitive scenarios). Schmitz and colleagues broke new ground with their study first describing resuscitation in microgravity. Scientific findings such as these have the potential to become part of current guideline recommendations, for example in the "CPR under special circumstances" chapter of the ERC [2], especially considering the increasing number of manned space flights. One logical further development would now be the integration of artificial intelligence to (a) either further improve the simulation scenarios, (b) further support teams during a simulated CPR, or (c) both. This individualized approach enhances competence and confidence in performing CPR, ultimately translating into improved patient outcomes.

2. Prehospital Care

The initial phase of cardiac arrest is most decisive for patients' outcomes. As such, innovations in prehospital care are essential for improving overall survival rates. Different mobile technologies such as the integration of automated external defibrillators (AEDs) [3] into public spaces and the utilization of drone technology for rapid AED delivery to remote locations are transforming the landscape of prehospital care [4]. Additionally, telemedicine has enabled real-time communication between emergency medical services (EMSs) and healthcare providers, allowing for the early identification of potential cardiac events and the initiation of care even before the patient reaches the hospital [5]. In this context, four publications dealt with the prehospital treatment of cardiac arrest victims. Out-of-hospital cardiac arrest (OHCA) has a high prevalence of obstructive coronary artery disease and total coronary occlusion. Macherey-Meyer and colleagues were able to demonstrate for the first time that prehospital loading with antiplatelets and anticoagulants did not increase bleeding rates and was associated with favorable survival. They also found overtreatment of non-ischemic victims as well as undertreatment of ischemic victims, concluding that loading without definite diagnosis of sustained ischemia remains debatable until more data are available. Several skills have been identified as critical for ensuring patient safety such as communication and teamwork. The Team Emergency Assessment Measure (TEAM) questionnaire is designed to rate the non-technical performance of emergency medical teams during emergencies, e.g., resuscitation or trauma management. Originally developed in Australia, it has today been translated into and validated in more than 10 languages [6].

Han et al. were able to show high reliability (Cronbach's alpha of 0.939; mean interitem correlation of 0.584) and a good concurrent validity (0.682), both indications of significant association (mean item–total correlation of 0.789), as well as excellent agreement (mean intra-class correlation coefficient of 0.804), making the TEAM approach a valid and reliable tool to evaluate the non-technical skills of a team of paramedics performing CPR. Regarding the selection of the target hospital, the research group of Jung and colleagues once again succeeded in highlighting the importance of the cardiac arrest centers (CACs) recommended in the current guidelines. Thus, patients in the CAC group had a significantly higher likelihood of good neurological recovery and survival to discharge compared to the non-CAC group. The fact that only around a quarter of the approximate 96,000 patients were transported to CACs is somewhat saddening. We remain hopeful that the results of this work will help to change this. Finally, Chiang et al. offered more insight into the ongoing debate about the role of mechanical CPR devices in OHCA, concluding that their use may benefit adults who have suffered OHCA in achieving ROSC and survival to admission. But they also concluded that due to the low certainty of evidence, more well-designed large-scale randomized controlled trials are needed to validate these findings.

3. Post-Resuscitation Care

Post-resuscitation care plays a crucial role in neurological outcome and overall recovery. As the incidence of OHCA is high and the survival rate is low, it remains a challenge to treat those who survive the first phase and regain spontaneous circulation. In a previous narrative review, the authors summarized the existing evidence on oxygen dosage, the role of noradrenaline in urine output and blood pressure, and blood pressure targets themselves. Furthermore, they offered the prospect of experimental approaches to improve neuroprognostication, which includes various approaches like bundles and novel biomarkers. While whole-blood transcriptome analysis has been shown to reliably predict neurological survival in two feasibility studies, Hinkelbein et al. were unable to prognosticate survival or non-survival after OHCA based on proteomics-based serum alterations in the human protein expression, at least not in the first 24 h after ROSC. However, since a good neurological outcome is essential, advancements in neuroprognostication as well as the integration of neuroimaging, biochemical markers, and electrophysiological assessments are vital to refine prognostic accuracy and thus aid clinicians in making informed decisions regarding the continuation or withdrawal of aggressive interventions [7]. Injuries related to CPR are a frequent finding in cardiac arrest victims. These include bony and parenchymal organ injuries [8]. The most common injuries frequently found are chest wall injuries [8], but if and to what extent these CPR-associated chest wall injuries contribute to a delay in the respiratory recovery of cardiac arrest survivors has not been sufficiently explored. Kunz and colleagues examined surviving intensive care unit (ICU) patients who had undergone CPR due to medical reasons in their single-center retrospective cohort study in relation to the existence of CPR-associated chest wall injuries, detected by chest radiography and computed tomography. Over a third of all included patients presented with chest wall injuries, including flail chest in 9%. Through the multivariable logistic regression analysis, the authors were able to identify flail chest to be independently associated with the need for tracheostomy (OR 15.5). In the linear regression analysis, pneumonia and fractured ribs were associated with an increased ICU length of stay, whereas flail chest and pneumonia were associated with a prolonged duration of mechanical ventilation. It was interesting to see that four patients with flail chest who underwent surgical rib stabilization could be weaned successfully from the ventilator afterwards. This means that surgical treatment of rib fractures could represent a valuable therapeutic option in this population. As the results of this study suggest, CPR-associated chest wall injuries, flail chest in particular, may impair the respiratory recovery of cardiac arrest survivors in the ICU. These findings make this study a valuable addition to the body of clinical data but need to be confirmed in larger trials.

4. Excursion: Controlled Automated Reperfusion of the Whole Body (CARL)

In the context mentioned above, the CARL system offers interesting and physiologically comprehensible and fascinating approaches, which have also been positively confirmed in initial reports. CARL therapy (or targeted extracorporeal CPR) consists of core elements such as the control of physical reperfusion conditions (blood pressure, blood flow, pulsatility, and blood temperature), the situational modification of the reperfusion solution, usually recirculating the blood, by adjusting the oxygen and carbon dioxide content, the pH value, the electrolyte content, and the osmolarity, as well as quickly available, comprehensive monitoring. The focus is on preparing the tissue damaged by the lack of oxygen for the resumption of the body's own blood circulation [9] (see also Figure 1). The CARL concept constitutes a new frontier in resuscitation science by focusing on the controlled restoration of blood flow following cardiac arrest, where a pulsatile flow is used instead of a continuous flow within the framework of an ECPR, aiming to minimize reperfusion injury and optimize organ recovery within an individualized therapeutic regimen. This approach involves the precise regulation of blood pressure, oxygenation, and perfusion rates during the reperfusion phase [9]. CARL represents a paradigm shift, challenging traditional beliefs about the immediate and aggressive restoration of blood flow. By carefully managing the reperfusion process, CARL seeks to mitigate the harmful effects associated with the abrupt reintroduction of oxygen to ischemic tissues. Ongoing research and clinical trials are exploring the potential of CARL to enhance survival rates and improve long-term outcomes in post-cardiac arrest patients. In this Special Issue, the research group led by Trummer published two experimental studies. The first study compared the CARL model directly to ECPR in refractory OHCA. By using CARL, not only were spontaneous rhythm conversions observed using a modified priming solution, but the application of potassium-induced secondary cardioplegia also proved to be a safe and effective method for sustained rhythm conversion. Finally, significantly fewer defibrillation attempts were needed, and cardiac arrhythmias were reduced during reperfusion via CARL. In their second animal model study, the authors were able to demonstrate a highly significant favorable neurological outcome for animals with head elevation during the first 20 min of post-resuscitation care, whereas histopathologic findings did not show corresponding differences between the groups. A possible explanation for the transient neurologic deficits potentially attributable to functions localized in the posterior perfusion area may be venous congestion and edema as modifiable contributing factors of neurologic injury following prolonged cardiac arrest.

We hope that the results of this interesting technique in humans are just as promising as those obtained so far in the animal model.

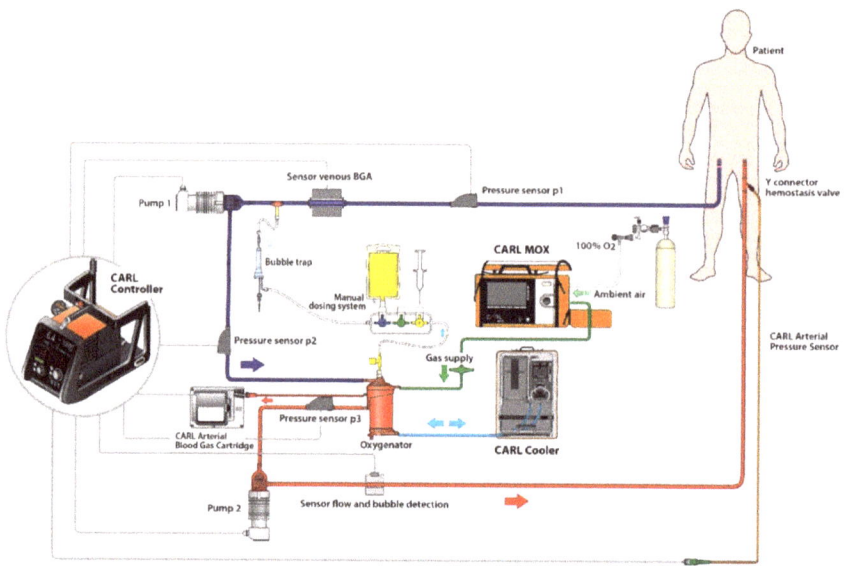

Figure 1. A schematic representation of the CARL (Controlled Automated Reperfusion of the Whole Body) operating principle. The right to use the image was granted by Prof. Dr. med. Georg Trummer as a consultant of Resuscitec GmbH for the "Medical" sector. BGA: blood gas, MOX: mobile oxygenator.

5. Pediatrics

While the principles of CPR remain consistent across age groups, pediatric resuscitation presents unique challenges and considerations. Recognizing the differences in anatomy, physiology, and the underlying causes of cardiac arrest in children is paramount for successful outcomes [10,11]. Educational programs must address the specific needs of healthcare providers dealing with pediatric populations, emphasizing the importance of age-appropriate techniques and interventions [10–12]. Birth asphyxia is a major cause of delivery room resuscitation. Subsequent organ failure and hypoxic–ischemic encephalopathy (HIE) account for 25% of all early post-natal deaths. In neonatal sepsis, the nSOFA (neonatal sequential organ failure assessment) considers platelet count as well as respiratory and cardiovascular dysfunction. In this Special Issue, Dathe et al. evaluated the nSOFA for the first time in cases of resuscitation regarding its potential as a useful predictor for in-hospital mortality in neonates ($\geq$36 + 0 weeks of gestation) following asphyxia with HIE and therapeutic hypothermia. The nSOfA scores for survivors were lower overall, as were their respiratory, cardiovascular, and hematologic sub-scores compared to non-survivors. The odds ratio for mortality was 1.6 [95% CI = 1.2–2.1] per one-point increase in the nSOFA and the optimal cut-off value of the nSOFA to predict mortality was 3.5 (sensitivity of 100.0%; specificity of 83.9%). With the help of their results, the authors were able to prove that an early nSOFA ($\leq$6 h of life) offers the possibility of identifying infants at risk of mortality. This is an important finding, since early accurate prognosis following asphyxia with HIE and therapeutic hypothermia is essential to guide decision making.

6. Conclusions

Cardiopulmonary resuscitation remains a dynamic field, constantly evolving to incorporate the latest clinical updates and perspectives. Simulation and education, post-resuscitation care, prehospital interventions, pediatric considerations, and emerging concepts like Controlled Automated Reperfusion of the Whole Body collectively contribute to the advancement of CPR practices. As we navigate this ever-changing landscape, collaboration between healthcare professionals, researchers, educators, and technology developers remains crucial. By staying informed and embracing innovation, the medical community can continue to refine and optimize CPR protocols, ultimately improving outcomes for individuals facing cardiac arrest. This Special Issue highlights many aspects of many areas of resuscitation (from preclinical to post-resuscitation) over a wide age range (from neonates to adults) in many different types of studies (from retrospective to prospective studies, and from original research to review papers and meta-analyses). In conclusion, the diverse array of topics covered in this Special Issue underscores the multifaceted nature of cardiopulmonary resuscitation, emphasizing the ongoing pursuit of excellence in saving lives across various age groups and clinical scenarios. We extend our gratitude to all contributors for their invaluable insights, and we look forward to the ongoing collaboration and innovation that will further advance the field of resuscitation medicine.

Conflicts of Interest: The authors declare no conflict of interest.

References

1. Arriaga, A.F.; Bader, A.M.; Wong, J.M.; Lipsitz, S.R.; Berry, W.R.; Ziewacz, J.E.; Hepner, D.L.; Boorman, D.J.; Pozner, C.N.; Smink, D.S.; et al. Simulation-Based Trial of Surgical-Crisis Checklists. *N. Engl. J. Med.* **2013**, *368*, 246–253. [CrossRef] [PubMed]
2. Lott, C.; Truhlář, A.; Alfonzo, A.; Barelli, A.; González-Salvado, V.; Hinkelbein, J.; Nolan, J.P.; Paal, P.; Perkins, G.D.; Thies, K.C.; et al. ERC Special Circumstances Writing Group Collaborators. European Resuscitation Council Guidelines 2021: Cardiac arrest in special circumstances. *Resuscitation* **2021**, *161*, 152–219. [CrossRef] [PubMed]
3. Olasveengen, T.M.; Semeraro, F.; Ristagno, G.; Castren, M.; Handley, A.; Kuzovlev, A.; Monsieurs, K.G.; Raffay, V.; Smyth, M.; Soar, J.; et al. European Resuscitation Council Guidelines 2021: Basic Life Support. *Resuscitation* **2021**, *161*, 98–114. [CrossRef]
4. Lim, J.C.L.; Loh, N.; Lam, H.H.; Lee, J.W.; Liu, N.; Yeo, J.W.; Ho, A.F.W. The Role of Drones in Out-of-Hospital Cardiac Arrest: A Scoping Review. *J. Clin. Med.* **2022**, *11*, 5744. [CrossRef]
5. Derkenne, C.; Jost, D.; Thabouillot, O.; Briche, F.; Travers, S.; Frattini, B.; Lesaffre, X.; Kedzierewicz, R.; Roquet, F.; de Charry, F.; et al. Paris Fire Brigade Cardiac Arrest Task Force. Improving emergency call detection of Out-of-Hospital Cardiac Arrests in the Greater Paris area: Efficiency of a global system with a new method of detection. *Resuscitation* **2020**, *146*, 34–42.
6. Karlgren, K.; Dahlström, A.; Birkestam, A.; Drevstam Norling, A.; Forss, G.; Andersson Franko, M.; Cooper, S.; Leijon, T.; Paulsson, C. The TEAM instrument for measuring emergency team performance: Validation of the Swedish version at two emergency departments. *Scand. J. Trauma. Resusc. Emerg. Med.* **2021**, *29*, 139. [CrossRef] [PubMed]
7. Nolan, J.P.; Sandroni, C.; Böttiger, B.W.; Cariou, A.; Cronberg, T.; Friberg, H.; Genbrugge, C.; Haywood, K.; Lilja, G.; Moulaert, V.R.M.; et al. European Resuscitation Council and European Society of Intensive Care Medicine guidelines 2021: Post-resuscitation care. *Intensive Care Med.* **2021**, *47*, 369–421. [CrossRef] [PubMed]
8. Ram, P.; Menezes, R.G.; Sirinvaravong, N.; Luis, S.A.; Hussain, S.A.; Madadin, M.; Lasrado, S.; Eiger, G. Breaking your heart-A review on CPR-related injuries. *Am. J. Emerg. Med.* **2018**, *36*, 838–842. [CrossRef] [PubMed]
9. Benk, C.; Trummer, G.; Pooth, J.S.; Scherer, C.; Beyersdorf, F. CARL—Kontrollierte Reperfusion des ganzen Körpers: Von der kardiopulmonalen Reanimation zur zielgerichteten eCPR [CARL-Controlled reperfusion of the whole body]. *Z. Herz Thorax Gefasschir.* **2022**, *36*, 100–106. [CrossRef] [PubMed]
10. Madar, J.; Roehr, C.C.; Ainsworth, S.; Ersdal, H.; Morley, C.; Rüdiger, M.; Skåre, C.; Szczapa, T.; Te Pas, A.; Trevisanuto, D.; et al. European Resuscitation Council Guidelines 2021: Newborn resuscitation and support of transition of infants at birth. *Resuscitation* **2021**, *161*, 291–326. [CrossRef] [PubMed]
11. Van de Voorde, P.; Turner, N.M.; Djakow, J.; de Lucas, N.; Martinez-Mejias, A.; Biarent, D.; Bingham, R.; Brissaud, O.; Hoffmann, F.; Johannesdottir, G.B.; et al. European Resuscitation Council Guidelines 2021: Paediatric Life Support. *Resuscitation* **2021**, *161*, 327–387. [CrossRef] [PubMed]
12. Greif, R.; Lockey, A.; Breckwoldt, J.; Carmona, F.; Conaghan, P.; Kuzovlev, A.; Pflanzl-Knizacek, L.; Sari, F.; Shammet, S.; Scapigliati, A.; et al. European Resuscitation Council Guidelines 2021: Education for resuscitation. *Resuscitation* **2021**, *161*, 388–407. [CrossRef] [PubMed]

Disclaimer/Publisher's Note: The statements, opinions and data contained in all publications are solely those of the individual author(s) and contributor(s) and not of MDPI and/or the editor(s). MDPI and/or the editor(s) disclaim responsibility for any injury to people or property resulting from any ideas, methods, instructions or products referred to in the content.

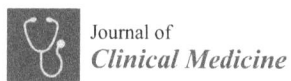

Article

Randomized Comparison of Two New Methods for Chest Compressions during CPR in Microgravity—A Manikin Study

Jan Schmitz [1,2,3,4,5,*], Anton Ahlbäck [6], James DuCanto [7], Steffen Kerkhoff [1,2,3,4], Matthieu Komorowski [8], Vanessa Löw [1], Thais Russomano [9], Clement Starck [4,10], Seamus Thierry [4,11], Tobias Warnecke [12] and Jochen Hinkelbein [1,2,3,4]

[1] Department of Anesthesiology and Intensive Care Medicine, University Hospital of Cologne, 50937 Cologne, Germany; steffen.kerkhoff@uk-koeln.de (S.K.); Vanessa.loew1@uk-koeln.de (V.L.); jochen.hinkelbein@uk-koeln.de (J.H.)
[2] Working Group Emergency Medicine and Air Rescue, German Society of Aviation and Space Medicine (DGLRM), 80331 Munich, Germany
[3] Working Group Standards, Recommendations, and Guidelines, German Society of Aviation and Space Medicine (DGLRM), 80331 Munich, Germany
[4] Space Medicine Group, European Society of Aerospace Medicine (ESAM), 50937 Cologne, Germany; clementstarck@gmail.com (C.S.); seam.thi@gmail.com (S.T.)
[5] Department of Sleep and Human Factors Research, Institute of Aerospace Medicine, German Aerospace Center, 51149 Cologne, Germany
[6] Department of Anesthesia and Intensive Care, Örebro University Hospital, 701 85 Örebro, Sweden; anton.ahlback@gmail.com
[7] Department of Anesthesiology, Aurora St. Luke's Medical Center, Milwaukee, WI 53215, USA; jducanto@mac.com
[8] Department of Surgery and Cancer, Faculty of Medicine, Imperial College London, London SW7 2AZ, UK; matthieu.komorowski@gmail.com
[9] Centre for Human and Applied Physiological Sciences, School of Basic and Medical Biosciences, Faculty of Life Sciences & Medicine, King's College London, London SE1 9RT, UK; trussomano@hotmail.com
[10] Anesthesiology and Intensive Care Department, University Hospital of Brest, 29609 Brest, France
[11] Anesthesiology Department, South Brittany General Hospital, 56322 Lorient, France
[12] Department of Anaesthesiology, Critical Care, Emergency Medicine and Pain Therapy, Klinikum Oldenburg, Medical Campus, University of Oldenburg, 26133 Oldenburg, Germany; tobiaswarnecke@web.de
* Correspondence: jan.schmitz1@uk-koeln.de

Citation: Schmitz, J.; Ahlbäck, A.; DuCanto, J.; Kerkhoff, S.; Komorowski, M.; Löw, V.; Russomano, T.; Starck, C.; Thierry, S.; Warnecke, T.; et al. Randomized Comparison of Two New Methods for Chest Compressions during CPR in Microgravity—A Manikin Study. *J. Clin. Med.* **2022**, *11*, 646. https://doi.org/10.3390/jcm11030646

Academic Editors: Timur Sellmann and Stephan Marsch

Received: 14 December 2021
Accepted: 25 January 2022
Published: 27 January 2022

Publisher's Note: MDPI stays neutral with regard to jurisdictional claims in published maps and institutional affiliations.

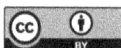

Copyright: © 2022 by the authors. Licensee MDPI, Basel, Switzerland. This article is an open access article distributed under the terms and conditions of the Creative Commons Attribution (CC BY) license (https:// creativecommons.org/licenses/by/ 4.0/).

Abstract: Background: Although there have been no reported cardiac arrests in space to date, the risk of severe medical events occurring during long-duration spaceflights is a major concern. These critical events can endanger both the crew as well as the mission and include cardiac arrest, which would require cardiopulmonary resuscitation (CPR). Thus far, five methods to perform CPR in microgravity have been proposed. However, each method seems insufficient to some extent and not applicable at all locations in a spacecraft. The aim of the present study is to describe and gather data for two new CPR methods in microgravity. Materials and Methods: A randomized, controlled trial (RCT) compared two new methods for CPR in a free-floating underwater setting. Paramedics performed chest compressions on a manikin (Ambu Man, Ambu, Germany) using two new methods for a free-floating position in a parallel-group design. The first method (Schmitz–Hinkelbein method) is similar to conventional CPR on earth, with the patient in a supine position lying on the operator's knees for stabilization. The second method (Cologne method) is similar to the first, but chest compressions are conducted with one elbow while the other hand stabilizes the head. The main outcome parameters included the total number of chest compressions (n) during 1 min of CPR (compression rate), the rate of correct chest compressions (%), and no-flow time (s). The study was registered on clinicaltrials.gov (NCT04354883). Results: Fifteen volunteers (age 31.0 ± 8.8 years, height 180.3 ± 7.5 cm, and weight 84.1 ± 13.2 kg) participated in this study. Compared to the Cologne method, the Schmitz–Hinkelbein method showed superiority in compression rates (100.5 ± 14.4 compressions/min), correct compression depth (65 ± 23%), and overall high rates of correct thoracic release after compression (66% high, 20% moderate, and 13% low). The Cologne method showed correct depth rates (28 ± 27%) but was associated with a lower mean compression rate (73.9 ± 25.5/min) and with lower rates of correct thoracic release (20% high, 7% moderate, and 73% low). Conclusions: Both methods are feasible without any equipment and could enable immediate CPR during cardiac arrest in microgravity, even in a single-helper scenario. The Schmitz–Hinkelbein method appears superior and could allow the delivery of high-quality CPR immediately after cardiac arrest with sufficient quality.

Keywords: CPR; microgravity; submerged model; spaceflight; resuscitation

1. Introduction

Space exploration and discovery will take humans far beyond low-Earth orbit (LEO). The National Aeronautics and Space Administration (NASA) and the European Space Agency (ESA) are preparing to send astronauts to the Moon (Artemis mission) to help prepare humanity for its next step—sending astronauts to Mars [1]. The journey will take up to 9 months each way causing extreme isolation and, therefore, resulting in total crew autonomy for almost 3 years [2,3].

During both Moon and Mars missions, there will be no possibility for crews to rapidly return to the ground in cases of an emergency; real-time assistance from Earth will be limited or impossible due to communication delays [4,5]. Given the delay of data transmission (up to 22 min per direction for the case of Mars), evacuation and telemedical support will not be possible/available in cases of a severe medical emergency [4,6].

During the journey in microgravity, the human body is subject to altered physiological conditions that are certain to significantly impact the astronaut's health [7]. Hemodynamic maladaptation resulting in hypotension, tachycardia, or even cardiac arrythmia with the risk of severe cardiovascular disease seems to be prevalent after exposure to microgravity [8,9]. Recent data also show that structural changes occur in the brain are associated with a decline in cognitive function resulting in spaceflight-associated neuro-optic syndrome [10,11]. Moreover, in the microgravity environment, the risk of trauma-associated injuries is significant [4,12]. Estimations from analogue populations suggest that one major medical event could occur for every 900-day mission [13]. Although no cardiac arrests have been reported to date, the theoretical risk of a dangerous cardiac or neurological event occurring in microgravity remains, even if it is low due to stringent screening and extensive training of astronauts. The risk of acute and life-threatening conditions also increases with mission duration and remoteness from Earth [4].

The European Resuscitation Council (ERC) basic life support guidelines highlight that cardiac arrest without immediate compensation with chest compressions will result in irreversible cerebral damage [14]. Current guidelines recommend a compression rate of 100–120/min with a compression depth of a minimum of 50 to a maximum 60 mm. Moreover, recently published guidelines on CPR in microgravity follow mainly ERC recommendations for CPR [15]. In recent years, research has been undertaken to develop methods of CPR in microgravity; thus far, five different methods have been described [2,6,16].

Regarding CPR quality, the Handstand method seems to be the most effective with respect to treating cardiac arrest, but with the major limitation that it needs a diameter between the operator and the compartment [2,6,16]. If the Handstand method is unapplicable in some scenarios, the Evetts–Russomano method is an acceptable alternative because CPR quality appears to be only slightly lower [16]. However, regardless of the method used, CPR quality in (simulated) microgravity is worse in comparison to ground-based CPR. Therefore, there is a need to develop new CPR methods.

The aim of the present study is to describe two new methods for CPR in microgravity and to analyze and compare the quality of CPR achieved.

2. Materials and Methods

We conducted a randomized parallel group trial (RCT) comparing two new methods for CPR in a free-floating underwater setting. Both methods require the operator to stabilize the patient on his/her thighs and deliver chest compressions using both arms in the first method (Schmitz–Hinkelbein method, SHM, Figure 1), or using one elbow in the Cologne method (CM, Figure 2).

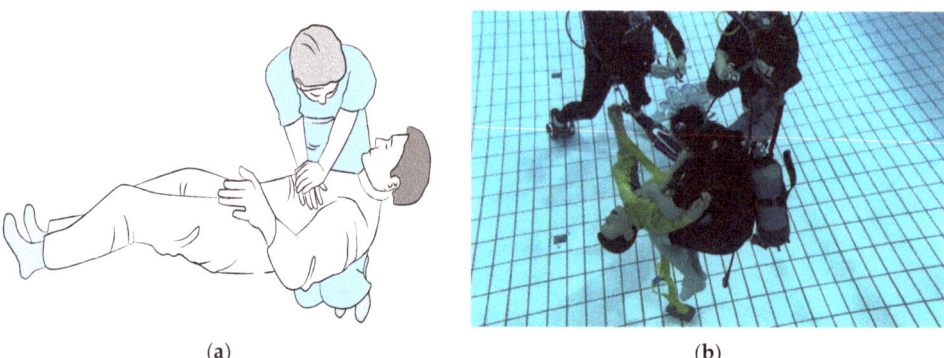

Figure 1. Graphic example (**a**) and execution in our submerged setting (**b**) of the Schmitz–Hinkelbein method (Graphic: Medizinfoto Köln, Photo: Jan Schmitz).

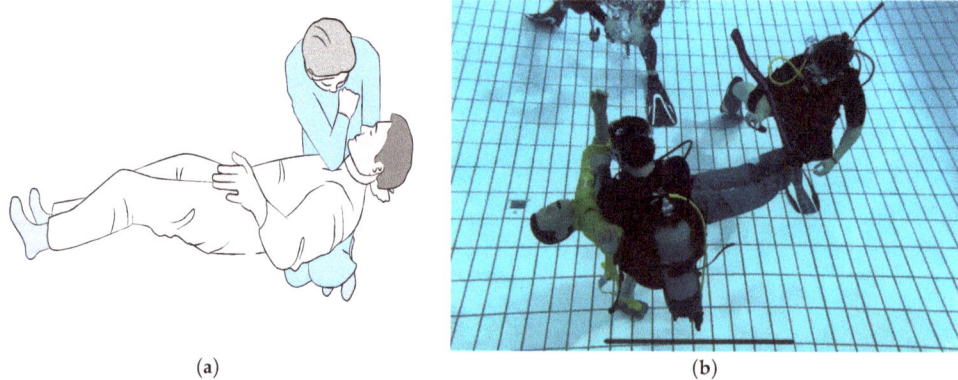

Figure 2. Graphic example (**a**) and execution in our submerged setting (**b**) of the Cologne method (Graphic: Medizinfoto Köln, Photo: Jan Schmitz).

2.1. Subjects

The participants were trained paramedics holding a valid diving certificate. The criteria for inclusion were EMT with valid diving certificates (SSI—Open Water Diver (OWD); CMAS *; PADI Open Water Diver; ISO 24801-2 (Autonomous Diver); or NAUI Scuba Diver) or equivalent licenses. The criteria for exclusion were any acute or chronic ear, nose, or throat disease. Figure 3 shows the enrollment process.

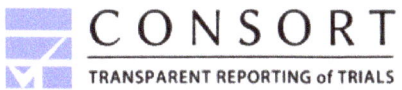

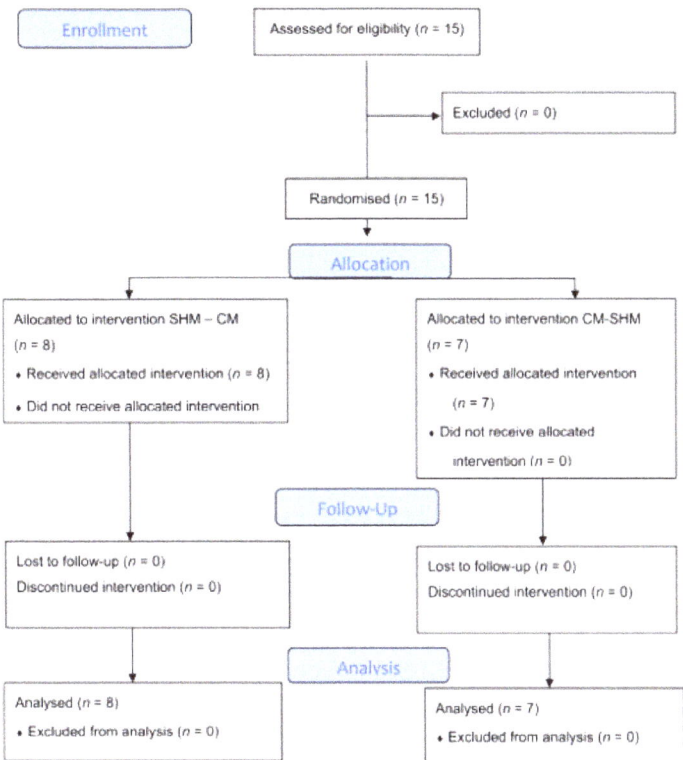

Figure 3. CONSORT flow diagram. SHM: Schmitz–Hinkelbein method; CM: Cologne method.

Written informed consent was obtained from all subjects before completing a short questionnaire to gather information about the participant's level of experience as an EMT and with CPR, as well as their total number of dives. Moreover, current health status was checked for acute or chronic ENT diseases.

2.2. Setting

All participants tested both CPR methods during a single dive. Chest compressions were performed using a full-body manikin (AmbuMan® Airway Wireless, Ambu Ltd., Bad Nauheim, Germany). The manikin was submerged and counterbalanced in a free-floating position approximately 1.5 m above the bottom of the pool (Figure 4). One dive instructor as well as one additional diver accompanied the trial: the first one to monitor the setting in case of emergency and to measure time, and the other to record the mechanical monitoring instrument showing the effectiveness of resuscitations.

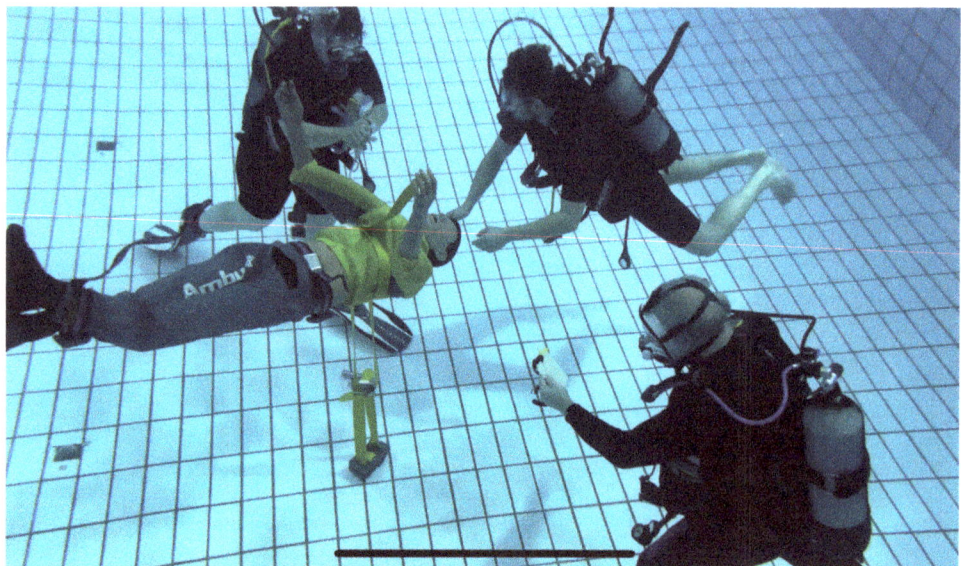

Figure 4. Submerged setting with manikin in free-floating position (Photo: J. Schmitz).

2.3. Randomisation

The method order was randomized with a coin toss prior to each dive.

(1) **Schmitz–Hinkelbein method**

In the first method (Schmitz–Hinkelbein method, SHM), the patient is in a supine position on the performer's knees for stabilization, similar to the CPR method performed on Earth. It is important that the rescuer flexes his/her hips properly to provide a stable base under the patient. Chest compressions are conducted using both hands according to CPR guidelines for normogravity (Figure 1).

(2) **Cologne method**

The second method (Cologne method, CM) is similar to the first, but chest compressions are conducted with the elbow. The free arm of the rescuer can be used to stabilize the patient (Figure 2).

2.4. Data Collection

Participants were asked to perform external chest compressions for at least 60 s for each method. The additional diver provided a hand signal to the operator to begin compressions and also timed the attempts. The sequence to perform each method was determined by an additional diver by flipping a coin prior to the dive and signaling the result by a hand signal while diving.

2.5. Video Analysis

As a consequence of the submerged model, technical evaluation of CPR parameters by software was not possible. Video clips of at least 60 s per method were recorded (using the manual compression screen on the manikin) with a GoPro® HERO4 (GoPro Inc., San Mateo, CA, USA) in a water-resistant case. All investigators were experienced in the performance of CPR and had undertaken preliminary training on a manikin during ground-based training/trials. In total, 30 videoclips were recorded (15 for each method). Recorded videoclips were screened and analyzed by two experienced emergency physicians independently.

2.6. The Primary Endpoint Was as Follows:

- Compression rate (defined as compression of the thorax) (per min).

2.7. The Secondary Endpoints Were as Follows:

- Number of chest compressions (n);
- Correct depth (defined as min. 50 to max. 60 mm of depth) (mm);
- Number of periods with no chest compression above 2 s (no-flow time) (n);
- Correct thoracic release between compressions (high = more than 66%; moderate = 33–65%; low = 0–32% of number of chest compressions with release of more than 4 cm according to indicator on manikin).

Data of primary and secondary endpoints were assessed and recorded independently. In cases of discrepancy, a third physician was consulted and majority counts were used.

2.8. Statistics

Case number determination (Cohen's d > 0.8, alpha 0.05 and statistical power 0.8) revealed a required number of participants of fifteen for each method. For statistical analyses, data were processed with Excel for Mac 16.32 (Microsoft©, Redmond, WC, USA). Data were checked for normal distribution with the Kolmogoroff–Smirnov test, and differences were tested with an unpaired t-test. Results were considered significant if $p < 0.05$. All findings are presented as means ± standard deviations (p-value) if not stated otherwise.

2.9. Ethics and Registration

This study was registered on ClinicalTrials.gov (NCT04354883, 21 April 2020) and authorized by the ethical committee of the University Hospital of Cologne (19-1069_1, date: 1 April 2019).

3. Results

3.1. Subjects

Demographic parameters for female (n = 5) and male (n = 10) paramedics differed significantly for weight (63.3 ± 6.5 kg (mean BMI: 21.7) vs. 84.5 ± 14.1 kg (mean BMI: 26.1); $p < 0.001$) and age (22 ± 2 years vs. 32 ± 9 years; $p < 0.001$) but not for height (female, 170.7 ± 6.7 cm vs. male, 180.1 ± 8.9 cm; $p < 0.001$). All subjects held a valid diving license (OWD: 25%, CMAS *: 15%, CMAS **: 10%, and other: 50%).

3.2. Compression Rate

Fifteen participants conducted the Schmitz–Hinkelbein method (SHM). The average compression rate was 111.1 ± 6.3/min. The correct compression rate, defined as 100–120 compressions min^{-1}, was achieved 90 ± 11% of the time.

Fifteen participants conducted the Cologne method (CM) with an average compression rate of 102 ± 8.3/min chest compressions per minute, and the expected compression rate was achieved 72 ± 23% of the time.

3.3. Chest Compression Depth

The expected 50–60 mm of chest compression depth was achieved 65 ± 23% of the time and 28 ± 27% of the time when performing SHM and CM, respectively.

3.4. Period of No Chest Compression >2 s (No-Flow Time)

Among the fifteen providers, a total of 6 and 4 periods of no-flow time were recorded, respectively.

3.5. Correct Thoracic Release between Compressions

For SHM, ten participants (66.6%) achieved a high rate of correct thoracic release, three participants (20%) showed a moderate rate of correct thoracic release, and two participants (13.3%) showed a low rate of correct thoracic release.

In performing CM, three participants (20%) showed a high rate of correct thoracic release, one participant (6.7%) showed a moderate rate of correct thoracic release, and eleven participants (73.7%) showed a low rate of correct thoracic release.

4. Discussion

The Schmitz–Hinkelbein method showed overall superior results for compression rate and compression depth associated with low rates of no-flow time and high rates of correct thoracic release in comparison to the second new method (CM).

4.1. General Considerations

The average compression rate for SHM was 111.1 ± 6.3 with a correct compression rate achieved $90 \pm 11\%$ of the time and fulfilled latest criteria for CPR-compression rate on Earth (100–120 compressions per minute) [14]. The average compression rate of the second new method was 102 ± 8 with a correct compression rate of $72 \pm 23\%$, which was quite low and did not reach criteria for CPR in normogravity [14].

In recent studies, the Handstand method (HS) proved to deliver the most effective chest compressions with regards to the 2021 ERC guidelines [14]. The recently published international guidelines for CPR in microgravity [15] recommend the ER method as the primary method for basic life support in microgravity because of its advantages in feasibility and independence of cabin diameter. Normally, emergency equipment is stored near the Crew Medical Restraint System; thus, transport of a patient undergoing CPR is possible.

Moreover, our two new methods for CPR can be applied as first-approach methods, enabling transport of the patient to the Crew Medical Restraint System (CMRS).

As soon as the patient has been restrained on the CMRS, HS should be applied if not limited by the dimensions of the spacecraft and provider height because it yields the best-quality manual chest compressions in microgravity thus far [17].

The feasibility of a CPR method (in space) is a fundamental component of the health system (crew). Although recent data show that, throughout Europe, there are important differences in Emergency Medical Service systems [18], it is well established that an early start on chest compressions (as soon as possible) is vitally important after cardiac arrest and is correlated with a higher probability of survival [10,19]. As a first approach, HS, ER and RBH are independent of any resources (and initially superior to those methods that require the patient to be restrained). Our new methods also do not require equipment After starting CPR in space, the patient should be restrained as soon as possible because of its substantial benefits. Taking into account the transport of the patient to locations of both medical equipment and the CMRS, as well as the time required to restrain the patient SHM could theoretically produce the best outcome [20].

Most current methods require equipment or methods of securing the patient and/or rescuer in order to begin CPR in the event of cardiac arrests. These methods need time to be implemented and will not be feasible in all future space vehicles because of differences in spacecraft diameter and availability of equipment. Methods for CPR have to be universally usable independent of room size or available equipment (e.g., patient restraining system), or should at least be able to guarantee high-quality CPR until needed equipment is retrieved

The advantages of the two new methods are mainly the usability for initial CPR as single-helper or two-helper methods, and as reliable methods for ensuring high-quality chest compressions that could increase the probability of surviving cardiac arrest [16].

A major limitation is always a lack of post-resuscitation care after cardiac arrest in space. A recent study showed data of an automatic external chest compression device (ACCD) evaluated during a parabolic flight in 2021. Although transportation costs will be extremely high for ACCD, the use of an ACCD allows continuous delivery of high-quality CC in microgravity and hypergravity conditions [17].

4.2. Number of Chest Compressions and Compression Rate

In order to maintain adequate cardiac output, the compression rate (CR) is crucial [17]. In comparison, the HS method achieved the highest average rate (115.4 ± 12.1/min). Almost every performed method met the minimum requirement in terms of compression rate: ER (104.6 ± 6.0/min), STD (100.0 ± 3.0/min), and SM (102.6 ± 12.1/min) [21]. Only the RBH method did not meet the required criteria (94.7 ± 5.4/min) according to universal CPR guidelines [18].

Our first evaluated method achieved an average rate (100.5 ± 14.4/min) and our second method did not meet the required criteria (73.9 ± 25.5/min). Thus, compression rates showed significant differences ($p < 0.001$) between these two methods in our study, and only SHM met required criteria according to universal CPR guidelines [18].

4.3. Compression Depth

Prior data showed that the HS method was, in terms of compression depth, superior (44.9 ± 3.3 mm) [22]. Furthermore, the RBH (39.8 ± 6.3 mm) [22] and ER methods (35.6 ± 6.7 mm) [18] showed good results. Similarly to CPR in normogravity, with the operator kneeling next to the patient, both conventional methods STD (19.8 ± 11.2 mm) and SM (30.7 ± 11.9 mm) showed insufficient chest compressions. Table 1 summarizes the mathematical estimation parameters of known CPR methods with the new methods evaluated in our study.

Table 1. Number of chest compression and depth rates of known methods [16] and evaluated methods in this study.

Method	Number of Chest Compressions (/min)	Correct Compression Depth (50–60 mm)
	New Methods	
Schmitz–Hinkelbein method	100.5 ± 14.4	0.65 ± 0.23
Cologne method	73.9 ± 25.5	0.28 ± 0.27
	Existing Methods	
Handstand method	115.4 ± 12.1	0.91 ± 0.07
Evetts–Russomano method	104.6 ± 5.4	0.74 ± 0.1
Reverse bear hug method	94.7 ± 5.4	0.82 ± 0.13
Side straddle method	100.0 ± 3.0	0.50 ± 0.28

Our two evaluated methods, both with a rescuer in a kneeling position next to the patient, showed improved depth rates. The first method (SHM) showed that almost two of three chest compressions (65 ± 23%; median 70%) had correct depths (50–60 mm). The second method showed worse depth rates with only one of four chest compressions (28.0 ± 2.7%; median 22%) with correct depth rates. The depth of chest compressions showed significant differences ($p < 0.001$) between these two methods in our study.

4.4. Limitations

Although compression rates primarily depend on which CPR method is used, compression depth depends not only on the method but also on the manikin used, the performers' demographics, and the method of simulated microgravity. Although data for gender differences were found to be not significant [23], different types of manikins with variable resistance may affect results in compression depth and correct thoracic release. To what extent the differently used manikin types could influence the quality of CPR is still unknown.

The resistance of water might have also influenced compression rates, because the second method was the only method that did not meet criteria for correct compression rate. Moreover, the impact of environment on physical strain may complicate comparability of different CPR methods for resuscitation in space, as recent data showed a significant reduction in quality of resuscitation during an alpine rescue mission scenario at high altitudes due to physical strength [24].

The ERC recommends a cycle of 2 min of continuous chest compressions [14]. As parabolic flight can only enable a cycle of up to 22 s, we found that a cycle of one minute can conclude data of endpoints as, i.e., criteria of chest compressions is counted on a per-minute basis. Exhaustion may increase with longer cycles of chest compressions.

There are different methods to simulate microgravity on earth. Some studies used a body suspension device (BSD) [21], which was developed by the John Ernsting Aerospace Physiology Laboratory, Microgravity Centre, Pontifical Catholic University of Rio Grande do Sul. In contrast to parabolic flights [22] with limited study time (max. 22 s per parabola), longer periods of continuous chest compressions are possible with a BSD. Due to the fact that some studies used parabolic flights to simulate microgravity, data for prolonged CPR can only be compared conditionally [25]. Moreover, there are no data concerning the exhaustion of the operator after more than 3 min of CPR in a microgravity environment.

Moreover, the height of the performers seems to influence the quality of chest compressions, as one recent study showed in a normogravity setting [26].

The relative success of the first CPR method (SHM) examined in this study suggests that it may be more appropriate than procedures currently known for CPR in space. Therefore, further empirical examination, such as evaluation of the first and second methods with electronic data collection during parabolic flights, should be of future interest.

5. Conclusions

Thus far, five different methods for CPR in microgravity have been described [17]. Regarding compression depth, no method achieved the requirements of the current guidelines [14]. The Schmitz–Hinkelbein method showed sufficient compression rate and depth and seemed promising, but it needs evaluation in an authentic microgravity setting, such as during a parabolic flight. In order to provide high-quality CPR in space, a combination of different methods can be applied. The first new method (SHM) evaluated in this study seems to have some advantages and can be applied as a first-approach method since chest compressions can be conducted immediately without any equipment. Moreover, the performance of this method can be practiced prior to space missions and is similar to performing CPR on Earth.

Author Contributions: J.H. and J.S. designed the study. Data collection and analysis were performed by J.H., V.L., T.W. and J.S. J.S. drafted the manuscript. A.A., J.D., S.K., M.K., V.L., T.R., C.S., S.T. and T.W. improved the manuscript by reviewing and providing critical comments. All authors have read and agreed to the published version of the manuscript.

Funding: Equipment was provided by the manufacturer (Ambu GmbH, Bad Nauheim, Germany) for free and was returned after the completion of the study. No other sponsoring was received.

Institutional Review Board Statement: The study was conducted according to the guidelines of the Declaration of Helsinki, and approved by the Ethics Committee of University Hospital of Cologne (19-1069_1, date 1 April 2019).

Informed Consent Statement: Informed consent was obtained from all subjects involved in the study.

Data Availability Statement: The data presented in this study are available on request from the corresponding author. The data are not publicly available due to privacy issues.

Conflicts of Interest: The authors declare no conflict of interest.

Abbreviations

BSD	Body Suspension Device
CMAS	Confederation Mondiale des Activites Subaquatiques
CM	Cologne method
CMO	Crew Medical Officer
CMRS	Crew Medical Restraint System
CPR	Cardiopulmonary Resuscitation
CD	Compression Depth
CR	Compression Rate
ER	Evetts–Russomano method
ESA	European Space Agency
ETI	Endotracheal Intubation
GA	General anesthesia
HS	Handstand method
ISS	International Space Station
LEO	Low-earth Orbit
NASA	National Aeronautics and Space Administration
PADI	Professional Association of Diving Instructors
OWD	Open Water Diver
RBH	Reverse bear hug method
RCT	Randomized Controlled Trial
SHM	Schmitz–Hinkelbein method
SSI	Scuba Schools International

References

1. Witze, A. Can NASA really return people to the Moon by 2024? *Nat. Cell Biol.* **2019**, *571*, 153–154. [CrossRef] [PubMed]
2. Hinkelbein, J.; Spelten, O. Going beyond anesthesia in space exploration missions: Emergency medicine and emergency medical care. *Aviat. Space Environ. Med.* **2013**, *84*, 747. [CrossRef] [PubMed]
3. Nicogossian, A. Medicine and space exploration. *Lancet* **2003**, *362*, s8–s9. [CrossRef]
4. Komorowski, M.; Fleming, S.; Mawkin, M.; Hinkelbein, J. Anaesthesia in austere environments: Literature review and considerations for future space exploration missions. *NPJ Microgravity* **2018**, *4*, 5. [CrossRef]
5. Nicogossian, A.E.; Pober, D.F.; Roy, S.A. Evolution of Telemedicine in the Space Program and Earth Applications. *Telemed. e-Health* **2001**, *7*, 1–15. [CrossRef]
6. Hinkelbein, J. Spaceflight: The final frontier for airway management? *Br. J. Anaesth.* **2020**, *125*, e5–e6. [CrossRef]
7. Tanaka, K.; Nishimura, N.; Kawai, Y. Adaptation to microgravity, deconditioning, and countermeasures. *J. Physiol. Sci.* **2017**, *67*, 271–281. [CrossRef]
8. Shen, M.; Frishman, W.H. Effects of Spaceflight on Cardiovascular Physiology and Health. *Cardiol. Rev.* **2019**, *27*, 122–126. [CrossRef]
9. Hughson, R.L.; Helm, A.; Durante, M. Heart in space: Effect of the extraterrestrial environment on the cardio-vascular system. *Nat. Rev. Cardiol.* **2018**, *15*, 167–180. [CrossRef]
10. Roberts, D.; Brown, T.; Nietert, P.; Eckert, M.; Inglesby, D.; Bloomberg, J.; George, M.; Asemani, D. Prolonged Microgravity Affects Human Brain Structure and Function. *Am. J. Neuroradiol.* **2019**, *40*, 1878–1885. [CrossRef]
11. Russomano, T.; Da Rosa, M.; A Dos Santos, M. Space motion sickness: A common neurovestibular dysfunction in microgravity. *Neurol. India* **2019**, *67*, S214–S218. [CrossRef]
12. Swaffield, T.P.; Neviaser, A.S.; Lehnhardt, K. Fracture Risk in Spaceflight and Potential Treatment Options. *Aerosp. Med. Hum. Perform.* **2018**, *89*, 1060–1067. [CrossRef] [PubMed]
13. Summers, R.L.; Johnston, S.L.; Marshburn, T.H.; Williams, D.R. Emergencies in space. *Ann. Emerg. Med.* **2005**, *46*, 177–184. [CrossRef] [PubMed]
14. Lott, C.; Truhlář, A.; Alfonzo, A.; Barelli, A.; González-Salvado, V.; Hinkelbein, J.; Nolan, J.P.; Paal, P.; Perkins, G.D.; Thies, K.-C.; et al. European Resuscitation Council Guidelines 2021: Cardiac arrest in special circumstances. *Resuscitation* **2021**, *161*, 152–219. [CrossRef] [PubMed]
15. Hinkelbein, J.; Kerkhoff, S.; Adler, C.; Ahlbäck, A.; Braunecker, S.; Burgard, D.; Cirillo, F.; De Robertis, E.; Glaser, E.; Haidl, T.K.; et al. Cardiopulmonary resuscitation (CPR) during spaceflight—A guideline for CPR in microgravity from the German Society of Aerospace Medicine (DGLRM) and the European Society of Aerospace Medicine Space Medicine Group (ESAM-SMG). *Scand. J. Trauma Resusc. Emerg. Med.* **2020**, *28*, 108. [CrossRef]

16. Forti, A.; van Veelen, M.J.; Squizzato, T.; Cappello, T.D.; Palma, M.; Strapazzon, G. Mechanical cardiopulmonary resuscitation in microgravity and hypergravity conditions: A manikin study during parabolic flight. *Am. J. Emerg. Med.* **2021**, *53*, 54–58 [CrossRef] [PubMed]
17. Braunecker, S.; Douglas, B.; Hinkelbein, J. Comparison of different techniques for in microgravity—A simple mathematic estimation of cardiopulmonary resuscitation quality for space environment. *Am. J. Emerg. Med.* **2015**, *33*, 920–924. [CrossRef]
18. Rehnberg, L.; Russomano, T.; Falcão, F.; Campos, F.; Evetts, S.N. Evaluation of a Novel Basic Life Support Method in Simulated Microgravity. *Aviat. Space Environ. Med.* **2011**, *82*, 104–110. [CrossRef]
19. Tjelmeland, I.B.M.; Masterson, S.; Herlitz, J.; Wnent, J.; Bossaert, L.; Rosell-Ortiz, F.; Alm-Kruse, K.; Bein, B.; Lilja, G.; Gräsner, J.-T. et al. Description of Emergency Medical Services, treatment of cardiac arrest patients and cardiac arrest registries in Europe. *Scand. J. Trauma Resusc. Emerg. Med.* **2020**, *28*, 1–16. [CrossRef]
20. Song, J.; Guo, W.; Lu, X.; Kang, X.; Song, Y.; Gong, D. The effect of bystander cardiopulmonary resuscitation on the survival of out-of-hospital cardiac arrests: A systematic review and meta-analysis. *Scand. J. Trauma Resusc. Emerg. Med.* **2018**, *26*, 86 [CrossRef]
21. Rehnberg, L.; Ashcroft, A.; Baers, J.H.; Campos, F.; Cardoso, R.B.; Velho, R.; Gehrke, R.D.; Dias, M.K.P.; Baptista, R.R.; Russomano T. Three Methods of Manual External Chest Compressions During Microgravity Simulation. *Aviat. Space Environ. Med.* **2014**, *85*, 687–693. [CrossRef] [PubMed]
22. Jay, G.D.; Lee, P.; Goldsmith, H.; Battat, J.; Maurer, J.; Suner, S. CPR effectiveness in microgravity: Comparison of three positions and a mechanical device. *Aviat. Space Environ. Med.* **2003**, *74*, 1183–1189. [PubMed]
23. Kordi, M.; Kluge, N.; Kloeckner, M.; Russomano, T. Gender influence on the performance of chest compressions in simulated hypogravity and microgravity. *Aviat. Space Environ. Med.* **2012**, *83*, 643–648. [CrossRef]
24. Egger, A.; Niederer, M.; Tscherny, K.; Burger, J.; Fuhrmann, V.; Kienbacher, C.; Roth, D.; Schreiber, W.; Herkner, H. Influence of physical strain at high altitude on the quality of cardiopulmonary resuscitation. *Scand. J. Trauma Resusc. Emerg. Med.* **2020**, *28*, 19 [CrossRef] [PubMed]
25. Kordi, M.; Cardoso, R.B.; Russomano, T. A preliminary comparison between methods of performing external chest compressions during microgravity simulation. *Aviat. Space Environ. Med.* **2011**, *82*, 1161–1163. [CrossRef] [PubMed]
26. Nakashima, Y.; Saitoh, T.; Yasui, H.; Ueno, M.; Hotta, K.; Ogawa, T.; Takahashi, Y.; Maekawa, Y.; Yoshino, A. Comparison of Chest Compression Quality Using Wing Boards versus Walking Next to a Moving Stretcher: A Randomized Crossover Simulation Study. *J. Clin. Med.* **2020**, *9*, 1584. [CrossRef] [PubMed]

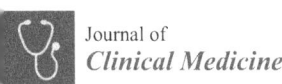

Article

Proteomics-Based Serum Alterations of the Human Protein Expression after Out-of-Hospital Cardiac Arrest: Pilot Study for Prognostication of Survivors vs. Non-Survivors at Day 1 after Return of Spontaneous Circulation (ROSC)

Jochen Hinkelbein [1,*,†], Lydia Kolaparambil Varghese Johnson [2,†], Nikolai Kiselev [3], Jan Schmitz [1], Martin Hellmich [4], Hendrik Drinhaus [1], Theresa Lichtenstein [5], Christian Storm [6] and Christoph Adler [7,8]

[1] Department of Anesthesiology and Intensive Care Medicine, Faculty of Medicine, University Hospital Cologne, 50937 Cologne, Germany; jan.schmitz1@uk-koeln.de (J.S.); hendrik.dinhaus@uk-koeln.de (H.D.)
[2] Faculty of Medicine and Surgery, Università degli Studi di Perugia, 05100 Terni, Italy; lydia.kolaparambil@gmail.com
[3] Clinic for Anesthesiology, Intensive Care Medicine, Preclinical Emergency Medicine and Pain Management, Sankt Katharinen Hospital Frechen, 50226 Frechen, Germany; n.kiselev@gmx.net
[4] Institute of Medical Statistics and Computational Biology (IMSB), Faculty of Medicine, University Hospital Cologne, University of Cologne, 50937 Cologne, Germany; martin.hellmich@uk-koeln.de
[5] Department of Psychiatry and Psychotherapy, Faculty of Medicine, University Hospital Cologne, University of Cologne, 50937 Cologne, Germany; theresa.lichtenstein@uk-koeln.de
[6] Medical Department, Division of Nephrology and Internal Intensive Care Medicine, Charité—Universitaetsmedizin Berlin, 10117 Berlin, Germany; christian.storm@charite.de
[7] Heart Centre, University Hospital Cologne, 50937 Cologne, Germany; christoph.adler@uk-koeln.de
[8] Fire Department City of Cologne, Institute for Security Science and Rescue Technology, 50737 Cologne, Germany
* Correspondence: jochen.hinkelbein@uk-koeln.de
† These authors contributed equally to this work.

Abstract: Background: Targeted temperature management (TTM) is considered standard therapy for patients after out-of-hospital cardiac arrest (OHCA), cardiopulmonary resuscitation (CPR), and return of spontaneous circulation (ROSC). To date, valid protein markers do not exist to prognosticate survivors and non-survivors before the end of TTM. The aim of this study is to identify specific protein patterns/arrays, which are useful for prediction in the very early phase after ROSC. Material and Methods: A total of 20 adult patients with ROSC (19 male, 1 female; 69.9 ± 9.5 years) were included and dichotomized in two groups (survivors and non-survivors at day 30). Serum samples were drawn at day 1 after ROSC (during TTM). Three panels (organ failure, metabolic, neurology, inflammation; OLINK, Uppsala, Sweden) were utilised. A total of four proteins were found to be differentially regulated (>2- or <−0.5-fold decrease; t-test). Bioinformatic platforms were utilised to analyse pathways and identify signalling cascades and to screen for potential biomarkers. Results: A total of 276 proteins were analysed and revealed only 11 statistically significant protein alterations (Siglec-9, LAYN, SKR3, JAM-B, N2DL-2, TNF-B, BAMBI, NUCB2, STX8, PTK7, and PVLAB). Following the Bonferroni correction, no proteins were found to be regulated as statistically significant. Concerning the protein fold change for clinical significance, four proteins (IL-1 alpha, N-CDase, IL5, CRH) were found to be regulated in a clinically relevant context. Conclusions: Early analysis at 1 day after ROSC was not sufficiently possible during TTM to prognosticate survival or non-survival after OHCA. Future studies should evaluate protein expression later in the course after ROSC to identify promising protein candidates.

Keywords: proteomics; CPR; protein expression; targeted temperature management; ROSC

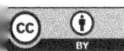

1. Introduction

Sudden cardiac arrest is a sword of Damocles causing around 20% of all deaths [1] in the world. Additionally, each year, 375,000 people in Europe [2] require immediate cardiopulmonary resuscitation (CPR) after out-of-hospital cardiac arrest (OHCA). Targeted temperature management (TTM) is considered as a grade IB recommendation [3] since 2010, as it improves mortality and the neurological outcomes significantly after the return of spontaneous circulation (ROSC). The case-fatality rate for patients after ROSC is still very high, arriving at a rate of around 71.5% after 1 year [4].

In this context, prognostication and predicting the outcome is of cardinal importance since brain injury is the determinant of morbidity and mortality in these patients [5]. According to the 2015 ERC guidelines [6], the earliest time to predict a poor neurological outcome using clinical examination in comatose patients is 72 h after cardiac arrest or 72 h after the restoration of normothermia in patients treated with TTM.

The majority of mortality after ROSC is due to hypoxic–ischemic brain injury (HIBI) [7]. In addition, a good prognostication is essential to minimise a falsely pessimistic prediction in comatose patients [8]. To date, multiple prognostic tests were evaluated for neurological prognostication [5], such as cranial computer tomography (CCT), detailed clinical neurological assessment, electroencephalography (EEG), and measurement of somatosensory-evocable potentials (SEPs). Nonetheless, these are not always accurate predictors for the neurological outcome and specifically for survival for several reasons, such as the sedation for induction. In addition, the maintenance of TTM decreases the validity of prognostication [7]. Enolase-2 (NSE) or S-100B serum markers are other possible methods. However, these markers alone do not provide a valid prognostication of the clinical outcome since they are influenced by multiple factors [9]. Ulterior limitations are based on the fact that prognostication cannot be made prior to the return of normothermia [6]. Additionally, to date, other reliable single-protein markers do not exist to prognosticate survivors and non-survivors prior to the end of TTM. However, the current guidelines recommend a multimodal strategy for prognostication.

In this prospective cohort study, serum proteins of survivors and non-survivors of OHCA are analysed by both proteomic and bioinformatic methods to identify proteins of interest, which could allow for prognostication if used in an array or as a set of proteins. This study aims to investigate the proteome in the context of TTM after cardiac arrest and to identify specific protein patterns that are employable in prognostication, which could be useful as a complete set for estimating survival.

2. Material and Methods

The main goal of this study was to identify protein markers that are useful for clinical outcome prediction in the early phase of treatment (i.e., 24 h after ROSC and during TTM) in patients after CPR and ROSC.

2.1. Study Design

This prospective observational study included 20 patients with cardiac causes, resuscitated from a non-traumatic, non-hypoxic-related, out-of-hospital cardiac arrest (OHCA), and treated with TTM, according to the standard protocol of the hospital for at least 24 h.

2.2. Patients

Adult patients, admitted for an OHCA after CPR, ROSC, and TTM were included in the study. Patients presenting hypoxia-related, traumatic or other causes were excluded from the study.

2.3. Sample Collection

In all patients, blood was drawn on day 0 (i.e., the day of CPR in the emergency department or ICU after arrival) and day 1 (i.e., after 24 h and during TTM). If no blood sample was available for one of both days, patients were excluded from the analysis

(Figure 1). Patients that are not eligible for TTM were also excluded from the study. Survivors and non-survivors were dichotomized on the 30th day after CPR to allocate patients to the two compared groups: Survivors vs. non-survivors.

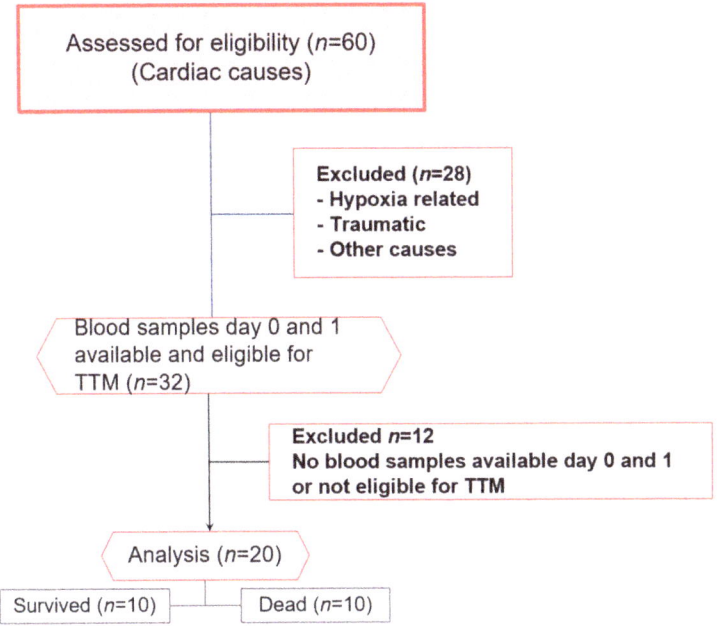

Figure 1. CONSORT flow chart for patients included and excluded in the study. Surviving and diseased patients ($n = 10$) were analysed.

For all ($n = 20$) patients, demographic and clinical variables were collected from the electronic files of the patients via the ORBIS software (AGFA HealthCare, Bonn, Germany). Blood samples were collected daily at the same time from an arterial line into serum tubes. After the acquisition, the serum was centrifuged at $5000 \times g$ for 5 min and stored at $-80\,°C$ until proteomic analysis at the end of the study.

2.4. TTM Therapy

In clinical routine, the ERC guideline recommendations [10] for the treatment of cardiac arrest and post-cardiac arrest care management were utilised. Briefly, patients were treated with TTM for 24 h, according to our standard operating procedure (SOP). The emergency medical service initiated peripheral cooling with ice packs to the femoral and/or neck area in patients with OHCA. The controlled cooling to a target temperature of 32–34 °C was continued in the intensive care unit (ICU) using an endovascular cooling device (Thermogard XP® catheter, Zoll Medical Corp., Chelmsford, MA, USA) and maintained for 24 h. TTM was terminated by rewarming through the same endovascular device at a controlled rate of 0.3 °C/h until the physiologic body temperature of 36.5 °C was reached. This temperature was maintained for further 48 h. The basic metabolic panel, magnesium, phosphorus, ionized calcium, CBC with differential, and PT/PTT were monitored every 6 h during the clinical routine.

2.5. Proteomic Analysis

The concept of proteomic and biostatistical analysis of proteins is defined as the separation, identification, and quantification of the entire protein of a cell, organism or tissue under specific conditions. Cardiac arrest leads to a critical whole body ischemia and in the case of ROSC, additional damage occurs during and after reperfusion. The so-called

Post-Cardiac Arrest Syndrome is a combination of pathophysiological processes, which is associated with post-cardiac arrest brain injury, post-cardiac arrest myocardial dysfunction and systemic ischemia/reperfusion response. To improve the complex interaction between the different organ systems, we decided to choose the following panels: Inflammation panel, organ damage panel, and neurology panel.

In summary, as a first step, statistically significantly regulated proteins were identified by OLINK and analysed by bioinformatic network analyses (GeneMania®, Toronto ON, Canada; http://www.genemania.org, accessed on 14 December 2021). Thereafter, these statistically significant proteins were grouped using a hierarchical cluster analysis (Perseus®, Martinsried, Germany). As a third step, proteins of similarly early upregulated clusters underwent further network analysis to evaluate possible corresponding proteins or functions. This approach, related to pooled proteomic data, is described in detail below

2.6. Sample Preparation

The collected and stored serum samples were sent to OLINK (Analysis Service, Uppsala, Sweden) on dry ice for further proteomic analysis to allow for the high-quality and blinded proteomic analysis by a certified laboratory. The preparation was conducted according to their quality-checked protocol (ISO/IEC 17025:2005). Four internal controls were added to each sample to monitor the quality of the assay performance, as well as the quality of individual samples. The quality control (QC) is performed in two steps Evaluation of each sample plate, based on the standard deviation of the internal controls and the median value of the controls. Ninety percent of the samples passed for the OLINK inflammation panel, 95% for the neurology panel, and 100% for the organ damage panel.

2.7. OLINK Panels

Three OLINK panels were used for the analysis: Inflammation panel, organ damage panel, and neurology panel. For each protein, a unique pair of oligonucleotide-labelled antibody probes binds to the targeted protein, and if the two probes are close, a new PCR target sequence is formed by a proximity-dependent DNA polymerization event. The resulting sequence is subsequently detected and quantified using the standard real-time PCR. Then, the data are normalized and transformed using internal extension controls and inter-plate controls, to adjust for intra- and inter-run variation. The final assay read-out is given in normalized protein expression (NPX), which is an arbitrary unit on a log2 scale where a high value corresponds to the higher protein expression. Each proximity extension assay (PEA) measurement has a lower detection limit (LOD) calculated based on negative controls that are included in each run, and measurements below LOD were removed from further analysis. All of the assay characteristics, including detection limits and measurements of assay performance and validations, are available from the manufacturer's webpage (http://www.olink.com, accessed on 14 December 2021). The analyses were based on 1 µL of serum for each panel of 92 assays [11]:

- The inflammation panel covers a wide range of inflammation-related protein biomarkers, which enables the analysis of 92 biomarkers through a multiplex immunoassay The panel is assembled to detect an assortment of traditional, as well as exploratory biomarkers within the inflammation research field.
- The organ damage panel investigates 92 biomarkers from 1 µL of the biological sample It provides the optimal dynamic range and focuses on proteins that are relevant for processes involved in the biological response to organ damage. The proteins analysed in this panel are important in processes of response to stress, regulation of cell proliferation, cell cycle, and cell death/apoptosis.
- The neurology panel consists of a proximity extension assay (PEA) technology, which tests 92 neurology-related protein biomarkers across 96 samples simultaneously without compromising on data quality.

2.8. Bioinformatic Analysis of Proteins

After the protein expression analysis by OLINK, the identified and altered proteins were used for further bioinformatic investigations to classify underlying networks, signalling cascades, and affected pathways. Biological functions of regulated proteins were identified using the functional network analysis.

- Heatmapper (http://www.heatmapper.ca/, accessed on 14 December 2021) is an online server, which allows for the visualization of the results of gene expression profiling and cluster analysis in the form of heat maps through a graphical interface [12]. It allows for the accurate inspection of combinations of dataset characteristics to identify correlations and clustering results, as well as sample-related characteristics (e.g., survival time and gene expression levels). This approach allows for the visualization, as well as the accurate and rapid interpretation of the data obtained by large scale gene expression profiling [13]. By organizing complex data as matrix, the visualization of these data is improved. Heat mapping reorders rows and columns of the dataset to place the data with similar profiles, which are close to each other. In a second step, ranges of similar values are assigned to specific colour codes [14]. A heat map performs two actions on a matrix: First, it reorders the rows and columns to ensure that rows (and columns) with similar profiles are closer to one another, causing these profiles to be more visible. Second, each entry in the data matrix is displayed as a colour, making it possible to view the patterns graphically [14].

- GeneMANIA (http://www.genemania.org/, accessed on 14 December 2021) is a tool that helps in predicting the interactions and functions of a list of genes in a network form or when feasible, in pathways [15,16]. GeneMANIA provides the possibility of customizing the network, allowing for the choice of data sources or highlighting specific functions, with a more comfortable graphic experience [16]. GeneMANIA knowledge is based on data from large databases, which comprehend Gene Expression Omnibus, BioGRID, EMBL-EBI, Pfam, Ensembl, Mouse Genome Informatics, the National Center for Biotechnology Information, InParanoid, and Pathway Commons [15,16]. A network of interactions is created and the strength of the interaction is weighed. In the case of no interaction, an association weight of zero is assigned, while in the case of interaction, a positive value reflecting the strength of the interaction and the reliability of the finding, is assigned [17]. For example, the association of a pair of genes in a gene expression dataset is the Pearson correlation coefficient of their expression levels across multiple conditions in an experiment. The more the genes are co-expressed, the higher the weight they are linked by, ranging up to 1.0, indicating a perfectly correlated expression [15].

- WebGestalt is a tool to interpret the lists of genes from large scale x-OMICS (proteomics, genomics) studies [18]. The proteins of interest were uploaded to the tool where user IDs are unambiguously mapped to unique Entrez gene IDs, and all of them are mapped from a selected platform genome. Through the GoSlim classification plot, it is possible to examine the distribution of the genes of interest across the major branches of the gene ontology (GO) biological process, cellular component, and molecular function ontologies [19]. Each biological process, cellular component, and molecular function category is represented by a red, blue, and green bar, respectively.

2.9. Statistics

A p-value of < 0.05 was considered as statistically significant. For the analysis of demographic parameters, the U-test was utilised. For the protein expression analysis (OLINK data), the t-test was primarily utilised and supplemented with a Bonferroni correction to avoid the type I error due to multiple testing ($n = 276$ tests). In addition to statistical significance, the fold changes (FC) in protein regulation were analysed to address clinical relevance. Proteins with a fold change ≥ 2.0 and ≤ -0.5 were considered clinically relevant and utilised for a second analysis approach.

The patients' sample size was calculated using the *t*-test. From a preliminary set of patients and protein changes, as well as the assumption of an alpha error of 5% and a beta-error of 80%, adult patients ($n = 20$) were considered sufficient for the analysis.

2.10. Ethical Registration

This prospective observational cohort study was approved by the Ethics Committee of the University of Cologne, Faculty of Medicine, Cologne, Germany (No. 14-053) and was registered with ClinicalTrials.gov (Identifier: NCT02247947).

3. Results

A total number of patients ($n = 20$) were included in this study (Figure 1). The mean patient age was 69.9 ± 9.5 years (survivors: 60.9 ± 3.8 years; deceased: 69.2 ± 12.2 years; each, $n = 10$; $p = 0.697$; Table 1). All of the studied patients had a cardiac cause, which primarily led to cardiac arrest.

Table 1. Demographics table reporting on the different analysed variables. All of the parameters are given as means +/−SD. For the analysis of demographic parameters, the U-test was utilised.

	Total	Survived	Dead	*p*-Value
Number of patients	$n = 20$	$n = 10$	$n = 10$	
Age	69.9 (9.5)	70.8 (3.8)	69.2 (12.3)	0.697
Gender				<0.001
Female	1 (5%)	0 (0%)	1 (10%)	
Male	19 (95%)	10 (100%)	9 (90%)	
Cause of cardiac arrest				
Myocardial infarction–no. (%)	14 (70)	8 (80)	6 (60)	0.620
Primary arrhythmia–no. (%)	6 (30)	2 (20)	4 (40)	0.620
Cardiac arrest characteristics				
No-flow time (min)	4.2 ± 2.9	3.0 ± 1.7	5.4 ± 3.6	0.030
Witnessed arrest by bystander–no. (%)	14 (70)	9 (90)	5 (50)	0.140
BLS provided by bystander–no. (%)	15 (75)	8 (80)	7 (70)	0.990
Dose of epinephrine during CPR (mg)	5.5 ± 4.2	4.8 ± 4.1	6.0 ± 4.2	0.060
Number of shocks	5.0 ± 4.2	4.7 ± 4.1	5.3 ± 4.3	0.730
Time to ROSC (min)	17 ± 11	15 ± 12	23 ± 15	0.080
ICU treatment				
Period of ICU hospitalization (days)	12 ± 12	14 ± 9	7 ± 6	0.04
Ventilation time (days)	11 ± 10	10 ± 12	7 ± 5	0.07

3.1. Proteomic Analysis

A total of 276 proteins were analysed with the three OLINK arrays and revealed 11 statistically significant protein alterations (neurology panel: $n = 5$ (proteins, Siglec-9, LAYN, SKR3, JAM-B, N2DL-2); inflammation panel: $n = 1$ (TNF-B); organ damage panel: $n = 5$ (BAMBI, NUCB2, STX8, PTK7, PVLAB)). After the application of Bonferroni correction, no proteins were found to be regulated as statistically significant. Concerning the protein fold change for clinical significance, a total of four proteins (IL-1 alpha, *n*-CDase, IL5, CRH) were found to be regulated with a fold change ≥ 2.0 or ≤ -0.5.

3.2. Bioinformatic Analysis

Bioinformatic analysis was conducted on both groups of proteins with a significant *t*-test (prior to the Bonferroni correction) and to the group of proteins with a significant fold change.

Heat map analysis for the four clinically relevant proteins in survivors and non-survivors showed no difference in clustering (Figure 2A,B). IL1A was downregulated, and CRH, IL5, and *n*-CDAS were upregulated in both groups. Concerning the analysis of the

11 statically significant proteins, clustering for regulation was different for the proteins in surviving and non-surviving patients (Figure 2C,D). Solely clustering of TNF-B was different between both groups and was allocated to another cluster.

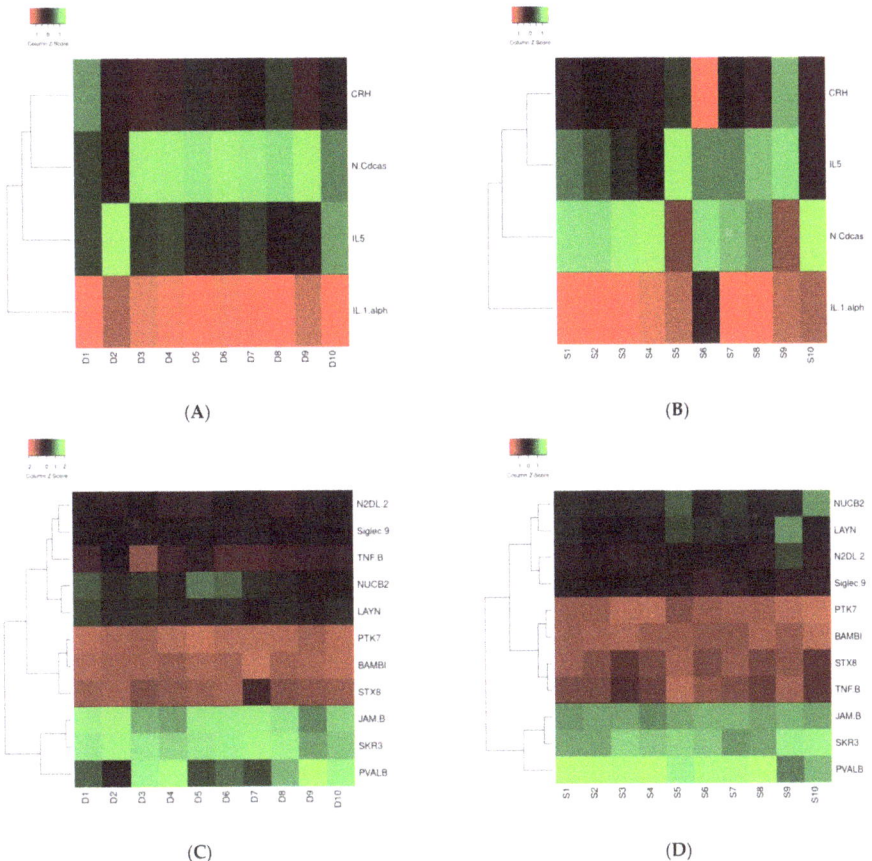

Figure 2. (**A**–**D**) Heat map of IL1A, ASAH2, IL5, and CRH ((**A**): Surviving patients; (**B**): Non-surviving patients) and TNF-B, Siglec-9, LAYN, SKR3, JAM-B, N2DL-2, BAMBI, NUCB2, STX8, PTK7, and PVALB ((**C**): Surviving patients; (**D**): Non-surviving patients) proteins in correlation with the survival and dead groups. The 11 proteins in the middle were found in the present study. Circulated proteins were identified as linked to the proteins of the present study, which is shown by the red lines.

From WebGestalt, all four proteins with >2/<−0.5-fold changes were shown to be involved in metabolic processes, response to stimuli, and cell communication (biological process category) (Figure 3). Three proteins were involved in extracellular space (cellular component category) and protein binding (molecular function category). The GeneMania software was utilized to examine the network and correlating proteins for each group.

Interleukin-1-alpha (IL1A), *n*-acylsphingosine amidohydrolase-2 (ASAH2), corticotropin-releasing hormone (CRH), and interleukin-5 (IL5) showed physical interactions with interleukin-1 receptor type 2 (IL1R2), interleukin-5 receptor subunit alpha (IL5RA), corticotropin-releasing hormone receptor-1 (CRHR1), corticotropin-releasing hormone receptor-2 (CRHR2), and other proteins (Figure 4A). Additionally, the pathway interaction of these proteins was studied. IL1A and IL5, in their pathways, present several important proteins, such as IL1R2, IL5RA, interleukin-1 receptor-associated kinase 4 (IRAK4), and cytokine receptor common subunit beta (CSF2RB) (Figure 4B).

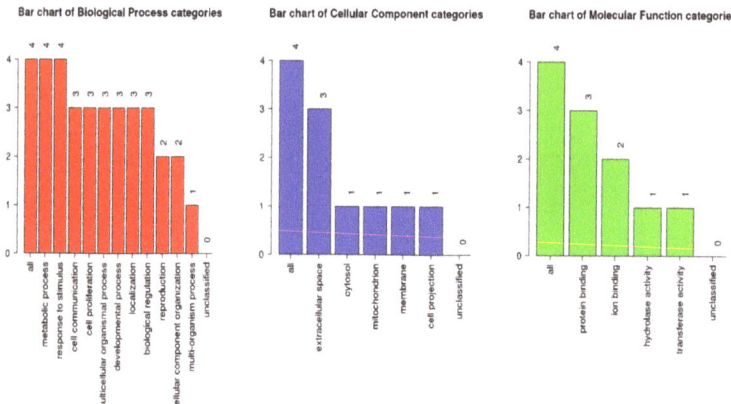

Figure 3. GOslim summary for the biological process, cellular component, and molecular function category for IL1A, ASAH2, IL5, and CRH proteins. Each of the functions is represented by a red, blue and green bar, respectively.

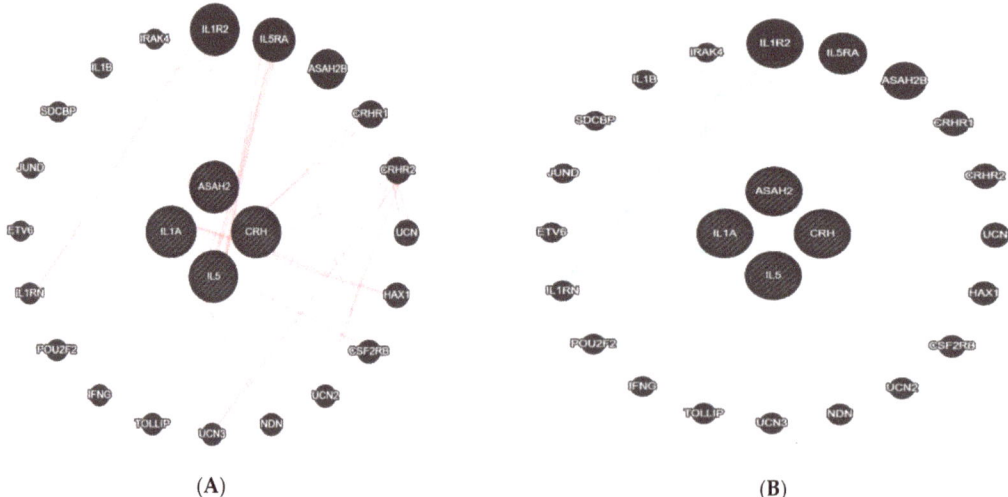

(A)   (B)

Figure 4. (**A**,**B**) Physical interaction table of IL1A, ASAH2, IL5, and CRH proteins. This figure shows the connection between the proteins found in the present analysis (within the circle) and the linked proteins as identified by GeneMania. The four proteins in the centre were found in the present study. All of the other encircled proteins in the periphery linked with red lines to the central proteins are the ones with a relevant physical interaction with the latter.

After the bioinformatic analysis, the 11 proteins that were found as statistically significant (*t*-test) had pathway interactions only with a few proteins, such as activin receptor type-1B (ACVR1B), junctional adhesion molecule 3 (JAM3), vesicle transport through interaction with T-SNAREs 1A and IB (VTI1A VTI1B), and inhibin subunit beta A (INHBA) (Figure 5A). The physical interactions of these genes included links with proteins, such as uromodulin (UMOD), phosphatidylinositol glycan anchor biosynthesis class K LTB (PIGK) SRY-box transcription factor 30 (SOX30), etc. (Figure 5B).

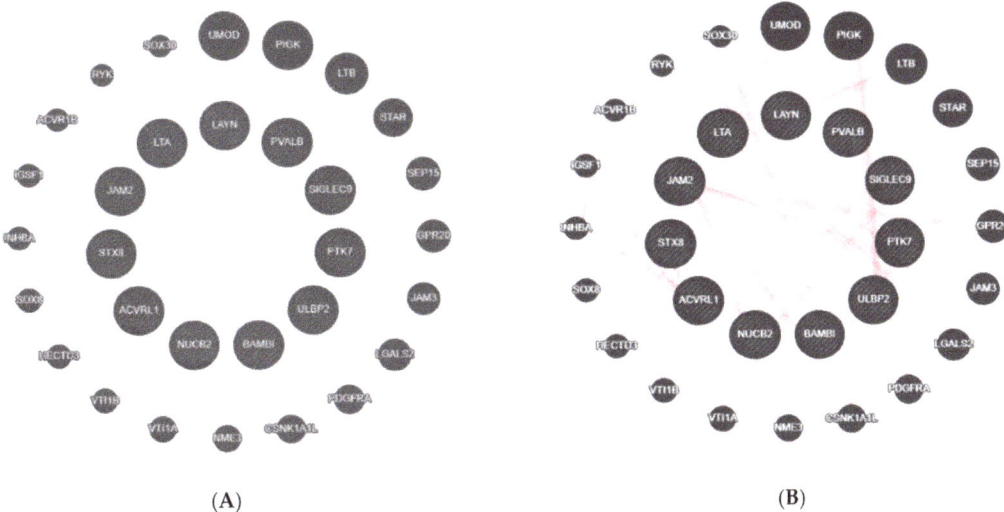

Figure 5. (**A**) shows the physical interaction table for TNF-B, Siglec-9, LAYN, SKR3, JAM-B, N2DL-2, BAMBI, NUCB2, STX8, PTK7, and PVALB. This figure shows the connection between the proteins found in the present analysis (within the circle) and the linked proteins as identified by GeneMania. The 11 central proteins were identified in the present study. All of the other encircled proteins in the periphery linked with blue lines to the central proteins are the ones with a relevant physical interaction with the latter. Interaction of proteins is visualized by blue lines. (**B**) shows pathway interactions for TNF-B, Siglec-9, LAYN, SKR3, JAM-B, N2DL-2, BAMBI, NUCB2, STX8, PTK7, and PVALB. The 11 proteins in the middle were found in the present study. The circulated proteins were identified as linked to the proteins of the present study, which is shown by the red lines.

4. Discussion

The aim of the present study was to identify protein biomarkers to facilitate the prognostication for survival in OHCA patients after CPR, ROSC, and TTM. Of the 276 proteins analysed from the three OLINK panels, four showed a clinically relevant regulation and 11 proteins showed statistical significance. However, after Bonferroni correction, the statistical significance was no longer demonstrated. Bioinformatic analysis revealed the pathways involved and the related proteins which were significantly altered.

4.1. Patient Population

For the present study, the patient group was dichotomized into surviving and non-surviving patients for the investigation of specific protein regulation patterns in each respective group. Since survival is most often used as a hard outcome parameter after CPR [20,21], it was chosen to separate the patient groups.

Concerning the demographic parameters of the patients, the ages of the patients were comparable between the survivors and non-survivors (70.8 vs. 69.2 years) and the mean age (69.9 years) is comparable to the age of patients that are presented in other papers regarding cardiac arrest and CPR [22,23]. In the present study, at least the age of the patients indicates that the patient group may be comparable to the other patients. However, the male:female proportion (19:1) is significantly different and gender aspects seem of low relevance for this specific aspect of protein expression. Nevertheless, the role of gender aspects seems to be controversially discussed [24].

4.2. Protein Identification

In the present study, four vs. 11 proteins were found to have a significantly different serum expression to discriminate survivors and non-survivors. Although significance was not achieved after Bonferroni correction, the proteins are of interest for a clinically relevant approach (fold >2 and <−0.5). The aim of this study was not to find single biomarkers for a definite answer, but a full set or array of proteins which could facilitate prognostication.

Of all the proteins found to be significantly regulated in the present study, TNFB seems to be most promising. TNFB was significantly downregulated in the non-survivors' group, which could be an early indicator of low survival. However, from the cluster analysis of all the other proteins analysed, up and downregulation was comparable on both groups.

In addition to the findings of the present study, a recent trial from Cakmak et al. [25] found that serum copeptin levels predict ROSC and the short-term prognosis of patients with OHCA. Therefore, the authors concluded that serum copeptin levels may serve as a guide in diagnostic decision making to predict ROSC in patients undergoing CPR and in determining the short-term prognosis of patients with ROSC. In this study, blood was drawn at patient admission. However, the aim of the present study was to identify protein alteration with a potential to predict the overall outcome after TTM, for use in a later protein expression profile.

4.3. Biological Processes and Cascades

Concerning the biological function and the associated cascades, proteins were mainly involved in the metabolic process and biological regulation with a protein binding function. In addition, the proteins originated from the membrane and extracellular space. Although this indication does not directly reveal the relevant proteins, it may give some suggestion for identifying the important proteins in this context. Since the present study was not designed to find these new or unknown proteins, it can provide a suggestion for which other proteins may be interesting for analysis in future studies. Moreover, this evidence provides insight into the function of the identified proteins in the metabolic and cellular processes, which might be relevantly affected, and consequently require attention for treatment.

4.4. Limitations

In the present study, three different panels, with each containing 96 different proteins, were used for the analysis. For a careful interpretation of the results, several limitations are noteworthy. First, the approach utilised specific proteins and not a broad analysis of potentially unknown proteins. Therefore, it was not possible to identify new biomarkers for prognostication. Second, this can be considered only as a first pilot study for future analysis, and only patients ($n = 20$) were examined. Potentially, if several hundred or thousands of patients are analysed, additional markers could be found. This study could be a solid base for future clinical studies, even if it has specific limitations.

5. Conclusions

The present study aimed to identify proteins associated with survival or death at day 30 after out-of-hospital cardiac arrest and ROSC. Although several proteins were identified to reveal statistical or clinical relevance, bioinformatic analyses unveiled no promising candidates. Therefore, early analysis at 24 h after ROSC was not sufficiently possible during TTM to prognosticate survival or non-survival after cardiac-induced OHCA. As a result, further studies are necessary to better evaluate protein expression after ROSC and to identify promising protein candidates for prognostication, e.g., 6 h post-ROSC. This study could be considered as a launching platform for future multi-centric studies.

Author Contributions: Data curation, M.H.; Formal analysis, J.H., L.K.V.J., J.S., M.H., T.L., C.S. and C.A.; Investigation, J.H., N.K., J.S. and H.D.; Methodology, J.H., L.K.V.J., C.S. and C.A.; Project administration, C.A.; Resources, N.K.; Supervision, J.H.; Validation, M.H., T.L. and C.A.; Writing—original draft, J.H., L.K.V.J., H.D., T.L. and C.A.; Writing—review & editing, J.H., J.S., M.H., H.D., T.L., C.S. and C.A. All authors have read and agreed to the published version of the manuscript.

Funding: This research received no external funding.

Institutional Review Board Statement: No. 14-053; NCT02247947.

Informed Consent Statement: Informed consent was obtained from all subjects involved in the study or the relatives, respectively.

Conflicts of Interest: The authors declare no conflict of interest.

Abbreviations

ACVR1B	Activin receptor type-1B
ASAH2	N-acylsphingosine amidohydrolase-2
BAMBI	Activin membrane-bound inhibitor homolog
CCT	Cranial computer tomography
CPR	Cardiopulmonary resuscitation
CRH	Corticotropin-releasing hormone
CRHR1	Corticotropin-releasing hormone receptor-1
CRHR2	Corticotropin-releasing hormone receptor-2
CSF2RB	Cytokine receptor common subunit beta
DNA	Desoxyribonucleid acid
EEG	Electroencephalography
ERC	European resuscitation council
FC	Fold change
GO	Gene ontology
HIBI	Hypoxic–ischemic brain injury
ICU	Intensive care unit
IL-1A	Interleukin-1-alpha
IL1R2	Interleukin-1 receptor type 2
IL5	Interleukin-5
IL5RA	Interleukin-5 receptor subunit alpha
INHBA	Inhibin subunit beta A
IRAK4	Interleukin-1 receptor-associated kinase 4
JAM-B	Junctional adhesion molecule B
JAM3	Junctional adhesion molecule 3
LAYN	Layilin
LOD	Lower detection limit
NPX	Normalized protein expression
NSE	Enolase-2
NUCB2	Nucleobindin-2
N2DL-2	NKG2D ligand-2
n-CDase	Neutral ceramidase
OHCA	Out-of-hospital cardiac arrest
PCR	Polymerase chain reaction
PEA	Proximity extension assay
PIGK	Phosphatidylinositol glycan anchor biosynthesis class K LTB
PT	Prothrombin time
PTK7	Tyrosin protein kinase 7
PTT	Partial thromboplastin time
QC	Quality control
ROSC	Return of spontaneous circulation
SEP	Somatosensory-evocable potentials
Siglec-9	Sialic acid-binding immunoglobulin-like lectin 9
SOP	Standard operating procedure
SOX30	SRY-box transcription factor 30
STX8	Syntaxin 8
TNF-B	Tumour necrosis factor
TTM	Targeted temperature management
UMOD	Uromodulin
VTI1A	Vesicle transport through interaction with T-SNAREs 1A
VTI1B	Vesicle transport through interaction with T-SNAREs 1B

References

1. Hayashi, M.; Shimizu, W.; Albert, C.M. The spectrum of epidemiology underlying sudden cardiac death. *Circ. Res.* **2015**, *116*, 1887–1906. [CrossRef] [PubMed]
2. The Hypothermia after Cardiac Arrest Study Group. Mild therapeutic hypothermia to improve the neurologic outcome after cardiac arrest. *N. Engl. J. Med.* **2002**, *346*, 549–556. [CrossRef] [PubMed]
3. Peberdy, M.A.; Callaway, C.W.; Neumar, R.W.; Geocadin, R.G.; Zimmerman, J.L.; Donnino, M.; Gabrielli, A.; Silvers, S.M.; Zaritsky A.L.; Merchant, A.; et al. Part 9: Post-cardiac arrest care: 2010 American Heart Association guidelines for cardiopulmonary resuscitation and emergency cardiovascular care. *Circulation* **2010**, *122*, S768–S786. [CrossRef] [PubMed]
4. Vane, M.F.; Carmona, M.J.C.; Pereira, S.M.; Kern, K.B.; Timerman, S.; Perez, G.; Vane, L.A.; Otsuki, D.A.; Auler, J.O., Jr. Predictors and their prognostic value for no ROSC and mortality after a non-cardiac surgery intraoperative cardiac arrest: A retrospective cohort study. *Sci. Rep.* **2019**, *9*, 14975–14979. [CrossRef] [PubMed]
5. Hawkes, M.A.; Rabinstein, A.A. Neurological prognostication after cardiac arrest in the era of target temperature management. *Curr. Neurol. Neurosci. Rep.* **2019**, *19*, 10. [CrossRef]
6. Callaway, C.W.; Donnino, M.W.; Fink, E.L.; Geocadin, R.G.; Golan, E.; Kern, K.B.; Leary, M.; Meurer, W.J.; Peberdy, M.A. Thompson, T.M.; et al. Part 8: Post–cardiac arrest care: 2015 American Heart Association guidelines update for cardiopulmonary resuscitation and emergency cardiovascular care. *Circulation* **2015**, *132*, S465–S482. [CrossRef]
7. Dragancea, I.; Rundgren, M.; Englund, E.; Friberg, H.; Cronberg, T. The influence of induced hypothermia and delayed prognostication on the mode of death after cardiac arrest. *Resuscitation* **2013**, *84*, 337–342. [CrossRef]
8. Sandroni, C.; D'Arrigo, S.; Nolan, J.P. Prognostication after cardiac arrest. *Crit. Care* **2018**, *22*, 150. [CrossRef]
9. Tiainen, M.; Roine, R.O.; Pettilä, V.; Takkunen, O. Serum neuron-specific enolase and S-100B protein in cardiac arrest patients treated with hypothermia. *Stroke* **2003**, *34*, 2881–2886. [CrossRef]
10. Nolan, J.P.; Soar, J.; Cariou, A.; Cronberg, T.; Moulaert, V.R.M.; Deakin, C.D.; Bottiger, B.W.; Friberg, H.; Sunde, K.; Sandroni, C European Resuscitation Council and European Society of Intensive Care Medicine guidelines for post-resuscitation care 2015 *Resuscitation* **2015**, *95*, 202–222. [CrossRef]
11. Petrera, A.; von Toerne, C.; Behler, J.; Huth, C.; Thorand, B.; Hilgendorff, A.; Hauck, S.M. Multi-platforms approach for serum proteomics: Complementarity of Olink PEA technology to mass spectrometry-based protein profiling. *J. Proteome Res.* **2021**, *20* 751–762. [CrossRef] [PubMed]
12. Babicki, S.; Arndt, D.; Marcu, A.; Liang, Y.; Grant, J.R.; Maciejewski, A.; Wishart, D.S. Heatmapper: Web-enabled heat mapping for all. *Nucleic Acids Res.* **2016**, *44*, W147–W153. [CrossRef] [PubMed]
13. Verhaak, R.G.W.; Sanders, M.A.; Bijl, M.A.; Delwel, R.; Horsman, S.; Moorhouse, M.J.; Van Der Spek, P.J.; Löwenberg, B.; Valk P.J.M. HeatMapper: Powerful combined visualization of gene expression profile correlations, genotypes, phenotypes and sample characteristics. *BMC Bioinform.* **2006**, *7*, 337. [CrossRef] [PubMed]
14. Key, M. A tutorial in displaying mass spectrometry-based proteomic data using heat maps. *BMC Bioinform.* **2012**, *13*, S10 [CrossRef] [PubMed]
15. Mostafavi, S.; Ray, D.; Warde-Farley, D.; Grouios, C.; Morris, Q. GeneMANIA: A real-time multiple association network integration algorithm for predicting gene function. *Genome Biol.* **2008**, *9*, S4. [CrossRef] [PubMed]
16. Warde-Farley, D.; Donaldson, S.L.; Comes, O.; Zuberi, K.; Badrawi, R.; Chao, P.; Franz, M.; Grouios, C.; Kazi, F.; Lopes, C.T.; et al The GeneMANIA prediction server: Biological network integration for gene prioritization and predicting gene function. *Nucleic Acids Res.* **2010**, *38*, W214–W220. [CrossRef]
17. Franz, M.; Rodriguez, H.; Lopes, C.; Zuberi, K.; Montojo, J.; Bader, G.D.; Morris, Q. GeneMANIA update 2018. *Nucleic Acids Res* **2018**, *46*, W60–W64. [CrossRef]
18. Liao, Y.; Wang, J.; Jaehnig, E.J.; Shi, Z.; Zhang, B. WebGestalt 2019: Gene set analysis toolkit with revamped UIs and APIs. *Nucleic Acids Res.* **2019**, *47*, W199–W205. [CrossRef]
19. Wang, J.; Vasaikar, S.; Shi, Z.; Greer, M.; Zhang, B. WebGestalt 2017: A more comprehensive, powerful, flexible and interactive gene set enrichment analysis toolkit. *Nucleic Acids Res.* **2017**, *45*, W130–W137. [CrossRef]
20. Jacobs, I.; Nadkarni, V.; Bahr, J.; Berg, R.A.; Billi, J.E.; Bossaert, L.; Cassan, P.; Coovadia, A.; D'Este, K.; Finn, J.; et al. Cardiac arrest and cardiopulmonary resuscitation outcome reports: Update and simplification of the Utstein templates for resuscitation registries: A statement for healthcare professionals from a task force of the International Liaison Committee on Resuscitation (American Heart Association, European Resuscitation Council, Australian Resuscitation Council, New Zealand Resuscitation Council, Heart and Stroke Foundation of Canada, InterAmerican Heart Foundation, Resuscitation Councils of Southern Africa) *Circulation* **2004**, *110*, 3385–3397.
21. Franek, O. "Survival incidence" should be an important parameter of cardiac arrest survival chance, beside to "survival rate" *Resuscitation* **2015**, *96*, 79. [CrossRef]
22. Andersen, L.W.; Holmberg, M.J.; Berg, K.M.; Donnino, M.W.; Granfeldt, A. In-hospital cardiac arrest: A review. *JAMA* **2019**, *321* 1200. [CrossRef] [PubMed]
23. Zelfani, S.; Manai, H.; Riahi, Y.; Daghfous, M. Out of hospital cardiac arrest: When to resuscitate. *Pan Afr. Med. J.* **2019**, *33*, 289 [CrossRef] [PubMed]

24. Safdar, B.; Stolz, U.; Stiell, I.; Cone, D.C.; Bobrow, B.J.; Deboehr, M.; Dreyer, J.; Maloney, J.; Spaite, D. Differential survival for men and women from out-of-hospital cardiac arrest varies by age: Results from the OPALS study. *Acad. Emerg. Med.* **2014**, *21*, 1503–1511. [CrossRef] [PubMed]
25. Cakmak, S.; Sogut, O.; Albayrak, L.; Yildiz, A. Serum copeptin levels predict the return of spontaneous circulation and the short-term prognosis of patients with out-of-hospital cardiac arrest: A randomized control study. *Prehosp. Disaster Med.* **2020**, *35*, 120–127. [CrossRef] [PubMed]

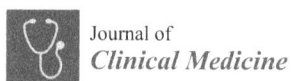

Article

Direct Transport to Cardiac Arrest Center and Survival Outcomes after Out-of-Hospital Cardiac Arrest by Urbanization Level

Eujene Jung [1,2], Young Sun Ro [3,4,5,*], Jeong Ho Park [3,4,5], Hyun Ho Ryu [1,2,5] and Sang Do Shin [3,4,5]

1. Department of Emergency Medicine, Chonnam National University Hospital, Gwangju 61469, Korea; 81823ej@hanmail.net (E.J.); oriryu@hanmail.net (H.H.R.)
2. Department of Emergency Medicine, Chonnam National University Medical School, Gwangju 61469, Korea
3. Department of Emergency Medicine, Seoul National University Hospital, Seoul 03080, Korea; timthe@gmail.com (J.H.P.); sdshin@snu.ac.kr (S.D.S.)
4. Department of Emergency Medicine, Seoul National University College of Medicine, Seoul 03080, Korea
5. Laboratory of Emergency Medical Services, Seoul National University Hospital Biomedical Research Institute, Seoul 03080, Korea
* Correspondence: ro.youngsun@gmail.com; Tel.: +82-2-2072-3257

Abstract: Current guidelines for post-resuscitation care recommend regionalized care at a cardiac arrest center (CAC). Our objectives were to evaluate the effect of direct transport to a CAC on survival outcomes of out-of-hospital cardiac arrests (OHCAs), and to assess interaction effects between CAC and urbanization levels. Adult EMS-treated OHCAs with presumed cardiac etiology between 2015 and 2019 were enrolled. The main exposure was the hospital where OHCA patients were transported by EMS (CAC or non-CAC). The outcomes were good neurological recovery and survival to discharge. Multivariable logistic regression analyses were conducted. Interaction analysis between the urbanization level of the location of arrest (metropolitan or urban/rural area) and the exposure variable was performed. Among the 95,931 study population, 23,292 (24.3%) OHCA patients were transported directly to CACs. Patients in the CAC group had significantly higher likelihood of good neurological recovery and survival to discharge than the non-CAC group (both $p < 0.01$, aORs (95% CIs): 1.75 (1.63–1.89) and 1.70 (1.60–1.80), respectively). There were interaction effects between CAC and the urbanization level for good neurological recovery and survival to discharge. Direct transport to CAC was associated with significantly better clinical outcomes compared to non-CAC, and the findings were strengthened in OHCAs occurring in nonmetropolitan areas.

Keywords: out-of-hospital cardiac arrest; post-resuscitation care; outcomes

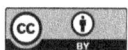

1. Introduction

Out-of-hospital cardiac arrest (OHCA) is a major global health problem, with high incidence and poor survival outcomes [1,2]. Despite extensive efforts to increase resuscitation and post-resuscitation care, mortality and disability rates remain high, with only 7–10% of OHCA patients surviving to discharge and only less than 5% of those patients discharging with favorable neurological recovery [2,3]. The emergency medical services (EMS) personnel are responsible for on-scene and during-transport resuscitation and transporting of OHCA patients to the appropriate hospital for post-resuscitation care [4].

Regional systems of care involving centralization of post-resuscitation care have been proposed to improve survival outcomes of OHCA, as OHCA is considered to be best treated in regional hospitals with highly resource-intensive treatments such as extracorporeal membrane oxygenation, percutaneous cardiac intervention (PCI), and targeted temperature management (TTM) [5,6]. Current guidelines for post-resuscitation care recommend regionalization to designated cardiac arrest centers (CAC) that can provide 24 h immediate PCI and can provide TTM [5,7]. However, in recent systematic review and meta-analysis studies, it was suggested that while transporting patients directly to a CAC did associate with improved clinical outcomes at hospital discharge, it did not improve 1-month survival outcomes [8,9]. Sudden cardiac arrest is one of the most time-sensitive diseases, and the increased transport time interval in bypassing the nearest hospital to reach the destination hospital may be detrimental for some OHCA patients with specific conditions [10].

It is hypothesized that the direct transport to a CAC would improve overall survival outcomes in OHCA patients, while that effect will vary depending on the urbanization level. The urbanization level affects the distribution of CAC as a surrogate indicator of community, EMS, and resources of hospital resuscitation, and is one of the potential risk factors for survival outcomes of OHCA [11]. The objectives of this study were to evaluate effects of the direct transport to a CAC on clinical outcomes of OHCA patients with presumed cardiac etiology, and to assess whether the effects vary across the urbanization level of the location where OHCA occurred.

2. Materials and Methods

2.1. Study Design and Setting

This is a cross-sectional study, using a nationwide, population-based prospective registry of OHCAs including all patients transported by EMS in Korea.

Korea has approximately 50 million people living in 100,210 km^2, and there are 17 provinces. These areas are subdivided into 229 counties for administrative purposes, including 69 counties in metropolitan cities (median population density: 9214 persons per km^2), 78 counties in urban cities (median population density: 598 persons per km^2), and 82 counties in rural areas (median population density: 65 persons per km^2) [12]. Of the 17 provinces, 7 provinces are metropolitan cities, and 10 provinces have a mix of urban cities and rural areas.

The EMS system of Korea is a government-based system operated by 17 provincial headquarters of the National Fire Agency. The EMS personnel perform basic life support on scene and during transport with advanced airway management and intravenous fluid administration. Since declaration of death in the field is not permitted for EMS providers, all EMS-treated OHCA victims are transported to the nearest emergency department (ED) based on the standard operation protocol.

In Korea, there are 402 EDs that are categorized into three levels by the government according to capacity and resources such as equipment, staffing, and size of the ED: level-1 EDs ($n = 38$), level-2 EDs ($n = 128$), and level-3 EDs ($n = 236$). All EDs generally perform acute cardiac management and post-resuscitation care in accordance with international standard guidelines such as the 2020 American Heart Association guidelines [13]. Most of the level-1 and level-2 EDs perform post-resuscitation care such as PCI and TTM. The Ministry of Health and Welfare has designated and operated cardiovascular disease regional centers but has not yet designated and/or certified cardiac arrest-specific regional centers.

2.2. Data Sources

This study identified a study population using the Korean nationwide OHCA registry, which captures all EMS-assessed OHCA patients across the country. The OHCA registry is a prospective observational registry that was launched in 2006 through a collaboration between the National Fire Agency and the Korean centers for Disease Control and Prevention (CDC). The registry includes ambulance run sheets, dispatch records, EMS cardiac arrest in-depth registry, and medical record reviews. The medical record reviewers from Korea CDC extract data regarding the etiology, hospital care, and outcomes based on the Utstein guidelines. The project quality management committee (QMC) is composed of emergency medicine physicians, cardiologists, epidemiologists, statistical experts, and medical record review experts. All of the items, including definitions, inclusion and exclusion criteria, examples, and warnings, are defined in the medical record review guidelines and were developed by the project QMC. Explanations on nationwide OHCA registry, detailed data collection process, and quality management protocols are reported in previous studies [14].

2.3. Study Population

This study included all EMS-treated OHCA patients aged 18 or over with presumed cardiac etiology between January 2015 and December 2019. Patients whose arrest occurred in an ambulance during transport or witnessed by EMS personnel were excluded. The cause of arrest was presumed to be cardiac if there was no evident noncardiac cause such as asphyxia, drowning, trauma, poisoning, and burn. The cause of arrest was measured by medical record reviewers with discharge summary abstracts or medical records written by the inpatient care doctors, based on the Utstein guidelines [15].

2.4. Main Outcomes

The primary and secondary outcomes were good neurological recovery and survival to discharge. Good neurological recovery was defined as cerebral performance category I (good cerebral performance; no neurologic disability) or II (moderate cerebral disability able to perform daily activities independently) at time of hospital discharge.

2.5. Measurements and Variables

The main exposure of this study is the type of hospital that patients are transported to by EMS providers, which is classified as either CAC or non-CAC. In this study, CAC was defined as a hospital that performed both PCI and TTM at least once each year during the study period for OHCA patients [5].

Patient arrest information, including age, sex, comorbidities (diabetes mellitus, hypertension, and heart disease), urbanization level of arrest location (metropolitan or urban/rural area), and place of arrest (public or private), were collected. Prehospital EMS information including witness status, bystander CPR, initial electrocardiogram rhythm (shockable or non-shockable), EMS time variables (response time interval (time from the call to ambulance arrival at the scene), scene time interval (time from ambulance arrival to departure from the scene), and transport time interval (time from departure to hospital arrival)), multitier response, prehospital airway management, and mechanical CPR were retrieved. Information concerning hospital outcome-related variables, including post-resuscitation care and clinical outcomes, were also collected.

2.6. Statistical Analysis

A descriptive analysis was conducted to compare the characteristics of patients transported to CAC and non-CAC. Categorical variables were shown by counts and proportion and tested by chi-square test. Continuous variables were shown by medians and quartiles and tested by Wilcoxon rank-sum test, since EMS time variables have a nonparametric distribution.

Both univariable and multivariable logistic regression analysis were performed to estimate the effect of direct transport to CACs on study outcomes. Crude and adjusted odds ratios (aORs) with 95% confidence intervals (CIs) were calculated. Finally, the interaction model between the transported hospital and urbanization level of arrest location (metropolitan area or urban/rural area) was conducted to estimate whether the effects of direct transport to CACs varies across urbanization levels that affect the distribution of CAC.

A sensitivity analysis was conducted for pulseless OHCA patients who did not achieve prehospital return of spontaneous circulation (ROSC), to examine whether the association between direct transport to CAGs and study outcomes were maintained.

All statistical analysis was performed using SAS version 9.4 (SAS Institute Inc., Cary NC, USA). $p < 0.05$ was considered statistically significant.

2.7. Ethics Statements

This study complies with the Declaration of Helsinki. This study was approved by the Institutional Review Board (IRB) of Seoul National University Hospital and the requirement for informed consent was waived due to the retrospective nature of this study (IRB No. SNUH-1103-153-357).

3. Results

Among 139,212 EMS-treated OHCA cases that occurred within the study period, 95,931 (68.9%) met the inclusion criteria. We excluded patients who were younger than 18 years old ($n = 3124$), who had noncardiac etiology ($n = 33,004$), and those whose arrest occurred during transport ($n = 7153$) (Figure 1).

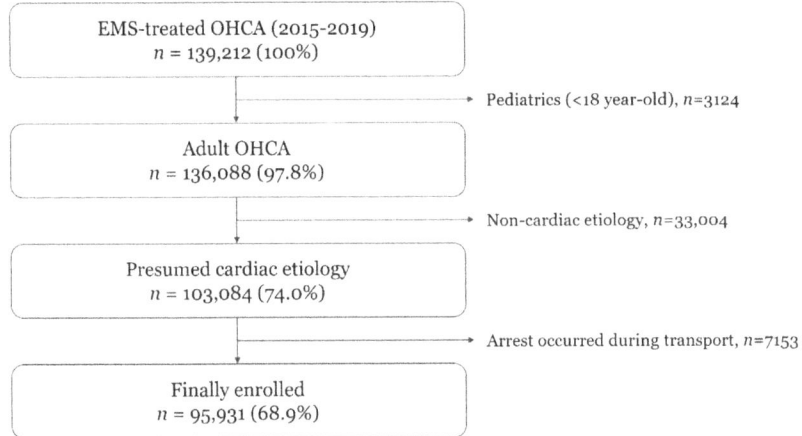

Figure 1. Patient flow. EMS, emergency medical services; OHCA, out-of-hospital cardiac arrest.

3.1. Demographic Findings

The demographics of the study population according to the transported hospitals are presented in Table 1. Of the 95,931 eligible patients, 23,292 (24.3%) and 72,639 (75.7%) OHCA patients were transported to CAC and non-CAC hospitals, respectively. The good neurological recovery and survival to discharge rates were 9.1% and 13.4% in the CAC group, and 4.7% and 7.4% in the non-CAC group, respectively (both p-value < 0.01). OHCAs in the CAC group occurred more frequently in metropolitan areas compared to the non-CAC group (67.1% vs. 32.1%, $p < 0.01$), and hospital treatments including TTM, PCI, and ECMO were also performed more frequently in the CAC group. The medians (interquartile ranges) of EMS transport time interval from scene to hospital were 7 (5–10) min in the CAC group and 6 (4–11) min in the non-CAC group ($p < 0.01$).

The demographics of OHCA patients according to the urbanization level of arrest location are summarized in Table 2. Of the eligible patients, 38,939 (40.6%) cases of OHCA occurred in metropolitan areas and 56,992 (59.4%) cases occurred in nonmetropolitan areas. OHCA cases occurring in metropolitan areas were transported more frequently to a CAC (40.1% vs. 13.5%, $p < 0.01$). Good neurological recovery and survival to discharge rates were 7.0% and 10.7% in the metropolitan group, and 5.0% and 7.6% in the urban/rural group, respectively (both p-value < 0.01).

3.2. Main Results

The results of multivariable logistic regression analyses are shown in Table 3. After adjustments for potential confounders, patients who were transported to CAC hospitals had significantly higher likelihood of good neurological recovery at hospital discharge and survival to discharge than those transported to non-CAC hospitals (aORs (95% CIs): 1.75 (1.63–1.89) and 1.70 (1.60–1.80), respectively).

Table 1. Characteristics of out-of-hospital cardiac arrest patients according to transported hospitals.

	Total	CAC	Non-CAC	p-Value
	n (%)	n (%)	n (%)	
Total	95,931 (100.0)	23,292 (100.0)	72,639 (100.0)	
Age, year				<0.01
19–65	31,722 (33.1)	8460 (36.3)	23,262 (32.0)	
65–120	64,209 (66.9)	14,832 (63.7)	49,377 (68.0)	
Sex, female	35,089 (36.6)	8110 (34.8)	26,979 (37.1)	<0.01
Comorbidity				
Diabetes mellitus	21,386 (22.3)	5922 (25.4)	15,464 (21.3)	<0.01
Hypertension	32,708 (34.1)	8988 (38.6)	23,720 (32.7)	<0.01
Heart disease	16,577 (17.3)	4523 (19.4)	12,054 (16.6)	<0.01
Metropolitan area	38,939 (40.6)	15,619 (67.1)	23,320 (32.1)	<0.01
Place of arrest, public	19,202 (20.0)	5070 (21.8)	14,132 (19.5)	<0.01
Arrest witnessed	44,429 (46.3)	11,659 (50.1)	32,770 (45.1)	<0.01
Bystander CPR	57,803 (60.3)	13,946 (59.9)	43,857 (60.4)	0.17
Initial shockable rhythm	16,237 (16.9)	4732 (20.3)	11,505 (15.8)	<0.01
Response time interval, min				<0.01
0–3	5123 (5.3)	1287 (5.5)	3836 (5.3)	
4–7	50,555 (52.7)	13,882 (59.6)	36,673 (50.5)	
8–	40,253 (42.0)	8123 (34.9)	32,130 (44.2)	
Median (IQR)	7 (5–9)	7 (5–10)	7 (5–10)	<0.01
Scene time interval, min				<0.01
0–10	28,566 (29.8)	5761 (24.7)	22,805 (31.4)	
11–15	33,584 (35.0)	8280 (35.5)	25,304 (34.8)	
16–	33,781 (35.2)	9251 (39.7)	24,530 (33.8)	
Median (IQR)	13 (10–18)	14 (11–18)	13 (10–17)	<0.01
Transport time interval, min				<0.01
0–3	17,312 (18.0)	3184 (13.7)	14,128 (19.4)	
4–7	39,459 (41.1)	10,588 (45.5)	28,871 (39.7)	
8–	39,160 (40.8)	9520 (40.9)	29,640 (40.8)	
Median (IQR)	6 (4–10)	7 (5–10)	6 (4–11)	<0.01
Multitier response	55,631 (58.0)	16,304 (70.0)	39,327 (54.1)	<0.01
EMS management				
Advanced airway	59,978 (62.5)	16,650 (71.5)	43,328 (59.6)	<0.01
Mechanical CPR	10,866 (11.3)	4138 (17.8)	6728 (9.3)	<0.01
ED level				<0.01
Level 1	17,778 (18.5)	10,032 (43.1)	7746 (10.7)	
Level 2	45,389 (47.3)	13,116 (56.3)	32,273 (44.4)	
Level 3	32,764 (23.2)	144 (0.6)	32,630 (44.9)	
Hospital treatment				
TTM	2938 (3.1)	1874 (8.0)	1064 (1.5)	<0.01
PCI	5879 (6.1)	2521 (10.8)	3358 (4.6)	<0.01
ECMO	936 (1.0)	476 (2.0)	460 (0.6)	<0.01
Survival outcomes				
Survival to discharge	8465 (8.8)	3120 (13.4)	5345 (7.4)	<0.01
Good neurological recovery	5563 (5.8)	2113 (9.1)	3450 (4.7)	<0.01

CAC, cardiac arrest center; CPR, cardiopulmonary resuscitation; IQR, interquartile range; ED, emergency department; TTM, targeted temperature management; PCI, percutaneous coronary intervention; ECMO, extracorporeal membrane oxygenation.

3.3. Interaction Analysis

In the interaction analysis, statistically significant interaction effects were found between transported hospital and urbanization level (Table 4). The aORs for the outcomes of the CAC group and non-CAC differed depending on the urbanization level of area of OHCA. The CAC hospitals had interaction effects for good neurological recovery at discharge (aORs (95% CIs): 1.51 (1.40–1.63) for patients in metropolitan areas vs. 1.98 (1.81–2.17) for patients in urban/rural areas, and survival to discharge (aORs (95% CIs):

1.63 (1.48–1.80) for patients in metropolitan areas vs. 1.91 (1.71–2.14) for patients in urban/rural areas (both p for interaction <0.01).

Table 2. Characteristics of out-of-hospital cardiac arrest patients according to urbanization level of arrest location.

	Total	Metropolitan	Urban/Rural	p-Value
	n (%)	n (%)	n (%)	
Total	95,931 (100.0)	38,939 (100.0)	56,992 (100.0)	
Cardiac arrest center				<0.01
Yes	23,292 (24.3)	15,619 (40.1)	7673 (13.5)	
No	72,639 (75.7)	23,320 (59.9)	49,319 (86.5)	
Age, year				<0.01
19–65	23,292 (24.3)	15,619 (40.1)	7673 (13.5)	
65–120	72,639 (75.7)	23,320 (59.9)	49,319 (86.5)	
Sex, female	64,209 (66.9)	25,674 (65.9)	38,535 (67.6)	<0.01
Comorbidity				
Diabetes mellitus	35,089 (36.6)	13,801 (35.4)	21,288 (37.4)	<0.01
Hypertension	21,386 (22.3)	9441 (24.2)	11,945 (21.0)	<0.01
Heart disease	32,708 (34.1)	14,135 (36.3)	18,573 (32.6)	<0.01
Place of arrest, public	19,202 (20.0)	8008 (20.6)	11,194 (19.6)	<0.01
Arrest witnessed	44,429 (46.3)	18,409 (47.3)	26,020 (45.7)	<0.01
Bystander CPR	57,803 (60.3)	22,538 (57.9)	35,265 (61.9)	<0.01
Initial shockable rhythm	16,237 (16.9)	7086 (18.2)	9151 (16.1)	0.01
Response time interval, min				<0.01
0–3	5123 (5.3)	2269 (5.8)	2854 (5.0)	
4–7	50,555 (52.7)	25,074 (64.4)	25,481 (44.7)	
8–	40,253 (42.0)	11,596 (29.8)	28,657 (50.3)	
Median (IQR)	7 (5–9)	6 (5–8)	8 (6–11)	<0.01
Scene time interval, min				<0.01
0–10	28,566 (29.8)	10,677 (27.4)	17,889 (31.4)	
11–15	33,584 (35.0)	15,132 (38.9)	18,452 (32.4)	
16–	33,781 (35.2)	13,130 (33.7)	20,651 (36.2)	
Median (IQR)	13 (10–18)	13 (10–17)	13 (10–18)	<0.01
Transport time interval, min				<0.01
0–3	17,312 (18.0)	7366 (18.9)	9946 (17.5)	
4–7	39,459 (41.1)	19,765 (50.8)	19,694 (34.6)	
8–	39,160 (40.8)	11,808 (30.3)	27,352 (48.0)	
Median (IQR)	6 (4–10)	6 (4–8)	7 (4–12)	<0.01
Multitier response	55,631 (58.0)	26,993 (69.3)	28,638 (50.2)	<0.01
EMS management				
Advanced airway	59,978 (62.5)	27,384 (70.3)	32,594 (57.2)	<0.01
Mechanical CPR	10,866 (11.3)	6947 (17.8)	3919 (6.9)	<0.01
ED level				<0.01
Level 1	17,778 (18.5)	7336 (18.8)	10,442 (18.3)	
Level 2	45,389 (47.3)	22,232 (57.1)	23,157 (40.6)	
Level 3	32,764 (23.2)	9371 (24.1)	23,393 (41.1)	
Hospital treatment				
TTM	2938 (3.1)	1745 (4.5)	1193 (2.1)	<0.01
PCI	5879 (6.1)	3185 (8.2)	2694 (4.7)	<0.01
ECMO	936 (1.0)	548 (1.4)	388 (0.7)	<0.01
Survival outcomes				
Survival to discharge	8465 (8.8)	4155 (10.7)	4310 (7.6)	<0.01
Good neurological recovery	5563 (5.8)	2711 (7.0)	2852 (5.0)	<0.01

CPR, cardiopulmonary resuscitation; IQR, interquartile range; ED, emergency department; TTM, targeted temperature management; PCI, percutaneous coronary intervention; ECMO, extracorporeal membrane oxygenation.

Table 3. Multivariable logistic regression models for study outcomes.

	Total	Outcome		Model 1	Model 2	Model 3
	n	n	%	aOR (95% CI)	aOR (95% CI)	aOR (95% CI)
Good neurological recovery						
Transported hospital						
Noncardiac center	72,639	3450	4.7	1.00	1.00	1.00
Cardiac center	23,292	2113	9.1	1.81 (1.70–1.90)	1.66 (1.55–1.79)	1.75 (1.63–1.89)
Urbanization level						
Urban/rural area	56,992	2852	5.0	1.00	1.00	1.00
Metropolitan area	38,939	2711	7.0	1.18 (1.12–1.26)	1.17 (1.09–1.25)	1.05 (0.98–1.13)
Survival to discharge						
Transported hospital						
Noncardiac center	72,639	5345	7.4	1.00	1.00	1.00
Cardiac center	23,292	3120	13.4	1.75 (1.67–1.85)	1.62 (1.53–1.72)	1.70 (1.60–1.80)
Urbanization level						
Urban/rural area	56,992	4310	7.6	1.00	1.00	1.00
Metropolitan area	38,939	4155	10.7	1.23 (1.18–1.30)	1.23 (1.16–1.30)	1.12 (1.05–1.18)

aOR, adjusted odds ratio; CI, confidence interval. Model 1: adjusted for age and sex. Model 2: adjusted for variables in Model 1, comorbidities (diabetes mellitus, hypertension, and heart disease), place of arrest, witness status, bystander CPR, and initial shockable rhythm. Model 3: adjusted for variables in Model 2, response time interval, scene time interval, transport time interval, multitier response, EMS airway management, and mechanical CPR.

Table 4. Interaction analysis between direct transport to cardiac arrest centers and urbanization level.

	Transported Hospital				p-for-Interaction
	Non-CAC	Cardiac Arrest Center			
		aOR	95% CI		
Good neurological recovery					
Urbanization level					<0.01
Metropolitan area	ref.	1.51	1.40	1.63	
Urban/rural area	ref.	1.98	1.81	2.17	
Survival to discharge					
Urbanization level					<0.01
Metropolitan area	ref.	1.63	1.48	1.80	
Urban/rural area	ref.	1.91	1.71	2.14	

CAC, cardiac arrest center; aOR, adjusted odds ratio; CI, confidence interval.

3.4. Sensitivity Analysis

The multivariable logistic regression analysis and interaction analysis were performed for pulseless OHCA patients who did not achieve prehospital ROSC (Tables 5 and S1). Pulseless OHCA patients who were transported to CAC hospitals had significantly higher likelihoods of good neurological recovery and survival to discharge (aORs (95% CIs) 1.49 (1.18–1.87) and 1.45 (1.30–1.61), respectively). In the interaction analysis, the CAC hospitals had interaction effects for good neurological recovery at discharge (aORs (95% CIs): 1.36 (1.04–1.77) for patients in metropolitan areas vs. 1.84 (1.22–2.79) for patients in urban/rural areas, and survival to discharge (aORs (95% CIs): 1.24 (1.09–1.42) for patients in metropolitan areas vs. 1.91 (1.60–2.27) for patients in urban/rural areas (both p for interaction < 0.01).

Table 5. Sensitivity analysis of pulseless OHCA patients who did not achieve prehospital ROSC.

	Transported Hospital			p-for-Interaction
	Non-CAC	Cardiac Arrest Center		
		aOR	95% CI	
Good neurological recovery				<0.01
Urbanization level				
Metropolitan area	ref.	1.36	1.04 1.77	
Urban/rural area	ref.	1.84	1.22 2.79	
Survival to discharge				<0.01
Urbanization level				
Metropolitan area	ref.	1.24	1.09 1.42	
Urban/rural area	ref.	1.91	1.60 2.27	

CAC, cardiac arrest center; aOR, adjusted odds ratio; CI, confidence interval.

4. Discussion

Using the Korean national OHCA database, this study discovered that adult OHCA patients with presumed cardiac etiology who were transported to CAC hospitals were more likely to have better survival outcomes compared to patients transported to non-CAC hospitals. In the interaction analysis, OHCAs occurring in urban/rural areas have better clinical outcomes from direct transport to a CAC hospital. These trends were maintained in the sensitivity analysis of pulseless OHCA patients who did not achieve prehospital ROSC. This research contributes to understanding the relationship between regionalization of post-resuscitation care and overall survival outcomes and will help develop strategies to improve survival outcomes in OHCAs that occur in urban/rural areas.

Regionalized systems of post-resuscitation care have been proposed to improve survival outcomes of OHCAs through centralization of highly resource-intensive treatments such as TTM, acute cardiac care including PCI, and multimodal neuro-intensive care. In recent systematic review and meta-analysis, direct transport of OHCA patients to CACs by EMS providers was associated with increased survival outcomes, despite very low certainty of evidence [8,9]. In meta-analysis studies, the definition of CAC varied from study to study, and the capability of PCI was essential, while availability for TTM was treated as important. Although the definition of CAC is used in various ways in different countries based on international guidelines [16], direct transport to a PCI-capable hospital increased overall survival and neurological outcomes of OHCAs [17,18]. Only 11% of OHCA patients who were transported to CAC hospitals had received PCI in this study. Even so, the good clinical outcomes of patients in the CAC group had probably been impacted by capability of PCI as well as the accumulated experience and ability of these CAC hospitals to treat OHCA patients [9].

However, direct transport of OHCA patients to CAC hospitals results in increased transport time interval for some patients [19]. A previous study related to prehospital transport time of OHCAs reported that delaying hospital arrival time by about 14 min counteracted the potential benefit of transporting them to a PCI-capable center [20,21]. Because current studies focusing on the relationship between distance from scene to hospital and clinical outcomes are mainly conducted in urban environments and limited to relatively short transport time intervals, there is insufficient evidence to agree to current guidelines stating to bypass the nearest hospital and transport to CAC hospitals in rural areas where transport distances may be substantially longer [22,23].

In the interaction analysis of the study, OHCAs occurring in nonmetropolitan areas had higher odds of survival outcomes with direct transport to a CAC hospital compared to OHCAs in metropolitan areas (p-for-interaction < 0.01). One hypothesis that may explain this result is that the clinical capabilities of non-CAC hospitals located in nonmetropolitan areas, including manpower, equipment, and facilities, are below those in metropolitan area. As the beneficial effects of regionalization of post-resuscitation care for OHCAs have been strengthened in urban/rural areas, CACs should be designated and invested in to achieve centralization of resource-intensive care to improve the survival outcomes of OHCAs in nonmetropolitan areas [24].

Characteristics of destination hospitals are associated with the clinical outcomes of OHCA, including level of EDs, urbanization level of location of hospitals, teaching status, and OHCA case volume [25–28]. In this study, direct transport of OHCA patients to a hospital where post-resuscitation care is capable showed favorable survival and neurological outcomes, and these results were reinforced in OHCA patients occurring in nonmetropolitan (urban/rural) areas. To improve the survival outcomes of OHCAs, it is considerable to designate and operate CACs to achieve a centralization of resource-intensive post-resuscitation care in nonmetropolitan areas.

This study has a number of limitations. First, since there were no designated cardiac arrest-specific regional centers in Korea, CAC was defined as a hospital that performed PCI and TTM in this study. The definition of CAC varied from study to study [8], which meant the definition would have affected the study results. The generalizability of findings of this study to other countries needs to be further evaluated. Second, the definition of urbanization level (metropolitan vs. urban/rural area) may not accurately reflect the level of medical resources because it is population-based and therefore such classification may have influenced the study results. Third, it is difficult to perform a geospatial analysis to evaluate the proportion of OHCA patients who were not transported to the nearest ED and their EMS transport time interval in this study. Fourth, this study is an observational retrospective analysis, which may have introduced some unmeasured confounders as is known with this study design. Lastly, while we used multivariable analysis, unmeasured and unmeasurable confounders may have influenced the clinical outcomes of the study.

5. Conclusions

Direct transport of OHCA patients to cardiac arrest centers was associated with significantly higher survival and favorable neurological outcomes compared to patients transported to non-CAC hospitals. Furthermore, the findings were consistent and strengthened in OHCAs occurring in nonmetropolitan areas. Designating and investing in CACs to achieve centralization of post-resuscitation care could improve the survival outcomes of OHCAs, especially in nonmetropolitan areas.

Supplementary Materials: The following supporting information can be downloaded at: https://www.mdpi.com/article/10.3390/jcm11041033/s1. Table S1: Sensitivity analysis of multivariable logistic regression model for pulseless out-of-hospital cardiac arrest patients who did not achieve prehospital ROSC.

Author Contributions: Conceptualization: E.J. and Y.S.R.; Data curation: E.J. and J.H.P.; Formal analysis: E.J.; Investigation: J.H.P. and S.D.S.; Methodology: Y.S.R. and S.D.S.; Software: E.J.; Supervision: Y.S.R., H.H.R. and S.D.S.; Validation: J.H.P., H.H.R. and S.D.S.; Visualization: E.J.; Writing—original draft: E.J.; Writing—review and editing: Y.S.R. All authors have read and agreed to the published version of the manuscript.

Funding: This research received no external funding.

Institutional Review Board Statement: This study complies with the Declaration of Helsinki. This study was approved by the Institutional Review Board (IRB) of Seoul National University Hospital and the requirement for informed consent was waived due to the retrospective nature of this study (IRB No. SNUH-1103-153-357).

Informed Consent Statement: Patient consent was waived due to anonymized data.

Data Availability Statement: The data of this study were obtained from the Korea Centers for Disease Control and Prevention, but restrictions apply to the availability of these data and so are not publicly available.

Conflicts of Interest: The authors declare no conflict of interest.

References

1. Atwood, C.; Eisenberg, M.S.; Herlitz, J.; Rea, T.D. Incidence of EMS-treated out-of-hospital cardiac arrest in Europe. *Resuscitation* **2005**, *67*, 75–80. [CrossRef] [PubMed]
2. Berdowski, J.; Berg, R.A.; Tijssen, J.G.; Koster, R.W. Global incidences of out-of-hospital cardiac arrest and survival rates: Systematic review of 67 prospective studies. *Resuscitation* **2010**, *81*, 1479–1487. [CrossRef] [PubMed]
3. Sasson, C.; Rogers, M.A.; Dahl, J.; Kellermann, A.L. Predictors of survival from out-of-hospital cardiac arrest: A systematic review and meta-analysis. *Circ. Cardiovasc. Qual. Outcomes* **2010**, *3*, 63–81. [CrossRef] [PubMed]
4. Hansen, C.M.; Kragholm, K.; Granger, C.B.; Pearson, D.A.; Tyson, C.; Monk, L.; Corbett, C.; Nelson, R.D.; Dupre, M.E.; Fosbøl, E.L. The role of bystanders, first responders, and emergency medical service providers in timely defibrillation and related outcomes after out-of-hospital cardiac arrest: Results from a statewide registry. *Resuscitation* **2015**, *96*, 303–309. [CrossRef] [PubMed]
5. Nolan, J.P.; Soar, J.; Cariou, A.; Cronberg, T.; Moulaert, V.R.; Deakin, C.D.; Bottiger, B.W.; Friberg, H.; Sunde, K.; Sandroni, C. European resuscitation council and European society of intensive care medicine 2015 guidelines for post-resuscitation care. *Intensive Care Med.* **2015**, *41*, 2039–2056. [CrossRef] [PubMed]
6. Berg, K.M.; Cheng, A.; Panchal, A.R.; Topjian, A.A.; Aziz, K.; Bhanji, F.; Bigham, B.L.; Hirsch, K.G.; Hoover, A.V.; Kurz, M.C. Part 7: Systems of Care: 2020 American Heart Association Guidelines for Cardiopulmonary Resuscitation and Emergency Cardiovascular Care. *Circulation* **2020**, *142*, S580–S604. [CrossRef]
7. Merchant, R.M.; Topjian, A.A.; Panchal, A.R.; Cheng, A.; Aziz, K.; Berg, K.M.; Lavonas, E.J.; Magid, D.J. Part 1: Executive Summary: 2020 American Heart Association Guidelines for Cardiopulmonary Resuscitation and Emergency Cardiovascular Care. *Circulation* **2020**, *142*, S337–S357. [CrossRef]
8. Yeung, J.; Matsuyama, T.; Bray, J.; Reynolds, J.; Skrifvars, M.B. Does care at a cardiac arrest centre improve outcome after out-of-hospital cardiac arrest? - A systematic review. *Resuscitation* **2019**, *137*, 102–115. [CrossRef] [PubMed]
9. Lipe, D.; Giwa, A.; Caputo, N.D.; Gupta, N.; Addison, J.; Cournoyer, A. Do Out-of-Hospital Cardiac Arrest Patients Have Increased Chances of Survival When Transported to a Cardiac Resuscitation Center? *J. Am. Heart Assoc.* **2018**, *7*, e011079. [CrossRef] [PubMed]
10. Cha, W.C.; Lee, S.C.; Do Shin, S.; Song, K.J.; Sung, A.J.; Hwang, S.S. Regionalisation of out-of-hospital cardiac arrest care for patients without prehospital return of spontaneous circulation. *Resuscitation* **2012**, *83*, 1338–1342. [CrossRef]
11. Yasunaga, H.; Miyata, H.; Horiguchi, H.; Tanabe, S.; Akahane, M.; Ogawa, T.; Koike, S.; Imamura, T. Population density, call-response interval, and survival of out-of-hospital cardiac arrest. *Int. J. Health Geogr.* **2011**, *10*, 26. [CrossRef] [PubMed]
12. Jung, E.; Ro, Y.S.; Ryu, H.H.; Shin, S.D.; Moon, S. Interaction Effects between COVID-19 Outbreak and Community Income Levels on Excess Mortality among Patients Visiting Emergency Departments. *J. Korean Med. Sci.* **2021**, *36*, e100. [CrossRef] [PubMed]
13. Magid, D.J.; Aziz, K.; Cheng, A.; Hazinski, M.F.; Hoover, A.V.; Mahgoub, M.; Panchal, A.R.; Sasson, C.; Topjian, A.A.; Rodriguez, A.J.; et al. Part 2: Evidence Evaluation and Guidelines Development: 2020 American Heart Association Guidelines for Cardiopulmonary Resuscitation and Emergency Cardiovascular Care. *Circulation* **2020**, *142*, S358–S365. [CrossRef] [PubMed]
14. Ro, Y.S.; Shin, S.D.; Lee, Y.J.; Lee, S.C.; Song, K.J.; Ryoo, H.W.; Ong, M.E.; McNally, B.; Bobrow, B.; Tanaka, H.; et al. Effect of Dispatcher-Assisted Cardiopulmonary Resuscitation Program and Location of Out-of-Hospital Cardiac Arrest on Survival and Neurologic Outcome. *Ann. Emerg. Med.* **2017**, *69*, 52–61. [CrossRef] [PubMed]
15. Perkins, G.D.; Jacobs, I.G.; Nadkarni, V.M.; Berg, R.A.; Bhanji, F.; Biarent, D.; Bossaert, L.L.; Brett, S.J.; Chamberlain, D.; de Caen, A.R.; et al. Cardiac Arrest and Cardiopulmonary Resuscitation Outcome Reports: Update of the Utstein Resuscitation Registry Templates for Out-of-Hospital Cardiac Arrest: A Statement for Healthcare Professionals from a Task Force of the International Liaison Committee on Resuscitation (American Heart Association, European Resuscitation Council, Australian and New Zealand Council on Resuscitation, Heart and Stroke Foundation of Canada, InterAmerican Heart Foundation, Resuscitation Council of Southern Africa, Resuscitation Council of Asia); and the American Heart Association Emergency Cardiovascular Care Committee and the Council on Cardiopulmonary, Critical Care, Perioperative and Resuscitation. *Circulation* **2014**, *132*, 1286–1300. [CrossRef]
16. Sinning, C.; Ahrens, I.; Cariou, A.; Beygui, F.; Lamhaut, L.; Halvorsen, S.; Nikolaou, N.; Nolan, J.P.; Price, S.; Monsieurs, K.; et al. The cardiac arrest centre for the treatment of sudden cardiac arrest due to presumed cardiac cause: Aims, function, and structure: Position paper of the ACVC association of the ESC, EAPCI, EHRA, ERC, EUSEM, and ESICM. *Eur. Heart J. Acute Cardiovasc. Care* **2020**, *9*, S193–S202. [CrossRef]
17. Stub, D.; Smith, K.; Bray, J.E.; Bernard, S.; Duffy, S.J.; Kaye, D.M. Hospital characteristics are associated with patient outcomes following out-of-hospital cardiac arrest. *Heart* **2011**, *97*, 1489–1494. [CrossRef]
18. Wnent, J.; Seewald, S.; Heringlake, M.; Lemke, H.; Brauer, K.; Lefering, R.; Fischer, M.; Jantzen, T.; Bein, B.; Messelken, M.; et al. Choice of hospital after out-of-hospital cardiac arrest–a decision with far-reaching consequences: A study in a large German city. *Crit. Care* **2012**, *16*, R164. [CrossRef]
19. Nichol, G.; Aufderheide, T.P.; Eigel, B.; Neumar, R.W.; Lurie, K.G.; Bufalino, V.J.; Callaway, C.W.; Menon, V.; Bass, R.R.; Abella, B.S.; et al. Regional systems of care for out-of-hospital cardiac arrest: A policy statement from the American Heart Association. *Circulation* **2010**, *121*, 709–729. [CrossRef]
20. Chien, C.Y.; Tsai, S.L.; Tsai, L.H.; Chen, C.B.; Seak, C.J.; Weng, Y.M.; Lin, C.C.; Ng, C.J.; Chien, W.C.; Huang, C.H. Impact of Transport Time and Cardiac Arrest Centers on the Neurological Outcome After Out-of-Hospital Cardiac Arrest: A Retrospective Cohort Study. *J. Am. Heart Assoc.* **2020**, *9*, e015544. [CrossRef]

21. Cournoyer, A.; Notebaert, É.; de Montigny, L.; Ross, D.; Cossette, S.; Londei-Leduc, L.; Iseppon, M.; Lamarche, Y.; Sokoloff, C. Potter, B.J. Impact of the direct transfer to percutaneous coronary intervention-capable hospitals on survival to hospital discharge for patients with out-of-hospital cardiac arrest. *Resuscitation* **2018**, *125*, 28–33. [CrossRef] [PubMed]
22. Davis, D.P.; Fisher, R.; Aguilar, S.; Metz, M.; Ochs, G.; McCallum-Brown, L.; Ramanujam, P.; Buono, C.; Vilke, G.M.; Chan, T.C. et al. The feasibility of a regional cardiac arrest receiving system. *Resuscitation* **2007**, *74*, 44–51. [CrossRef] [PubMed]
23. Spaite, D.W.; Bobrow, B.J.; Vadeboncoeur, T.F.; Chikani, V.; Clark, L.; Mullins, T.; Sanders, A.B. The impact of prehospital transport interval on survival in out-of-hospital cardiac arrest: Implications for regionalization of post-resuscitation care. *Resuscitation* **2008** *79*, 61–66. [CrossRef]
24. Girotra, S.; Chan, P.S.; Bradley, S.M. Post-resuscitation care following out-of-hospital and in-hospital cardiac arrest. *Heart (Br Card. Soc.)* **2015**, *101*, 1943–1949. [CrossRef]
25. Carr, B.G.; Goyal, M.; Band, R.A.; Gaieski, D.F.; Abella, B.S.; Merchant, R.M.; Branas, C.C.; Becker, L.B.; Neumar, R.W. A national analysis of the relationship between hospital factors and post-cardiac arrest mortality. *Intensive Care Med.* **2009**, *35*, 505–511 [CrossRef] [PubMed]
26. Shin, S.D.; Suh, G.J.; Ahn, K.O.; Song, K.J. Cardiopulmonary resuscitation outcome of out-of-hospital cardiac arrest in low-volume versus high-volume emergency departments: An observational study and propensity score matching analysis. *Resuscitation* **2011** *82*, 32–39. [CrossRef] [PubMed]
27. Søholm, H.; Wachtell, K.; Nielsen, S.L.; Bro-Jeppesen, J.; Pedersen, F.; Wanscher, M.; Boesgaard, S.; Møller, J.E.; Hassager, C. Kjaergaard, J. Tertiary centres have improved survival compared to other hospitals in the Copenhagen area after out-of-hospital cardiac arrest. *Resuscitation* **2013**, *84*, 162–167. [CrossRef]
28. Ro, Y.S.; Shin, S.D.; Song, K.J.; Park, C.B.; Lee, E.J.; Ahn, K.O.; Cho, S.I. A comparison of outcomes of out-of-hospital cardiac arrest with non-cardiac etiology between emergency departments with low- and high-resuscitation case volume. *Resuscitation* **2012**, *83* 855–861. [CrossRef]

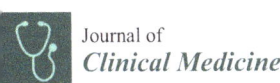

Review

Comparison between Prehospital Mechanical Cardiopulmonary Resuscitation (CPR) Devices and Manual CPR for Out-of-Hospital Cardiac Arrest: A Systematic Review, Meta-Analysis, and Trial Sequential Analysis

Cheng-Ying Chiang [1,†], Ket-Cheong Lim [1,†], Pei Chun Lai [2], Tou-Yuan Tsai [3,4], Yen Ta Huang [5,*] and Ming-Jen Tsai [1,*]

1. Department of Emergency Medicine, Ditmanson Medical Foundation Chia-Yi Christian Hospital, Chiayi City 600, Taiwan; chvv7552@gmail.com (C.-Y.C.); limkc20@gmail.com (K.-C.L.)
2. Education Center, National Cheng Kung University Hospital, College of Medicine, National Cheng Kung University, Tainan 704, Taiwan; debbie0613.lai@gmail.com
3. School of Medicine, Tzu Chi University, Hualien 970, Taiwan; 96311123@gms.tcu.edu.tw
4. Department of Emergency Medicine, Dalin Tzu Chi Hospital, Buddhist Tzu Chi Medical Foundation, Chiayi City 622, Taiwan
5. Department of Surgery, National Cheng Kung University Hospital, College of Medicine, National Cheng Kung University, Tainan 704, Taiwan
* Correspondence: uncleda.huang@gmail.com (Y.T.H.); tshi33@gmail.com (M.-J.T.)
† These authors contributed equally to this work.

Abstract: In pre-hospital settings, efficient cardiopulmonary resuscitation (CPR) is challenging; therefore, the application of mechanical CPR devices continues to increase. However, the evidence of the benefits of using mechanical CPR devices in pre-hospital settings for adult out-of-hospital cardiac arrest (OHCA) is controversial. This meta-analysis compared the effects of mechanical and manual CPR applied in the pre-hospital stage on clinical outcomes after OHCA. Cochrane Library, PubMed, Embase, and ClinicalTrials.gov were searched from inception until October 2021. Studies comparing mechanical and manual CPR applied in the pre-hospital stage for survival outcomes of adult OHCA were eligible. Data abstraction, quality assessment, meta-analysis, trial sequential analysis (TSA), and grading of recommendations, assessment, development, and evaluation were conducted. Seven randomized controlled and 15 observational studies were included. Compared to manual CPR, pre-hospital use of mechanical CPR showed a positive effect in achieving return of spontaneous circulation (ROSC) and survival to admission. No difference was found in survival to discharge and discharge with favorable neurological status, with inconclusive results in TSA. In conclusion, pre-hospital use of mechanical CPR devices may benefit adult OHCA in achieving ROSC and survival to admission. With low certainty of evidence, more well-designed large-scale randomized controlled trials are needed to validate these findings.

Keywords: cardiac arrest; resuscitation; cardiopulmonary resuscitation; mechanical; pre-hospital; out of hospital cardiac arrest

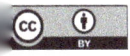

1. Introduction

Out-of-hospital cardiac arrest (OHCA) is a universal concern [1]. The global incidence is approximately 30–97 individuals per 100,000 person-years [2,3]. Although the management of OHCA has progressed, the survival rate remains poor, around 3.1% to 20.4% across the world [2,4]. Achieving survival from OHCA relies on implementing the integral chain of survival [5]. It includes early activation of the emergency medical services (EMS) system, provision of high-quality cardiopulmonary resuscitation (CPR), early defibrillation, advanced resuscitation, post-cardiac arrest care, and recovery [5]. Early administration of high-quality CPR plays an important role in achieving return of spontaneous circulation (ROSC) and preserving brain perfusion following ROSC [5]. However, efficient CPR in prehospital settings is challenging, especially when moving patients and during ambulance transport. The safety of EMS crews is also an issue when performing CPR, such as in a moving ambulance or resuscitating patients with coronavirus disease 2019 (COVID-19). Hence, the use of mechanical CPR devices in prehospital settings continues to increase and is recommended by professional societies in resuscitating COVID-19 patients [6,7].

However, the effect of mechanical CPR devices on the clinical outcomes of OHCA remains controversial and lacks evidence regarding the benefits of mechanical CPR for OHCA patients compared to manual CPR [8–12]. Zhu et al. conducted a meta-analysis in 2019, including nine randomized controlled trials (RCTs) and six non-RCTs, and found no significant differences in the resuscitative effects between mechanical and manual CPR in OHCA patients [8]. Similar result was found in Liu et al. in 2019 comparing manual CPR and mechanical CPR with the Lund University Cardiac Assist System (LUCAS) device [11]. Previous meta-analyses pooled the studies with "in-hospital" and "pre-hospital" use of mechanical CPR devices and concluded that mechanical CPR is not superior to manual CPR for OHCA. However, the resources in in-hospital settings are likely to be better than those in the pre-hospital stage, e.g., more personnel for maintaining the good quality of CPR, and a more spacious environment, and better equipment and medication. Hence, it is reasonable that studies investigating the "in-hospital" use of mechanical CPR for OHCA patients did not show benefits compared to manual CPR [13–16]. A further issue is whether previous meta-analyses had sufficient statistical power. Recently, increasing evidence including large-scale cohort and RCTs has shown the benefit of prehospital use of mechanical CPR devices [17–19]. Hence, a new Systemic Review and Meta-Analysis (SRMA) is needed to analyze the benefit between the use of manual CPR and mechanical CPR applied specifically in a "pre-hospital" setting. The aim of this study was to conduct a systematic review, meta-analysis, and trial sequential analysis of the published literature on the "prehospital" use of mechanical CPR devices compared to manual CPR for adult OHCA.

2. Materials and Methods

This SRMA was conducted according to the latest statement of the Preferred Reporting Items for Systematic Reviews and Meta-Analysis (PRISMA) [20]. Our protocol was registered on PROSPERO (CRD42021286570).

2.1. Inclusion Criteria

Studies were included if the participants were adult patients with OHCA, the intervention was the use of an automated mechanical CPR device in the prehospital stage (including at the scene of cardiac arrest or during ambulance transport), the comparison was with manual CPR, and the outcome indicators were survival-related outcomes. Primary outcomes were rates of ROSC and survival to hospital admission, which most directly reflect the effect and quality of CPR performed in the prehospital stage. The secondary outcomes, such as survival to discharge or 30 days, and survival to discharge with favorable neurological status (defined as Cerebral Performance Category: 1–2, Modified Rankin Scale: 0–2, or Glasgow coma scale ≥ 13), were likely influenced by post-resuscitation care. Any study with at least one of the aforementioned outcome measurements was included, comprising RCTs and non-RCTs.

2.2. Exclusion Criteria

Excluded studies: Studies that recruited patients with in-hospital cardiac arrest (IHCA) or OHCA who received mechanical CPR after arriving at the emergency department (ED) but not in the pre-hospital stage; studies including OHCA younger than 18 years, animal studies, simulation studies, or cardiac arrest caused by hypothermia, drowning, trauma, and toxic substances with a unique pathophysiology; studies using non-automated mechanical CPR devices, such as non-powered active devices; studies evaluating the harm, cost-effectiveness, or user ability as outcomes; and studies that were not the full-length article or without detailed description in the methodology. Articles with related studies, such as subgroup analysis that were published from the same institutions or individuals were excluded, but the most comprehensive one was retained. We also excluded studies designed to cross-over the implementation of manual CPR and mechanical CPR in individual participants.

2.3. Search Methods

We searched the PubMed, Embase, Cochrane Library, and ClinicalTrials.gov with the keywords of "cardiac arrest," "heart arrest," "cardiopulmonary resuscitation," "CPR," "chest compression," "mechanical," "Lucas," "Autopulse," and "Load distributing band" from inception until 27 October 2021. No language restrictions were imposed. The detailed search strategy is presented in Supplementary Table S1. We reviewed the references of eligible papers, similar articles recommended by the PubMed algorithm, and published systematic reviews to identify candidate trials that were not listed in the original database.

2.4. Selection of Studies

Two investigators independently screened the titles and abstracts of the studies identified from the database searches. We obtained the full-text articles for the review for more thorough screening and eligibility assessment using the same inclusion and exclusion criteria. Disagreements were resolved through consensus, and a third reviewer was involved if there was no agreement.

2.5. Data Extraction

Two investigators extracted data in an independent, consistent fashion using a preformed format. Data extraction included the name of the first author, year of publication, country where the study was conducted, study design, sample size, type of mechanical CPR device, total number of participants per treatment arm, and number of participants achieving the set primary and secondary outcomes. For RCTs, the data from the intention-to-treat analysis were chosen for data extraction. For non-RCTs, matched case-control data were extracted, if applicable.

2.6. Literature Quality Evaluation

Two authors independently assessed the risk of bias (RoB) for included studies by using a revised Cochrane risk of bias tool for randomized trials (RoB 2.0) for RCTs [21] and risk of bias in non-randomized studies of interventions (ROBINS-I) tool for non-RCTs [22].

2.7. Statistical Analysis

We performed a meta-analysis of the data using Review Manager version 5.41 (Cochrane Collaboration). A random-effects model was used to calculate summary statistics due to anticipated heterogeneity. Forest plots with odds ratios (ORs) and 95% confidence intervals (CIs) were analyzed using the Mantel-Haenszel (M-H) method for dichotomous data. Statistical significance was set at $p < 0.05$. Heterogeneity among studies was measured using I^2 statistics. If I^2 was higher than 50%, substantial heterogeneity was indicated. Sensitivity analyses of fixed-effect model, different study designs, studies with low RoB and subgroup analyses of different types of mechanical CPR devices and geographic locations where the study was conducted were performed.

2.8. Trial Sequential Analysis

Trial sequential analysis (TSA) was applied to quantify the statistical reliability of data by repetitive and cumulative testing for meta-analyses [23]. We conducted this analysis using TSA software version 0.9.5.10 Beta (Copenhagen Trial Unit, Center for Clinical Intervention Research, Copenhagen, Denmark). We applied a two-sided test, set Type I error of 5% and power of 80% and assumed a 10% relative risk reduction for mechanical

CPR. The O'Brien–Fleming monitoring boundaries were applied for hypothesis testing and a random-effects model with the Biggerstaff-Tweedie method was used [24]. The incidence of the control arm was filled in the "overall events/total cases" of the measured outcome in the manual CPR group of the enrolled studies. A Z-curve was constructed using cumulative evidence of trials over time. Either the Z-curve crossed the O'Brien-Fleming boundaries before the estimated required information size (RIS) was reached or the Z-curve was higher than 1.96 when the accumulated size was larger than RIS were considered true positives. Otherwise, a true negative was considered if the Z-curve entered the futility area. A total sample size that did not reach the RIS was defined as underpower.

2.9. Grading of the Certainty of Evidence

The quality of the overall certainty of evidence (CoE) was assessed using the Grading of Recommendations Assessment, Development, and Evaluation (GRADE) methodology for each outcome [25]. The level of CoE was high, moderate, low, or very low. GRADEpro software (https://gradepro.org) was used.

3. Results

3.1. Results of the Literature Search

In total, 3350 articles were identified: from PubMed, 1106; EMBASE, 1970; Cochrane Library, 233; ClinicalTrials.gov, 41, and 835 articles were excluded because of duplication. A total of 2515 articles were screened by reading titles and abstracts. In total, 2454 articles were excluded that did not meet the inclusion criteria, and 61 articles retrieved for full-text screening. Among them, 14 articles were excluded because they were not full articles. Of 47 articles assessed for eligibility, 21 articles were included, after excluding articles investigating different populations (IHCA and aircraft rescue) ($n = 14$), in-hospital use of mechanical CPR device ($n = 3$), different outcomes ($n = 6$), crossover study ($n = 1$), and no raw data for retrieval ($n = 2$). In addition, from grey literature, five articles were identified from citation searching, and one article was included in the review. In total, 22 studies were included. A flowchart according to the PRISMA statement [20] is shown in Figure 1.

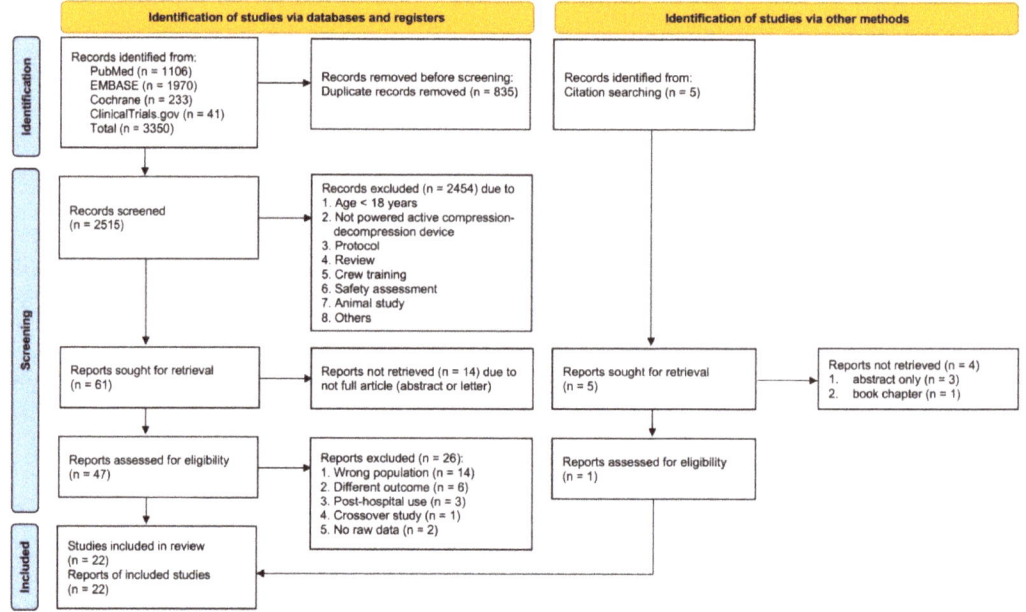

Figure 1. Flow diagram of preferred reporting items for systematic reviews and meta-analysis (PRISMA) 2020.

Table 1 summarizes the characteristics of the included studies. Seven RCTs and 15 non-RCTs with a total of 85,975 OHCAs were included in the meta-analysis. It included studies published between 2006 and 2021, conducted in 16 countries across the continents of North America, Asia, Oceania, and Europe. In terms of automatic CPR devices, LUCAS was applied in 12 studies [18,19,26–35], AutoPulse was applied in seven studies [36–42], and three studies involved both devices [17,43,44].

3.2. Risk of Bias Assessment

For the seven enrolled RCTs including three individual RCTs and four cluster-RCTs, the overall RoB were judged as "low" in four trials [33–36], "some concerns" in two trials [19,37], and "high" in 1 trial [38] (Supplementary Table S2). The majority of RoBs arose from the domain of the randomization process. In this domain, one trial was judged as "high" because the allocation sequence concealment was not clear and with baseline difference between intervention groups [38]; two trials were judged as "some concerns" because of baseline differences between intervention groups [19,37]. From the timing of identification or recruitment of participants in a cluster-randomized trial, one cluster RCT was judged as "high," because the participants were recruited after sending to the hospital (not before randomization of clusters) [38]. For the 15 included non-RCTs, the overall RoB were judged as "moderate" in 10 studies [17,18,26,27,29,31,39–41,44] and "serious" in 5 studies [28,30,32,42,43] (Supplementary Table S3). The majority of RoB arose from bias due to confounding factors (Domain 1 in ROBINS-I). However, this was inevitable because of non-randomized settings. In this case, ten non-RCTs that used appropriate analysis to control the important confounding factors were judged as "moderate" in this domain [17,18,26,27,29,31,39–41,44], but the other five non-RCTs did not and were judged as "serious [28,30,32,42,43]". One study was judged as "no information" for no detailed information on the selection of participants, deviations from intended interventions, and the treatment of missing data [28].

3.3. Outcomes

3.3.1. Primary Outcome: Return of Spontaneous Circulation

In this case, 18 of the included studies reported the outcomes of ROSC in patients with OHCA. There were 7 RCTs and 11 non-RCTs, with a total of 39,675 participants (Figure 2). The pooled estimates from both RCTs and non-RCTs revealed benefits of mechanical CPR over manual CPR in the ROSC outcome (OR = 1.32, 95% CI: 1.11–1.58). Heterogeneity among the studies was high (I^2 = 88%) (Figure 2A). In the subgroup analyses of RCTs and non-RCTs, a statistical difference between the prehospital use of mechanical CPR device and manual CPR was found in the non-RCTs (OR = 1.48; 95% CI: 1.12–1.97) but not in the RCTs (OR = 1.04; 95% CI: 0.90–1.20). The heterogeneity among the RCTs and non-RCTs was high (I^2 = 61% and 89%, respectively) (Figure 2A). We performed TSA to examine the results. However, the cumulative Z-curve crossed the O'Brien-Fleming boundaries before the RIS (41686 participants for required power) was reached (Figure 2B). A true-positive result indicated that the cumulative power from the available literature supports the association between ROSC achievement and prehospital use of mechanical CPR devices.

Table 1. Summary of the included studies.

Author	Year of Publication	Country	N	Study Period	Definite Study Design	Nationwide Study	Type of Mechanical Device	CPR Guideline	Witnessed Arrest	Shockable Rhythm
Randomized studies										
Anantharaman	2017	Singapore	1191	2011–2012	Cluster RCT	No	LUCAS	2010 ILCOR	52% man, 62% mech	17% man, 23% mech
Gao	2016	China	133	2011–2012	Cluster RCT	No	Autopulse	2010 AHA	59% man, 67% mech	13% man, 13% mech
Hallstrom	2006	USA and Canada	767	2004–2005	Cluster RCT	No	Autopulse	2000 AHA	49% man, 44% mech	32% man, 31% mech
Perkins	2015	UK	4471	2010–2013	Cluster RCT	No	LUCAS	2005/2010 ERC	62% man, 61% mech	22% man, 23% mech
Rubertsson	2014	Sweden, UK, The Netherlands	2589	2008–2013	Individually RCT	No	LUCAS	2005 ERC	72% man, 73% mech	30% man, 29% mech
Smekal	2011	Sweden	148	2005–2007	Individually RCT	No	LUCAS	2000 ERC	74% man, 68% mech	27% man, 27% mech
Wik	2014	Norway	4231	2009–2011	Individually RCT	No	Autopulse	2005 ERC/AHA	48% man, 47% mech	24% man, 21% mech
Non-randomized studies										
Axelsson	2006	Sweden	210	2003–2005	Prospective cohort	No	LUCAS	2000 AHA	100% man, 100% mech	32% man, 30% mech
Axelsson	2013	Sweden	1165	2007–2011	Retrospective cohort	No	LUCAS	Not reported	72% man, 73% mech	25% man, 26% mech
Casner	2005	USA	162	2003	Retrospective cohort	No	Autopulse	Not reported	Not reported	28% man, 33% mech
Chen	2021	Taiwan	552	2018–2020	Retrospective cohort	No	LUCAS	2015 AHA	53% man, 48% mech	21% man, 26% mech
Jennings	2012	Australia	286	2006–2010	Retrospective cohort	No	Autopulse	Not reported	72% man, 71% mech	36% man, 30% mech
Jung	2019	Korea	30,921	2016–2017	Prospective cohort	Yes	LUCAS/Autopulse	Not reported	47% man, 47% mech	14% man, 14% mech
Maule	2007	België	290	2004–2006	Retrospective cohort	No	LUCAS	Not reported	Not reported	Not reported
Newberry	2018	USA	2999	2013–2015	Retrospective cohort	No	LUCAS	Not reported	43% man, 37% mech	14% man, 12% mech
Ong	2006	USA	783	2001–2005	Prospective cohort	No	Autopulse	Not reported	47% man, 52% mech	20% man, 23% mech
Satterlee	2013	USA	572	2008–2010	Retrospective cohort	No	LUCAS	Not reported	61% man, 53% mech	18% man, 21% mech
Savastano	2019	Italy	1401	2015–2017	Prospective cohort	No	Autopulse	Not reported	70% man, 86% mech	14% man, 43% mech
Schmidbauer	2017	Sweden	13,922	2011–2015	Prospective cohort	Yes	LUCAS	2010 ERC	66% man, 67% mech	22% man, 23% mech
Seewald	2019	Germany	17,957	2007–2014	Retrospective cohort	Yes	LUCAS/Autopulse	Not reported	56% man, 62% mech	25% man, 33% mech
Ujvárosy	2018	Hungary	287	2010–2013	Retrospective cohort	No	LUCAS	Not reported	Not reported	Not reported
Zeiner	2015	Austria	938	2013–2014	Prospective cohort	No	LUCAS/Autopulse	Not reported	54% man, 56% mech	22% man, 34% mech

RCT: randomised controlled trial; AHA: American Heart Association; ERC: European Resuscitation Council; ILCOR: International Liaison Committee on Resuscitation Guidelines, man: manual; mech: mechanical; CPR: cardiopulmonary resuscitation.

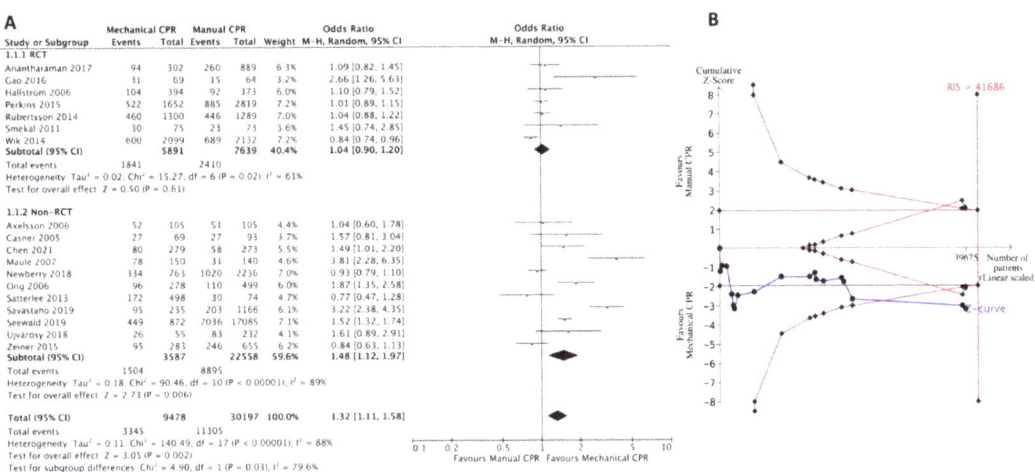

Figure 2. Forest plot (**A**) and trial sequential analysis (**B**) for return of spontaneous circulation between mechanical CPR device and manual CPR. CPR: cardiopulmonary resuscitation; CI: confidence interval; RCT: randomized controlled trial; RIS: required information size.

3.3.2. Primary Outcome: Survival to Hospital Admission

Six RCTs, and 10 non-RCTs reported survival to hospital admission, with a total of 38,829 patients (Figure 3A). A statistically significant difference indicated that the use of a mechanical CPR device was associated with survival to hospital admission in comparison with manual CPR (OR = 1.23, 95% CI: 1.04–1.47; I^2 = 84%). The subgroup analysis showed a significant difference between the two groups in non-RCTs (OR = 1.35; 95% CI: 1.03–1.76, I^2 = 85%) but not in RCTs (OR = 1.00; 95% CI: 0.86–1.16, I^2 = 55%). The TSA showed that the Z-curve crossed into the futility area after the first 13 articles (Figure 3B, arrow). After enrolling the last three articles, the cumulative Z-curve finally crossed the O'Brien-Fleming boundaries before the RIS (sample size = 38942) was reached (Figure 3B). A true-positive result supported the association between achievement of survival to hospital admission and prehospital use of mechanical CPR devices.

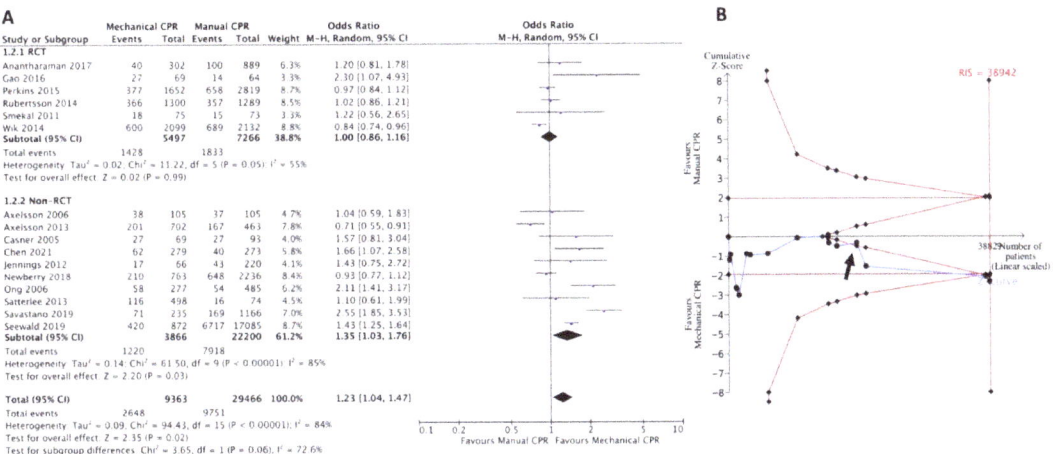

Figure 3. Forest plot (**A**) and trial sequential analysis (**B**) for survival to hospital admission between mechanical CPR device and manual CPR. CPR: cardiopulmonary resuscitation; CI: confidence interval; RCT: randomized controlled trial; RIS: required information size.

3.3.3. Secondary Outcome: Survival to Discharge

Seven RCTs and nine non-RCTs with 66,133 OHCAs were enrolled for analysis (Figure 4A). No significant benefit for survival to discharge was found when applying the mechanical CPR device compared to manual CPR (OR = 0.87; 95% CI: 0.87–1.06). There was high heterogeneity among the enrolled studies (I^2 = 78%). The subgroup analysis revealed consistent results in both RCTs (OR = 0.91; 95% CI: 0.75–1.10, I^2 = 38%) and non-RCTs (OR = 0.83; 95% CI: 0.59–1.16, I^2 = 86%). TSA assessment showed that the RIS of 261,712 participants could not be acquired from the pooled studies (Figure 4B). In addition, the accumulative Z-curve neither crossed the O'Brien-Fleming monitoring boundary nor entered the inner border of the futility boundary. An inconclusive result was indicated.

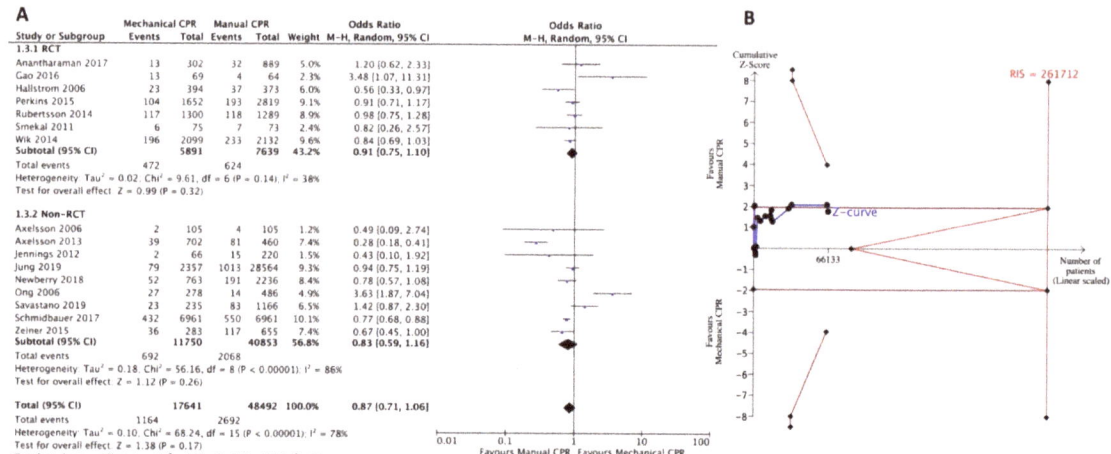

Figure 4. Forest plot (**A**) and trial sequential analysis (**B**) for survival to discharge between mechanical CPR device and manual CPR. CPR: cardiopulmonary resuscitation; CI: confidence interval; RCT randomized controlled trial; RIS: required information size.

3.3.4. Secondary Outcome: Survival to Discharge with Favorable Neurologic Status

The pooled results did not show a significant difference for discharge with favorable neurologic status between the use of mechanical CPR device and manual CPR. The pooled OR was 0.82 (95% CI: 0.64–1.07) (Figure 5A). The heterogeneity was high (I^2 = 68%) Subgroup analysis showed similar results in both RCTs (OR = 0.81; 95% CI: 0.61–1.08 I^2 = 60%) and non-RCTs (OR = 0.91; 95% CI: 0.54–1.52; I^2 = 78%). The estimated RIS was 303,182 in TSA (Figure 5B). The Z-curve showed similar trends as that for survival to discharge, indicating an inconclusive result.

3.4. Subgroup and Sensitivity Analysis

Subgroup analysis of primary outcomes found that mechanical CPR devices were significantly associated with achievement of ROSC in European studies. Mechanical CPR device was significantly associated with achievement of survival to hospital admission in Asian studies. In secondary outcomes, the subgroups that were significantly associated with lower OR in achieving survival to discharge were LUCAS and the location subgroup of Europe (Table 2). Sensitivity analyses of primary and secondary outcomes are shown in Supplementary Table S4. In terms of ROSC, sensitivity analyses of fixed-effect model, non-RCTs, and studies with low RoB showed findings consistent with those of our primary analysis. In terms of survival to hospital admission, analyses of fixed-effect model and non-RCTs showed results similar to those of the primary analysis.

Table 2. Subgroup analyses of pooled odds ratios of primary and secondary survival outcomes of OHCA.

Subgroups	ROSC				Survival to Hospital Admission				Survival to Discharge				Survival to Discharge with Favorable Neurologic Status			
	No. of Studies	Pooled OR (95% CI)	p	I^2 (%)	No. of Studies	Pooled OR (95% CI)	p	I^2 (%)	No. of Studies	Pooled OR (95% CI)	p	I^2 (%)	No. of Studies	Pooled OR (95% CI)	p	I^2 (%)
Type of mechanical CPR device																
LUCAS	10	1.19 (0.99–1.43)	0.06	74%	9	1.00 (0.88–1.13)	0.94	43%	8	0.74 (0.57–0.97)	0.03	78%	4	0.86 (0.67–1.12)	0.27	48%
Autopulse	6	1.65 (0.97–2.79)	0.06	94%	6	1.67 (0.97–2.84)	0.06	91%	6	1.24 (0.71–2.18)	0.45	83%	4	1.13 (0.47–2.73)	0.79	83%
LUCAS + Autopulse	2	1.15 (0.64–2.04)	0.65	92%	1	1.43 (1.25–1.64)	<0.001	NA	2	0.83 (0.60–1.15)	0.26	52%	2	0.61 (0.42–0.88)	0.009	27%
Geographic location																
Europe	10	1.37 (1.06–1.78)	0.02	92%	8	1.12 (0.88–1.42)	0.36	90%	9	0.77 (0.61–0.97)	0.02	79%	4	0.79 (0.61–1.02)	0.07	62%
North America	5	1.16 (0.85–1.60)	0.34	76%	4	1.33 (0.84–2.11)	0.22	79%	3	1.13 (0.45–2.84)	0.79	90%	3	0.93 (0.32–2.73)	0.89	88%
Asia	3	1.46 (0.97–2.20)	0.07	63%	3	1.51 (1.10–2.09)	0.01	23%	3	1.26 (0.72–2.18)	0.42	59%	3	0.95 (0.55–1.64)	0.86	35%
Oceania	0	NA	NA	NA	1	1.43 (0.75–2.72)	0.28	NA	1	0.43 (0.10–1.92)	0.27	NA	0	NA	NA	NA

CPR: cardiopulmonary resuscitation, OR: odds ratio, OHCA: out-of-hospital cardiac arrest, NA: not applicable, ROSC: return of spontaneous circulation.

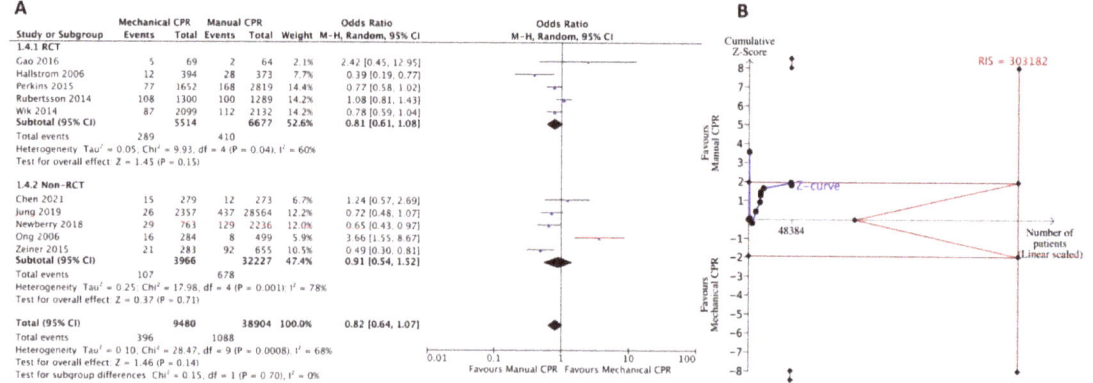

Figure 5. Forest plot (**A**) and trial sequential analysis (**B**) for survival to discharge with favorable neurologic status between mechanical CPR device and manual CPR. CPR: cardiopulmonary resuscitation; CI: confidence interval; RCT: randomized controlled trial; RIS: required information size.

3.5. GRADE Assessment

The GRADE assessment demonstrated an overall very low CoE in the four survival outcomes (Table 3). We downgraded the overall CoE in the RoB, inconsistency, and imprecision domains. In the overall RoB, we judged as "very serious" the four outcomes because non-RCTs were enrolled with a "Moderate" overall RoB. We rated down the CoE in the domain of inconsistency in the four outcomes because high heterogeneity was consistently found. We did not rate down the CoE in the domain of indirectness because each enrolled study faced the same direction in each endpoint and compared mechanical CPR and manual CPR directly. We downgraded the domain of imprecision in the outcomes of survival to discharge and survival to discharge with favorable neurologic status because of inconclusive results and insufficient sample size in TSA. Publication bias was not observed for all the endpoints (Supplementary Figure S1).

Table 3. GRADE assessment.

Mechanical CPR Compared to Manual CPR for Out-of-Hospital Cardiac Arrest							
Certainty Assessment						Summary of Findings	
No. of Participants (Studies)	Risk of Bias	Inconsistency	Indirectness	Imprecision	Publication Bias	Overall Certainty of Evidence	Anticipated Absolute Effects Risk Difference
ROSC 39,675 (7 RCTs, 11 non-RCTs)	very serious [a]	serious [b]	not serious	not serious	none	⊕◯◯◯ Very Low	67 more per 1000 (from 25 more to 112 more)
Survival to hospital admission 38,829 (6 RCTs, 10 non-RCTs)	very serious [a]	serious [b]	not serious	not serious	none	⊕◯◯◯ Very Low	47 more per 1000 (from 9 fewer to 90 more)
Survival to discharge 66,133 (7 RCTs, 9 non-RCTs)	very serious [a]	serious [b]	not serious	serious [c]	none	⊕◯◯◯ Very Low	7 fewer per 1000 (from 15 fewer to 3 more)
Survival to discharge with favorable neurologic status 48,384 (5 RCTs, 5 non-RCTs)	very serious [a]	serious [b]	not serious	serious [c]	none	⊕◯◯◯ Very Low	5 fewer per 1000 (from 10 fewer to 2 more)

[a] Non-RCTs enrolled with moderate overall risk of bias and RCTs enrolled with some concern overall risk of bias. [b] High heterogeneity ($I^2 > 50\%$) between studies was found. [c] Insufficient sample size or inconclusive result, analyzed by trial sequential analysis. CPR: cardiopulmonary resuscitation; ROSC: return of spontaneous circulation; ED: emergency department.

4. Discussion

To date, 10 systematic reviews have been published to compare the effects of manual CPR and mechanical CPR on cardiac arrest [8–12,45–49]. Among them, five systematic reviews focused on OHCA [8,10,11,45,48], four systematic reviews, including one Cochrane review, enrolled both OHCA and IHCA [9,12,46,49], and one review involved in IHCA [47]. Among the five systematic reviews involving pure OHCA, only one systematic review (in 2011) focused on the prehospital use of mechanical CPR, suggesting that there was insufficient evidence to support mechanical CPR device use in OHCA in prehospital settings [48]. Considering the differences in medical support, etiology of cardiac arrest, survival probability between OHCA and IHCA, and diversity in the environment and medical and personnel resources between prehospital and in-hospital settings, a new SRMA is needed to provide updated evidence for the effects of mechanical CPR devices for adult OHCA in prehospital settings. In this SRMA with 85,975 OHCAs from seven RCTs and 15 non-RCTs, we first applied TSA and GRADE assessments which have not been assessed in previous SRMA. We found that mechanical CPR use in prehospital settings had higher odds of achieving ROSC (OR = 1.32; 95% CI: 1.11–1.58) and survival to hospital admission (OR = 1.23; 95% CI: 1.04–1.47) than manual CPR. TSA showed that although the RIS was not reached, there was a true statistical significance. However, because of the inclusion of non-RCTs and the inconsistency between studies, the overall CoE was very low. Moreover, according to the current evidence, we did not have enough power to assess the outcomes of survival to discharge and discharge with favorable neurologic status.

In the prehospital setting, lack of personnel, competing resuscitation tasks, fatigue, and the challenge of continuing CPR while moving the patient to the ambulance or in a moving ambulance posed obstacles. The median CPR pause time during extrication was shorter when mechanical CPR was applied (39 s, interquartile range [IQR] 29–47 s) than manual CPR (270 s, IQR 201–387 s) [50]. Safety concerns for both the patient and the rescuer have also been explored in the delivery of manual CPR in a moving vehicle [51,52]. Moreover, acceleration forces during ambulance transport affect the quality of the manual CPR [53]. Theoretically, the application of mechanical CPR in prehospital settings should improve CPR quality. This difference compared to manual CPR is not reflected in the survival outcome of OHCA [8,45]. Since 2019, several observational studies have evaluated the resuscitative effects of mechanical and manual CPR on OHCA in prehospital settings [17,18,39,44]. Three of them reported that short-term outcomes such as ROSC or survival to admission were associated with the use of mechanical CPR [17,18,39]. These findings were not included in the previous SRMA. In our TSA (Figures 2B and 3B), after accumulating recent cohort studies, we found that the cumulative Z-curve finally crossed into the O'Brien-Fleming boundaries and showed the true-positive effects of mechanical CPR. This overturns the conclusion of no benefit for short-term survival outcomes in the use of mechanical CPR in the recent SRMA [8,45]. For the outcomes of ROSC and survival to hospital admission, the requirement of adequate sample size for statistical power was not met. More studies, especially large-scale high-quality RCTs, are required for any interpretation.

For the long-term survival outcomes, survival to discharge or discharge with favorable neurologic status, although not statistically significant and with insufficient statistical power to draw conclusions, the results showed the opposite trend to the short-term outcomes (Figures 4 and 5). Another study showed that the majority of OHCA patients who can survive to discharge were patients with initial shockable rhythm [54]. For patients with shockable rhythm, early defibrillation may be equal or more important than CPR. Our previous study demonstrated that the benefit of mechanical CPR to achieve ROSC was more evident in OHCA patients with non-shockable rhythm but not in shockable rhythm [18]. Savastano et al. also found that mechanical CPR devices positively affect survival to discharge for witnessed cardiac arrests with non-shockable rhythm but with a neutral effect for patients with shockable rhythm [39]. A possible explanation may be that, as found in previous RCTs, the first shock delivery was delayed when applying a mechanical CPR device. The AutoPulse Assisted Prehospital International Resuscitation trial conducted by Hallstrom et al. found the mean time to first shock in ventricular fibrillation was prolonged by 2.1 min in the mechanical CPR group [37]. In the LUCAS in Cardiac Arrest

(LINC) trial and the Circulation Improving Resuscitation Care (CIRC) trial, the delay in first shock delivery was 1–1.5 min longer with the device than with manual CPR [34,36]. In most RCTs, mechanical CPR administration was performed prior to cardiac rhythm assessment or delivery of the first shock [19,34–37]. Whether the delay of the first shock affects the survival outcome of OHCA with shockable rhythm needs to be further explored. However, selective use of mechanical CPR devices for patients with non-shockable rhythm or performing manual CPR first, and then switching to mechanical CPR after delivering the first shock may be a direction for further research.

In the subgroup analysis, we found that heterogeneity comes from the different study designs, and the survival benefit from mechanical CPR on short-term outcomes was from non-RCTs. There were several reasons for the synthesis of RCTs and non-RCTs for analysis. First, non-specific description of randomization sequence was noticed, and the baseline difference between groups could be identified in most cluster-RCTs [19,37,38]. Second, in individual RCTs, the randomization process was carried out once cardiac arrest was identified at the scene by the rescuers. The delay in applying mechanical CPR device may be present during the randomization and may influence the survival outcome in patients who were allocated to the mechanical CPR group [33,34,36]. Third, it is impossible for rescuers to blind the methods of CPR. Fourth, for the included non-RCTs, except for the unavoidable confounding bias, almost all considered observational studies were of high quality with low RoB (Supplementary Table S3). The above findings make the RCTs and non-RCTs comparable. Moreover, the statistical power was inadequate if only the RCTs were enrolled. Hence, we merged the evidence from both RCTs and non-RCTs and conducted a subgroup analysis according to the different study designs. Moreover, in the GRADE assessment, we downgraded the RoB and presented the faithful CoE accordingly (Table 3) [55].

This SRMA has several limitations. First, as mentioned for sufficient statistical power, we had to synthesize RCTs and non-RCTs for analysis. This also occurred in the previous SRMA. Instead, we downgraded the RoB in the GRADE assessment to carefully interpret the findings. Second, there was noticeable heterogeneity. However, the heterogeneity could be partially explained by the different study designs. There was still unobservable between-study heterogeneity, especially in terms of long-term survival outcomes. Third, post-arrest care is associated with long-term outcome [54,56]. However, the lack of post-arrest management characteristics in most studies precluded further analysis. Fourth, our meta-analysis did not demonstrate an association between complications and different manners of CPR. A network meta-analysis by Khan et al. in 2018 showed that, compared with mechanical CPR, manual CPR led to less pneumothorax and hematoma [46]. Our study cannot assess the impact of CPR-related complications on survival outcomes.

5. Conclusions

This SRMA suggests that prehospital use of mechanical CPR devices may benefit adult OHCA patients to achieve ROSC and survival to hospital admission. However, long-term outcomes such as survival to discharge or discharge with favorable neurological status remain inconclusive. Our finding provides the evidence and echoes the recommendations in the latest guideline of adult advanced life support, which suggest use of mechanical CPR device when high-quality manual CPR is not practical or compromises provider safety, such as during transportation to hospital in an ambulance [57]. Owing to the between-study heterogeneity and the evidence that mainly came from non-RCTs, it is necessary to conduct large-scale, high-quality randomized studies and investigate the different effects of mechanical CPR on OHCA with shockable and non-shockable rhythms.

Supplementary Materials: The following supporting information can be downloaded at: https://www.mdpi.com/article/10.3390/jcm11051448/s1, Supplementary Table S1: The used search term in the databases; Supplementary Table S2: Summary of the Cochrane risk-of-bias tool for randomized trials (RoB 2.0); Supplementary Table S3: Summary of the risk of bias in non-randomized studies—of interventions (ROBINS-I) assessment; Supplementary Table S4: Sensitivity analyses of pooled odds ratios of primary and secondary survival outcomes of OHCA; Supplementary Figure S1: Funnel plots of (A) Return of spontaneous circulation, (B) Survival to hospital admission, (C) Survival to discharge, and (D) Survival to discharge with favorable neurologic status

Author Contributions: Conceptualization, design, validation, software, and formal analysis, M.-J.T., C.-Y.C. and Y.T.H.; writing of the original draft of the manuscript, C.-Y.C., K.-C.L. and M.-J.T.; review, editing, and supervision of the manuscript, M.-J.T., P.C.L., T.-Y.T. and Y.T.H. All authors have read and agreed to the published version of the manuscript.

Funding: This research received no external funding.

Institutional Review Board Statement: Not applicable.

Informed Consent Statement: Not applicable.

Data Availability Statement: Data are available from the corresponding authors upon reasonable request.

Conflicts of Interest: The authors declare no conflict of interest.

References

1. Kudenchuk, P.J.; Sandroni, C.; Drinhaus, H.R.; Böttiger, B.W.; Cariou, A.; Sunde, K.; Dworschak, M.; Taccone, F.S.; Deye, N.; Friberg, H.; et al. Breakthrough in Cardiac Arrest: Reports From the 4th Paris International Conference. *Ann. Intensive Care* **2015**, *5*, 22. [CrossRef] [PubMed]
2. Kiguchi, T.; Okubo, M.; Nishiyama, C.; Maconochie, I.; Ong, M.E.H.; Kern, K.B.; Wyckoff, M.H.; McNally, B.; Christensen, E.F.; Tjelmeland, I.; et al. Out-of-Hospital Cardiac Arrest Across the World: First Report From the International Liaison Committee on Resuscitation (ILCOR). *Resuscitation* **2020**, *152*, 39–49. [CrossRef] [PubMed]
3. Berdowski, J.; Berg, R.A.; Tijssen, J.G.; Koster, R.W. Global Incidences of Out-of-Hospital Cardiac Arrest and Survival Rates: Systematic Review of 67 Prospective Studies. *Resuscitation* **2010**, *81*, 1479–1487. [CrossRef] [PubMed]
4. Yan, S.; Gan, Y.; Jiang, N.; Wang, R.; Chen, Y.; Luo, Z.; Zong, Q.; Chen, S.; Lv, C. The Global Survival Rate Among Adult Out-of-Hospital Cardiac Arrest Patients Who Received Cardiopulmonary Resuscitation: A Systematic Review and Meta-Analysis. *Crit. Care* **2020**, *24*, 61. [CrossRef]
5. Merchant, R.M.; Topjian, A.A.; Panchal, A.R.; Cheng, A.; Aziz, K.; Berg, K.M.; Lavonas, E.J.; Magid, D.J.; Adult Basic and Advanced Life Support, Pediatric Basic and Advanced Life Support, Neonatal Life Support, Resuscitation Education Science, and Systems of Care Writing Groups. Circulation 2020-Part 1: Executive summary: 2020 American Heart Association guidelines for cardiopulmonary resuscitation and emergency cardiovascular care. *Circulation* **2020**, *142*, S337–S357. [CrossRef]
6. Kahn, P.A.; Dhruva, S.S.; Rhee, T.G.; Ross, J.S. Use of Mechanical Cardiopulmonary Resuscitation Devices for Out-of-Hospital Cardiac Arrest, 2010–2016. *JAMA Netw. Open.* **2019**, *2*, e1913298. [CrossRef]
7. Edelson, D.P.; Sasson, C.; Chan, P.S.; Atkins, D.L.; Aziz, K.; Becker, L.B.; Berg, R.A.; Bradley, S.M.; Brooks, S.C.; Cheng, A.; et al. Interim Guidance for Basic and Advanced Life Support in Adults, Children, and Neonates With Suspected or Confirmed COVID-19: From the Emergency Cardiovascular Care Committee and Get With the Guidelines-Resuscitation Adult and Pediatric Task Forces of the American Heart Association. *Circulation* **2020**, *141*, e933–e943. [CrossRef]
8. Zhu, N.; Chen, Q.; Jiang, Z.; Liao, F.; Kou, B.; Tang, H.; Zhou, M. A Meta-Analysis of the Resuscitative Effects of Mechanical and Manual Chest Compression in Out-of-Hospital Cardiac Arrest Patients. *Crit. Care* **2019**, *23*, 100. [CrossRef]
9. Wang, P.; Brooks, S. Cochrane Corner: Are Mechanical Compressions Better Than Manual Compressions in Cardiac Arrest? *Heart* **2020**, *106*, 559–561. [CrossRef]
10. Bonnes, J.L.; Brouwer, M.A.; Navarese, E.P.; Verhaert, D.V.; Verheugt, F.W.; Smeets, J.L.; de Boer, M.J. Manual Cardiopulmonary Resuscitation Versus CPR Including a Mechanical Chest Compression Device in Out-of-Hospital Cardiac Arrest: A Comprehensive Meta-Analysis From Randomized and Observational Studies. *Ann. Emerg. Med.* **2016**, *67*, 349–360.e3. [CrossRef]
11. Liu, M.; Shuai, Z.; Ai, J.; Tang, K.; Liu, H.; Zheng, J.; Gou, J.; Lv, Z. Mechanical Chest Compression With LUCAS Device Does Not Improve Clinical Outcome in Out-of-Hospital Cardiac Arrest Patients: A Systematic Review and Meta-Analysis. *Medicine* **2019**, *98*, e17550. [CrossRef] [PubMed]
12. Li, H.; Wang, D.; Yu, Y.; Zhao, X.; Jing, X. Mechanical Versus Manual Chest Compressions for Cardiac Arrest: A Systematic Review and Meta-Analysis. *Scand. J. Trauma Resusc. Emerg. Med.* **2016**, *24*, 10. [CrossRef] [PubMed]
13. Hayashida, K.; Tagami, T.; Fukuda, T.; Suzuki, M.; Yonemoto, N.; Kondo, Y.; Ogasawara, T.; Sakurai, A.; Tahara, Y.; Nagao, K.; et al. Mechanical Cardiopulmonary Resuscitation and Hospital Survival Among Adult Patients With Nontraumatic Out-of-Hospital Cardiac Arrest Attending the Emergency Department: A Prospective, Multicenter, Observational Study in Japan (SOS-KANTO

[Survey of Survivors after Out-Of-Hospital Cardiac Arrest in Kanto Area] 2012 Study). *J. Am. Heart Assoc.* **2017**, *6*, e007420. [CrossRef] [PubMed]
14. Kim, H.T.; Kim, J.G.; Jang, Y.S.; Kang, G.H.; Kim, W.; Choi, H.Y.; Jun, G.S. Comparison of in-Hospital Use of Mechanical Chest Compression Devices for Out-of-Hospital Cardiac Arrest Patients: AUTOPULSE vs LUCAS. *Medicine* **2019**, *98*, e17881. [CrossRef]
15. Lin, C.K.; Huang, M.C.; Feng, Y.T.; Jeng, W.H.; Chung, T.C.; Lau, Y.W.; Cheng, K.I. Effectiveness of Mechanical Chest Compression for Out-of-Hospital Cardiac Arrest Patients in an Emergency Department. *J. Chin. Med. Assoc.* **2015**, *78*, 360–363. [CrossRef]
16. Ogawa, Y.; Shiozaki, T.; Hirose, T.; Ohnishi, M.; Nakamori, Y.; Ogura, H.; Shimazu, T. Load-Distributing-Band Cardiopulmonary Resuscitation for Out-of-Hospital Cardiac Arrest Increases Regional Cerebral Oxygenation: A Single-Center Prospective Pilot Study. *Scand. J. Trauma Resusc. Emerg. Med.* **2015**, *23*, 99. [CrossRef]
17. Seewald, S.; Obermaier, M.; Lefering, R.; Bohn, A.; Georgieff, M.; Muth, C.M.; Gräsner, J.T.; Masterson, S.; Scholz, J.; Wnent, J. Application of Mechanical Cardiopulmonary Resuscitation Devices and Their Value in Out-of-Hospital Cardiac Arrest: A Retrospective Analysis of the German Resuscitation Registry. *PLoS ONE* **2019**, *14*, e0208113. [CrossRef]
18. Chen, Y.R.; Liao, C.J.; Huang, H.C.; Tsai, C.H.; Su, Y.S.; Liu, C.H.; Hsu, C.F.; Tsai, M.J. The Effect of Implementing Mechanical Cardiopulmonary Resuscitation Devices on Out-of-Hospital Cardiac Arrest Patients in an Urban City of Taiwan. *Int. J. Environ. Res. Public Health* **2021**, *18*, 3636. [CrossRef]
19. Anantharaman, V.; Ng, B.L.; Ang, S.H.; Lee, C.Y.; Leong, S.H.; Ong, M.E.; Chua, S.J.; Rabind, A.C.; Anjali, N.B.; Hao, Y. Prompt Use of Mechanical Cardiopulmonary Resuscitation in Out-of-Hospital Cardiac Arrest: The MECCA Study Report. *Singap. Med. J.* **2017**, *58*, 424–431. [CrossRef]
20. Page, M.J.; McKenzie, J.E.; Bossuyt, P.M.; Boutron, I.; Hoffmann, T.C.; Mulrow, C.D.; Shamseer, L.; Tetzlaff, J.M.; Akl, E.A.; Brennan, S.E.; et al. The PRISMA 2020 Statement: An Updated Guideline for Reporting Systematic Reviews. *BMJ* **2021**, *372*, n71. [CrossRef]
21. Sterne, J.A.C.; Savović, J.; Page, M.J.; Elbers, R.G.; Blencowe, N.S.; Boutron, I.; Cates, C.J.; Cheng, H.Y.; Corbett, M.S.; Eldridge, S.M.; et al. RoB 2: A Revised Tool for Assessing Risk of Bias in Randomised Trials. *BMJ* **2019**, *366*, l4898. [CrossRef] [PubMed]
22. Sterne, J.A.; Hernán, M.A.; Reeves, B.C.; Savović, J.; Berkman, N.D.; Viswanathan, M.; Henry, D.; Altman, D.G.; Ansari, M.T.; Boutron, I.; et al. Robins-I: A Tool for Assessing Risk of Bias in Non-Randomised Studies of Interventions. *BMJ* **2016**, *355*, i4919. [CrossRef] [PubMed]
23. Brok, J.; Thorlund, K.; Wetterslev, J.; Gluud, C. Apparently Conclusive Meta-Analyses May Be Inconclusive-Trial Sequential Analysis Adjustment of Random Error Risk Due to Repetitive Testing of Accumulating Data in Apparently Conclusive Neonatal Meta-Analyses. *Int. J. Epidemiol.* **2009**, *38*, 287–298. [CrossRef]
24. Kang, H. Trial Sequential Analysis: Novel Approach for Meta-Analysis. *Anesth. Pain Med.* **2021**, *16*, 138–150. [CrossRef] [PubMed]
25. Guyatt, G.H.; Oxman, A.D.; Vist, G.E.; Kunz, R.; Falck-Ytter, Y.; Alonso-Coello, P.; Schünemann, H.J.; GRADE Working Group. GRADE: An Emerging Consensus on Rating Quality of Evidence and Strength of Recommendations. *BMJ* **2008**, *336*, 924–926. [CrossRef]
26. Axelsson, C.; Herrera, M.J.; Fredriksson, M.; Lindqvist, J.; Herlitz, J. Implementation of Mechanical Chest Compression in Out-of-Hospital Cardiac Arrest in an Emergency Medical Service System. *Am. J. Emerg. Med.* **2013**, *31*, 1196–1200. [CrossRef]
27. Axelsson, C.; Nestin, J.; Svensson, L.; Axelsson, A.B.; Herlitz, J. Clinical Consequences of the Introduction of Mechanical Chest Compression in the EMS System for Treatment of Out-of-Hospital Cardiac Arrest-A Pilot Study. *Resuscitation* **2006**, *71*, 47–55. [CrossRef]
28. Maule, Y. Mechanical External Chest Compression: A New Adjuvant Technology in Cardiopulmonary Resuscitation. *Urgences Accueil.* **2007**, *7*, 4–7.
29. Newberry, R.; Redman, T.; Ross, E.; Ely, R.; Saidler, C.; Arana, A.; Wampler, D.; Miramontes, D. No Benefit in Neurologic Outcomes of Survivors of Out-of-Hospital Cardiac Arrest With Mechanical Compression Device. *Prehosp. Emerg. Care* **2018**, *22*, 338–344. [CrossRef]
30. Satterlee, P.A.; Boland, L.L.; Johnson, P.J.; Hagstrom, S.G.; Page, D.I.; Lick, C.J. Implementation of a Mechanical Chest Compression Device as Standard Equipment in a Large Metropolitan Ambulance Service. *J. Emerg. Med.* **2013**, *45*, 562–569. [CrossRef]
31. Schmidbauer, S.; Herlitz, J.; Karlsson, T.; Axelsson, C.; Friberg, H. Use of Automated Chest Compression Devices After Out-of-Hospital Cardiac Arrest in Sweden. *Resuscitation* **2017**, *120*, 95–102. [CrossRef] [PubMed]
32. Ujvárosy, D.; Sebestyén, V.; Pataki, T.; Ötvös, T.; Lőrincz, I.; Paragh, G.; Szabó, Z. Cardiovascular Risk Factors Differently Affect the Survival of Patients Undergoing Manual or Mechanical Resuscitation. *BMC Cardiovasc. Disord.* **2018**, *18*, 227. [CrossRef] [PubMed]
33. Smekal, D.; Johansson, J.; Huzevka, T.; Rubertsson, S. A Pilot Study of Mechanical Chest Compressions With the LUCAS™ Device in Cardiopulmonary Resuscitation. *Resuscitation* **2011**, *82*, 702–706. [CrossRef] [PubMed]
34. Rubertsson, S.; Lindgren, E.; Smekal, D.; Östlund, O.; Silfverstolpe, J.; Lichtveld, R.A.; Boomars, R.; Ahlstedt, B.; Skoog, G.; Kastberg, R.; et al. Mechanical Chest Compressions and Simultaneous Defibrillation vs Conventional Cardiopulmonary Resuscitation in Out-of-Hospital Cardiac Arrest: The LINC Randomized Trial. *JAMA* **2014**, *311*, 53–61. [CrossRef]
35. Perkins, G.D.; Lall, R.; Quinn, T.; Deakin, C.D.; Cooke, M.W.; Horton, J.; Lamb, S.E.; Slowther, A.M.; Woollard, M.; Carson, A.; et al. Mechanical Versus Manual Chest Compression for Out-of-Hospital Cardiac Arrest (PARAMEDIC): A Pragmatic, Cluster Randomised Controlled Trial. *Lancet* **2015**, *385*, 947–955. [CrossRef]

6. Wik, L.; Olsen, J.A.; Persse, D.; Sterz, F.; Lozano, M.; Brouwer, M.A.; Westfall, M.; Souders, C.M.; Malzer, R.; van Grunsven, P.M.; et al. Manual vs. Integrated Automatic Load-Distributing Band CPR With Equal Survival After out of Hospital Cardiac Arrest. The Randomized CIRC Trial. *Resuscitation* **2014**, *85*, 741–748. [CrossRef]
7. Hallstrom, A.; Rea, T.D.; Sayre, M.R.; Christenson, J.; Anton, A.R.; Mosesso, V.N.; Van Ottingham, L.; Olsufka, M.; Pennington, S.; White, L.J.; et al. Manual Chest Compression vs Use of an Automated Chest Compression Device During Resuscitation Following Out-of-Hospital Cardiac Arrest: A Randomized Trial. *JAMA* **2006**, *295*, 2620–2628. [CrossRef]
8. Gao, C.; Chen, Y.; Peng, H.; Chen, Y.; Zhuang, Y.; Zhou, S. Clinical Evaluation of the AutoPulse Automated Chest Compression Device for Out-of-Hospital Cardiac Arrest in the Northern District of Shanghai, China. *Arch. Med. Sci.* **2016**, *12*, 563–570. [CrossRef]
9. Savastano, S.; Baldi, E.; Palo, A.; Raimondi, M.; Belliato, M.; Compagnoni, S.; Buratti, S.; Cacciatore, E.; Canevari, F.; Iotti, G.; et al. Load Distributing Band Device for Mechanical Chest Compressions: An Utstein-Categories Based Analysis of Survival to Hospital Discharge. *Int. J. Cardiol.* **2019**, *287*, 81–85. [CrossRef]
10. Ong, M.E.; Ornato, J.P.; Edwards, D.P.; Dhindsa, H.S.; Best, A.M.; Ines, C.S.; Hickey, S.; Clark, B.; Williams, D.C.; Powell, R.G.; et al. Use of an Automated, Load-Distributing Band Chest Compression Device for Out-of-Hospital Cardiac Arrest Resuscitation. *JAMA* **2006**, *295*, 2629–2637. [CrossRef]
11. Jennings, P.A.; Harriss, L.; Bernard, S.; Bray, J.; Walker, T.; Spelman, T.; Smith, K.; Cameron, P. An Automated CPR Device Compared With Standard Chest Compressions for Out-of-Hospital Resuscitation. *BMC Emerg. Med.* **2012**, *12*, 8. [CrossRef] [PubMed]
12. Casner, M.; Andersen, D.; Isaacs, S.M. The Impact of a New CPR Assist Device on Rate of Return of Spontaneous Circulation in Out-of-Hospital Cardiac Arrest. *Prehosp. Emerg. Care* **2005**, *9*, 61–67. [CrossRef] [PubMed]
13. Zeiner, S.; Sulzgruber, P.; Datler, P.; Keferböck, M.; Poppe, M.; Lobmeyr, E.; van Tulder, R.; Zajicek, A.; Buchinger, A.; Polz, K.; et al. Mechanical Chest Compression Does Not Seem to Improve Outcome After Out-Of Hospital Cardiac Arrest. A Single Center Observational Trial. *Resuscitation* **2015**, *96*, 220–225. [CrossRef] [PubMed]
14. Jung, E.; Park, J.H.; Lee, S.Y.; Ro, Y.S.; Hong, K.J.; Song, K.J.; Ryu, H.H.; Shin, S.D. Mechanical Chest Compression Device for Out-of-Hospital Cardiac Arrest: A Nationwide Observational Study. *J. Emerg. Med.* **2020**, *58*, 424–431. [CrossRef]
15. Sheraton, M.; Columbus, J.; Surani, S.; Chopra, R.; Kashyap, R. Effectiveness of Mechanical Chest Compression Devices Over Manual Cardiopulmonary Resuscitation: A Systematic Review With Meta-Analysis and Trial Sequential Analysis. *West. J. Emerg. Med.* **2021**, *22*, 810–819. [CrossRef]
16. Khan, S.U.; Lone, A.N.; Talluri, S.; Khan, M.Z.; Khan, M.U.; Kaluski, E. Efficacy and Safety of Mechanical Versus Manual Compression in Cardiac Arrest—A Bayesian Network Meta-Analysis. *Resuscitation* **2018**, *130*, 182–188. [CrossRef] [PubMed]
17. Couper, K.; Yeung, J.; Nicholson, T.; Quinn, T.; Lall, R.; Perkins, G.D. Mechanical Chest Compression Devices at in-Hospital Cardiac Arrest: A Systematic Review and Meta-Analysis. *Resuscitation* **2016**, *103*, 24–31. [CrossRef]
18. Ong, M.E.; Mackey, K.E.; Zhang, Z.C.; Tanaka, H.; Ma, M.H.; Swor, R.; Shin, S.D. Mechanical CPR Devices Compared to Manual CPR During Out-of-Hospital Cardiac Arrest and Ambulance Transport: A Systematic Review. *Scand. J. Trauma Resusc. Emerg. Med.* **2012**, *20*, 39. [CrossRef]
19. Wang, P.L.; Brooks, S.C. Mechanical Versus Manual Chest Compressions for Cardiac Arrest. *Cochrane Database Syst. Rev.* **2018**. [CrossRef]
20. Lyon, R.M.; Crawford, A.; Crookston, C.; Short, S.; Clegg, G.R. The Combined Use of Mechanical CPR and a Carry Sheet to Maintain Quality Resuscitation in Out-of-Hospital Cardiac Arrest Patients During Extrication and Transport. *Resuscitation* **2015**, *93*, 102–106. [CrossRef]
21. Becker, L.R.; Zaloshnja, E.; Levick, N.; Li, G.; Miller, T.R. Relative Risk of Injury and Death in Ambulances and Other Emergency Vehicles. *Accid. Anal. Prev.* **2003**, *35*, 941–948. [CrossRef]
22. Kahn, C.A.; Pirrallo, R.G.; Kuhn, E.M. Characteristics of Fatal Ambulance Crashes in the United States: An 11-Year Retrospective Analysis. *Prehosp. Emerg. Care* **2001**, *5*, 261–269. [CrossRef] [PubMed]
23. Kurz, M.C.; Dante, S.A.; Puckett, B.J. Estimating the Impact of Off-Balancing Forces Upon Cardiopulmonary Resuscitation During Ambulance Transport. *Resuscitation* **2012**, *83*, 1085–1089. [CrossRef] [PubMed]
24. Hassager, C.; Nagao, K.; Hildick-Smith, D. Out-of-Hospital Cardiac Arrest: In-Hospital Intervention Strategies. *Lancet* **2018**, *391*, 989–998. [CrossRef]
25. Schünemann, H.J.; Cuello, C.; Akl, E.A.; Mustafa, R.A.; Meerpohl, J.J.; Thayer, K.; Morgan, R.L.; Gartlehner, G.; Kunz, R.; Katikireddi, S.V.; et al. [GRADE guidelines, 105–114] [GRADE guidelines, 105–114]. GRADE Guidelines: 18. How Robins-I and Other Tools to Assess Risk of Bias in Nonrandomized Studies Should Be Used to Rate the Certainty of a Body of Evidence. *J. Clin. Epidemiol.* **2019**, *111*, 105–114. [CrossRef]
26. Chang, H.C.; Tsai, M.S.; Kuo, L.K.; Hsu, H.H.; Huang, W.C.; Lai, C.H.; Shih, M.C.; Huang, C.H. Factors Affecting Outcomes in Patients With Cardiac Arrest Who Receive Target Temperature Management: The Multi-Center TIMECARD Registry. *J. Formos. Med. Assoc.* **2022**, *121*, 294–303. [CrossRef]
27. Soar, J.; Böttiger, B.W.; Carli, P.; Couper, K.; Deakin, C.D.; Djärv, T.; Lott, C.; Olasveengen, T.; Paal, P.; Pellis, T.; et al. European Resuscitation Council Guidelines 2021: Adult Advanced Life Support. *Resuscitation* **2021**, *161*, 115–151. [CrossRef]

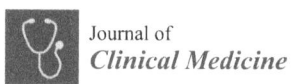

Article

Chest Compression-Related Flail Chest Is Associated with Prolonged Ventilator Weaning in Cardiac Arrest Survivors

Kevin Kunz [1,*], Sirak Petros [1], Sebastian Ewens [2], Maryam Yahiaoui-Doktor [3], Timm Denecke [2], Manuel Florian Struck [4,†] and Sebastian Krämer [5,†]

1. Medical Intensive Care Unit, University Hospital Leipzig, 04103 Leipzig, Germany; sirak.petros@medizin.uni-leipzig.de
2. Department of Diagnostic and Interventional Radiology, University Hospital Leipzig, 04103 Leipzig, Germany; sebastian.ewens@gmail.com (S.E.); timm.denecke@medizin.uni-leipzig.de (T.D.)
3. Medical Faculty, Institute for Medical Informatics, Statistics and Epidemiology, University of Leipzig, 04107 Leipzig, Germany; maryam.yahiaoui@imise.uni-leipzig.de
4. Department of Anesthesiology and Intensive Care Medicine, University Hospital Leipzig, 04103 Leipzig, Germany; manuelflorian.struck@medizin.uni-leipzig.de
5. Department of Visceral, Transplant, Thoracic and Vascular Surgery, Division of Thoracic Surgery, University Hospital Leipzig, 04103 Leipzig, Germany; sebastian.kraemer@medizin.uni-leipzig.de
* Correspondence: kevin.kunz2@medizin.uni-leipzig.de
† These authors contributed equally to this work.

Abstract: Chest compressions during cardiopulmonary resuscitation (CPR) may be associated with iatrogenic chest wall injuries. The extent to which these CPR-associated chest wall injuries contribute to a delay in the respiratory recovery of cardiac arrest survivors has not been sufficiently explored. In a single-center retrospective cohort study, surviving intensive care unit (ICU) patients, who had undergone CPR due to medical reasons between 1 January 2018 and 30 June 2019, were analyzed regarding CPR-associated chest wall injuries, detected by chest radiography and computed tomography. Among 109 included patients, 38 (34.8%) presented with chest wall injuries, including 10 (9.2%) with flail chest. The multivariable logistic regression analysis identified flail chest to be independently associated with the need for tracheostomy (OR 15.5; 95% CI 2.77–86.27; $p = 0.002$). The linear regression analysis identified pneumonia (β 11.34; 95% CI 6.70–15.99; $p < 0.001$) and the presence of rib fractures (β 5.97; 95% CI 1.01–10.93; $p = 0.019$) to be associated with an increase in the length of ICU stay, whereas flail chest (β 10.45; 95% CI 3.57–17.33; $p = 0.003$) and pneumonia (β 6.12; 95% CI 0.94–11.31; $p = 0.021$) were associated with a prolonged duration of mechanical ventilation. Four patients with flail chest underwent surgical rib stabilization and were successfully weaned from the ventilator. The results of this study suggest that CPR-associated chest wall injuries, flail chest in particular, may impair the respiratory recovery of cardiac arrest survivors in the ICU. A multidisciplinary assessment may help to identify patients who could benefit from a surgical treatment approach.

Keywords: cardiopulmonary resuscitation; chest wall injury; flail chest; ventilator weaning; surgical rib stabilization

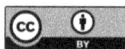

1. Introduction

According to the current Advanced Life Support guidelines, cardiopulmonary resuscitation (CPR) requires a chest compression depth of 5–6 cm, at a rate of 100–120 compressions per minute [1,2]. This may result in iatrogenic thoracic injuries, which have been commonly identified in studies of postmortem findings, whereas fatal injuries have not been found [3–8].

The European Resuscitation Council guidelines for post-resuscitation care and the European Society of Cardiology position paper on cardiac arrest centers do not give recommendations regarding the management of CPR-associated thoracic injuries, other than to perform chest radiography to identify possible pneumothorax [2,9]. There are neither studies to reveal whether thoracic injuries in CPR survivors influence the clinical course, nor if the management of these injuries may lead to an improvement in weaning from the ventilator.

Recently, several promising case series on the use of surgical stabilization of CPR-associated rib fractures have been published [10–12]. To summarize our own experience, and as a result of the paucity of reported data, this study aimed to analyze the consequences of CPR-related thoracic injuries on the course of respiratory recovery, during intensive care unit (ICU) treatment in CPR survivors.

2. Materials and Methods

In this study, ICU survivors of non-traumatic cardiac arrests were analyzed retrospectively, based on the medical records of the University Hospital of Leipzig, Germany. The analysis included patients who were treated in the medical ICU after CPR between January 2018 and June 2019. The patients who died during their hospital stay were excluded.

Demographic and clinical data were obtained from the patients' charts and digital health records. The chest radiography and computed tomography (CT) scans, performed after CPR, were reassessed by a board-certified radiologist, with a focus on thoracic injuries (MEDOS RIS version 9.3.3008, Nexus MagicWeb version VA60C_0115, Visage Imaging, PACS: syngo.plaza, Siemens Healthcare, Erlangen, Germany). The taxonomy of chest injuries was carried out according to the Chest Wall Injury Society collaborators [13]. "Flail segment" described three or more ribs fractured in two or more places. The term "anterior flail segment" was used if a minimum of three rib or costal cartilage fractures were detected on both sides, while "flail chest" described the paradoxical motion observed during clinical examination.

The statistical analysis included tests for the normal distribution of metric variables, such as the Shapiro–Wilk test. The metric data are presented either with mean and standard deviation or with median and 25% and 75% quartiles, based on their distributions. The metric data of the groups were compared with the Mann–Whitney U test, while the categorical data were compared by means of the chi-square test and Fisher's exact test. A logistic regression analysis was performed to identify the independent predictors of the need for tracheostomy, and a linear regression analysis with analysis of variance (ANOVA) was conducted to identify the predictors of the length of ICU stay and the duration of mechanical ventilation. Either odds ratios (ORs) or beta weights with 95% confidence intervals (CIs) were provided, and a p-value < 0.05 was considered to be statistically significant. The statistical analysis was performed using SPSS for Windows version 25 (IBM, Armonk, NY, USA).

3. Results

From a total of 316 patients who were treated in the medical ICU after CPR, 111 patients met the inclusion criteria, of which 109 had complete data and were the subjects of the study (Figure 1).

The demographic characteristics of the patients and the radiologically detected injuries are presented in Tables 1 and 2, respectively. Chest radiography was performed on 76 patients (69.7%), while a thoracic CT scan was performed on 44 patients (40.4%).

The median CPR duration was significantly longer among patients with out-of-hospital cardiac arrest (OHCA) than among those with in-hospital cardiac arrest (IHCA) (14 vs. 2.5 min; $p < 0.001$). The mean number of rib fractures in the patients with at least one detected fracture was 6.7 ± 3.7. Flail chest was detected in 10 patients (9.2%), while an anterior flail segment was observed in 15 patients (16.5%). Pneumothorax was observed in three patients, and there were no cases of hemothorax. Sternal fractures or an anterior flail segment were more frequent among patients with OHCA, compared to those with IHCA ($p = 0.048$).

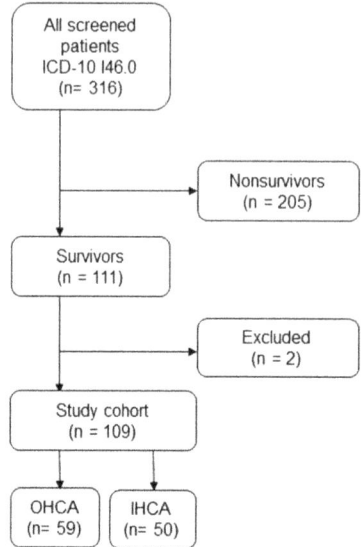

Figure 1. Study flowchart.

Table 1. Demographic characteristics of 109 patients with CPR-related chest injuries.

Variable	Value
OHCA, n (%)	59 (54.1%)
Male, n (%)	67 (61.5%)
Age, years	69 (56–77)
Height, cm	173 (165–180)
Weight, kg	80 (71–85)
BMI, kg/m^2	26.24 (23.60–29.31)
Heart failure, n (%)	44 (40.4%)
COPD, n (%)	15 (13.8%)
Pneumonia, n (%)	55 (50.5%)
eCPR, n (%)	2 (1.8%)
ACCD, n (%)	7 (6.4%)
CPR duration, min	5 (2.25–15)
ICU LOS, days	7 (3–18)
Mechanical ventilation, days	5 (2–14)
Tracheostomy, n (%)	21 (19.3%)

Data are presented as numbers (percentages) or medians (IQR). CPR, cardiopulmonary resuscitation; BMI, body mass index; COPD, chronic obstructive pulmonary disease; eCPR, extracorporeal CPR; ACCD, automated chest compression device; OHCA, out-of-hospital cardiac arrest; ICU LOS, intensive care unit length of stay.

Table 2. CPR-related thoracic injuries, detected by thoracic CT imaging or chest radiography.

	Number (%)
Rib fractures	34 (31.2%)
Unilateral	9 (8.3%)
Bilateral	25 (22.9%)
Anterior flail segment	18 (16.5%)
Sternal fracture	15 (13.8%)
Hemothorax	0
Pneumothorax	3 (2.8%)
No relevant chest injuries	71 (65.1%)

CPR, cardiopulmonary resuscitation; CT, computed tomography.

Seventy-six (69.7%) of the included patients were intubated (78% of the OHCA group) and mechanically ventilated during CPR. Seventy-one patients (93.4%) were successfully weaned from the ventilator during their ICU stay, while four patients remained mechanically ventilated until they were transferred to a rehabilitation unit. Due to extubation failure, 21 (19.3%) patients underwent percutaneous dilatational tracheostomy to facilitate weaning from mechanical ventilation.

The patients with flail chest had a significantly longer CPR duration, longer length of ICU stay, more days on mechanical ventilation, and higher rates of tracheostomy and pneumonia (Table 3).

Table 3. Characteristics of patients with and without CPR-related flail chest.

Variable	Flail Chest (n = 10)	No Flail Chest (n = 99)	p-Value
Male	9 (90%)	58 (58.6%)	0.048
Age, years	64.5 (61–68.25)	69 (55–77)	0.862
Height, cm	180 (170–185)	172 (165–180)	0.580
Weight, kg	80 (75–94.75)	79 (70–85)	0.236
BMI, kg/m^2	26.86 (24.64–29.24)	26.24 (23.38–29.39)	0.702
Heart failure, n (%)	4 (40%)	40 (40.4%)	0.628
COPD, n (%)	1 (10%)	14 (14.1%)	0.586
Pneumonia, n (%)	10 (100%)	45 (45.5%)	0.001
eCPR, n (%)	1 (10%)	1 (1%)	0.176
ACCD, n (%)	1 (10%)	6 (6.1%)	0.500
CPR duration, min	19 [10–21]	5 (2–15)	0.009
ICU LOS, days	25 (19.5–33.75)	6 (3–15)	<0.001
Mechanical ventilation, days	18.5 (14–28)	4 (2–10)	0.001
Tracheostomy, n (%)	8 (80%)	13 (13.1%)	<0.001

Date are presented as numbers (percentages) or medians (IQR). BMI, body mass index; COPD, chronic obstructive pulmonary disease; ACCD, automated chest compression device; CPR, cardiopulmonary resuscitation; eCPR, extracorporeal CPR; ICU LOS, intensive care unit length of stay.

The multivariable logistic regression analysis (Nagelkerke R-squared 0.321; Hosmer–Lemeshow $p = 0.545$) showed that flail chest was an independent predictor of the need for tracheostomy (OR 15.5; 95% CI 2.77–86.72; $p = 0.002$) (Table 4).

Table 4. Associations with the need for tracheostomy in logistic regression analysis.

Variable	Univariable OR (95% CI)	p-Value	Multivariable OR (95% CI)	p-Value
Age	1.01 (0.97–1.04)	0.783		
BMI	1.00 (0.93–1.07)	0.950		
Heart failure	1.16 (0.42–2.99)	0.831		
COPD	2.44 (0.73–8.01)	0.146		
Pneumonia	-	0.997		
Flail chest	26.46 (5.05–138.56)	<0.001	15.50 (2.77–86.72)	0.002
Duration of CPR	1.03 (1.00–1.06)	0.04	1.02 (0.98–1.05)	0.339
Rib fractures	5.19 (0.97–1.04)	0.001	0.36 (0.11–1.13)	0.080
Anterior flail segment	0.40 (0.13–1.22)	0.106		

OR, odds ratio; CI, confidence interval; BMI, body mass index, COPD, chronic obstructive pulmonary disease; CPR, cardiopulmonary resuscitation.

Furthermore, the multivariable linear regression analysis (ANOVA $p < 0.001$; adjusted R-Square 0.363) showed that pneumonia (β 11.34; 95% CI 6.70–15.99; $p < 0.001$) or the detection of multiple rib fractures (β 5.97; 95% CI 1.01–10.93; $p = 0.019$) independently influenced the length of ICU stay (Table 5).

Another multivariable linear regression analysis (ANOVA $p < 0.001$; adjusted R-Square 0.290) showed that flail chest (β 10.45; 95% CI 3.57–17.33; $p = 0.003$) and pneumonia (β 6.12; 95% CI 0.94–11.31; $p = 0.021$) significantly prolonged the duration of mechanical ventilation (Table 6).

Table 5. Associations with the length of ICU stay in linear regression analysis.

Variable	Univariable β (95% CI)	p-Value	Multivariable β (95% CI)	p-Value
Age	−0.69 (3.57–17.33)	0.442		
BMI	0.33 (0.94–11.31)	0.110		
Heart failure	1.40 (−0.34–9.44)	0.604		
COPD	7.46 (3.57–17.33)	0.050		
Pneumonia	14.99 (0.94–11.31)	<0.001	11.34 (6.70–15.99)	<0.001
Flail chest	17.81 (−0.34–9.44)	<0.001	7.85 (−0.59–15.76)	0.052
Duration of CPR	0.27 (3.57–17.33)	0.040	0.06 (−0.10–0.22)	0.489
Rib fractures	11.84 (0.94–11.31)	<0.001	5.97 (1.01–10.93)	0.019
Anterior flail segment	6.09 (−0.34–9.44)	0.086		

β, beta weight; CI, confidence interval; BMI, body mass index; COPD, chronic obstructive pulmonary disease; CPR, cardiopulmonary resuscitation.

Table 6. Associations with mechanical ventilation in linear regression analysis.

Variable	Univariable β (95% CI)	p-Value	Multivariable β (95% CI)	p-Value
Age	0.16 (−0.02–0.33)	0.750		
BMI	−0.09 (−0.53–0.35)	0.690		
Heart failure	−0.71 (−6.03–4.62)	0.791		
COPD	3.30 (−3.68–10.27)	0.349		
Pneumonia	9.17 (3.67–14.71)	0.01	6.12 (0.94–11.31)	0.021
Flail chest	14.58 (7.87–21.8)	<0.001	10.45 (3.57–17.33)	0.003
Duration of CPR	0.10 (−0.07–0.27)	0.236		
Rib fractures	8.35 (3.32–13.39)	0.001	4.55 (−0.34–9.44)	0.068
Anterior flail segment	2.44 (−3.70–8.58)	0.431		

β, beta weight; CI, confidence interval; BMI, body mass index; COPD, chronic obstructive pulmonary disease; CPR, cardiopulmonary resuscitation.

Four survivors failed to show adequate progression in weaning from the ventilator after receiving a tracheostomy, for a number of reasons, including flail chest. In a case-by-case decision, the treating physician, together with a thoracic surgeon, identified patients who would undergo surgical stabilization of their rib fractures, who were eventually weaned from mechanical ventilation (Table 7; Figure 2).

Table 7. Case characteristics of patients who underwent surgical rib fixation.

Variable	Patient 1	Patient 2	Patient 3	Patient 4
Age	61 years	53 years	61 years	66 years
Sex	male	male	male	male
BMI [kg/m^2]	24.7	24.7	29.2	22.5
Reason for CPR	Pulmonary embolism	Myocardial infarction	Myocardial infarction	Hypoxia
Relevant comorbidities	Aspiration pneumonia	Aspiration pneumonia	Influenza pneumonia Acinetobacter pneumonia	Aspiration pneumonia Heart failure COPD
Duration of CPR	65 min	20 min	15 min	21 min
Length of ICU stay	45 days	27 days	69 days	18 days
Mechanical ventilation	37 days	18 days	59 days	16 days
Number of fractured ribs	9 ribs	8 ribs	7 ribs	14 ribs
Anterior flail segment	Yes	Yes	Yes	Yes

BMI, body mass index; CPR, cardiopulmonary resuscitation; ICU, intensive care unit; COPD, chronic obstructive pulmonary disease.

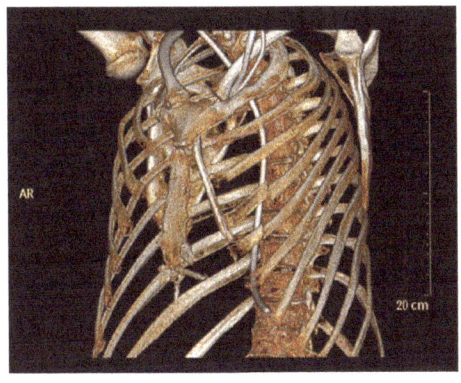
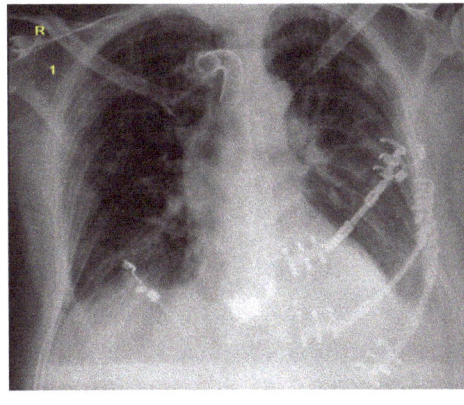

Figure 2. Chest CT reconstruction of a patient with multiple rib fractures and flail chest after 65 min of CPR, including the use of extracorporeal CPR, due to massive pulmonary embolism. (**a**) The patient underwent surgical rib fixation for stabilization (**b**) and was finally weaned from the ventilator after 37 days of mechanical ventilation.

4. Discussion

The results of this study suggest that the CPR-associated thoracic injury pattern among survivors of non-traumatic cardiac arrest may prolong the weaning process from the ventilator and ICU stay.

Rib fractures were the most frequently detected thoracic bone damage in our study. Most previous studies on injuries after CPR utilized necropsy, postmortem CT scans, or both, with the primary aim of demonstrating the differences between injuries caused by manual chest compressions and automated chest compression devices [3,4,6,8]. A recently published study, regarding CPR-associated thoracic injuries, included patients after OHCA, who received chest CT imaging after CPR. The median number of rib fractures was comparable with our results. An association between the detection of rib fractures and a prolonged length of ICU stay was found in the patients, which supports our results [12].

The frequency of clinically detected flail chest in our cohort was almost twice as high as that reported in a previous publication that was conducted almost half a century ago, which could be the result of higher survival rates [14]. The patients with flail chest had a higher rate of pneumonia, longer ICU stay and mechanical ventilation, and higher tracheostomy rates, compared with patients without flail chest. On the other hand, pneumonia and the detection of a rib fracture prolonged the overall length of ICU stay, while flail chest did not. Taken together, rib fractures, and especially multiple rib fractures that lead to flail chest, seem to influence post-resuscitation care in the ICU.

Regarding the treatment options after CPR-associated chest injuries, the present study was not designed to confirm whether early surgical rib fixation could influence the outcome. In this study, we present a series of four cases, in which surgical rib fractures might have contributed to improved respiratory function.

Recent data have shown improvements in the numeric pain score of patients with multiple rib fractures after surgical stabilization [15]. The Eastern Association for the Surgery of Trauma recommends rib fixation in patients with flail chest, to reduce the need for tracheostomy, increase the number of ventilator-free days, and reduce the length of ICU and hospital stays [16]. Whether patients with traumatic flail chest clearly benefit from surgical therapy remains controversial. Overall, surgical interventions have shown promising long-term outcomes and low complication rates [17–19]. However, these data refer to traumatic chest injuries and reflect a different patient cohort, in comparison to survivors of cardiac arrest with specific patterns of injuries. In a study of 61 ventilator-dependent patients with flail chest (including 7 CPR survivors), surgical rib fixation was associated with a shortened ICU stay and improved cost effectiveness [20].

Due to a considerable lack of data regarding the effect of surgical rib fixation on the course of the weaning process, more research is urgently needed. Future research should provide evidence of whether this procedure will remain a rare treatment option, or if it has the potential to change clinical practice patterns. This could particularly affect hospitals without cardiothoracic surgery departments, and the referral and capacity management of certified cardiac arrest centers.

As a result of this study, we have introduced a multidisciplinary assessment of CPR survivors with promising rehabilitation potential and a relevant probability of flail chest-related weaning failure, and whether they might benefit from surgical rib fixation. This assessment includes intensivists, respiratory therapists and thoracic surgeons.

Limitations

Retrospective single-center studies, with a limited number of patients, may result in selection bias. Less than half of the included patients underwent chest CT after CPR, which may have led to diagnostic bias, because the diagnostic accuracy of plane chest radiography for bone lesions is lower than CT [21]. Furthermore, deceased patients were not included in this study, who may have presented with other injury characteristics and different results.

5. Conclusions

Our results suggest that CPR-related injuries may impair the respiratory recovery of cardiac arrest survivors. The presence of flail chest may be associated with the need for tracheostomy, prolonged mechanical ventilation and pneumonia, whereas multiple rib fractures and pneumonia may contribute to longer ICU stays. A multidisciplinary assessment, including intensivists, respiratory therapists and thoracic surgeons, may help to identify the patients who may benefit from surgical rib fixation and chest stabilization, which has to be confirmed in future studies.

Author Contributions: Conceptualization, K.K. and S.K.; methodology, K.K., S.P. and S.K.; software, S.P. and M.Y.-D.; validation, K.K., T.D., M.F.S. and M.Y.-D.; formal analysis, K.K. and M.Y.-D.; investigation, K.K. and S.E.; resources, K.K. and S.P.; data curation, K.K. and S.E.; writing—original draft preparation, K.K., M.F.S. and S.K.; writing—review and editing, K.K., S.E., S.P. and T.D.; visualization, K.K., S.E. and S.K.; supervision, S.P., M.F.S. and S.K.; project administration, S.K. All authors have read and agreed to the published version of the manuscript.

Funding: This research received no external funding.

Institutional Review Board Statement: The study was conducted in accordance with the Declaration of Helsinki, and approved by the Ethics Committee of the University of Leipzig (172/20-ek; 7 May 2020).

Informed Consent Statement: Patient consent was waived, due to the retrospective nature of the study.

Data Availability Statement: The data supporting the findings of this study are available from the corresponding author, upon reasonable request.

Acknowledgments: We acknowledge support from the German Research Foundation (DFG) and the University of Leipzig, within the program of Open Access Publishing.

Conflicts of Interest: The authors declare no conflict of interest.

References

1. Olasveengen, T.M.; Semeraro, F.; Ristagno, G.; Castren, M.; Handley, A.; Kuzovlev, A.; Monsieurs, K.G.; Raffay, V.; Smyth, M.; Soar, J.; et al. European Resuscitation Council Guidelines 2021: Basic Life Support. *Resuscitation* **2021**, *161*, 98–114. [CrossRef] [PubMed]
2. Nolan, J.P.; Sandroni, C.; Böttiger, B.W.; Cariou, A.; Cronberg, T.; Friberg, H.; Genbrugge, C.; Haywood, K.; Lilja, G.; Moulaert, V.R.M.; et al. European Resuscitation Council and European Society of Intensive Care Medicine Guidelines 2021: Post-resuscitation care. *Resuscitation* **2021**, *161*, 220–269. [CrossRef] [PubMed]
3. Thompson, M.; Langlois, N.E.I.; Byard, R.W. Flail Chest Following Failed Cardiopulmonary Resuscitation. *J. Forensic Sci.* **2017**, *62*, 1220–1222. [CrossRef] [PubMed]
4. Ondruschka, B.; Baier, C.; Bayer, R.; Hammer, N.; Dreßler, J.; Bernhard, M. Chest compression-associated injuries in cardiac arrest patients treated with manual chest compressions versus automated chest compression devices (LUCAS II)—A forensic autopsy-based comparison. *Forensic Sci. Med. Pathol.* **2018**, *14*, 515–525. [CrossRef] [PubMed]
5. Lardi, C.; Egger, C.; Larribau, R.; Niquille, M.; Mangin, P.; Fracasso, T. Traumatic injuries after mechanical cardiopulmonary resuscitation (LUCAS2): A forensic autopsy study. *Int. J. Leg. Med.* **2015**, *129*, 1035–1042. [CrossRef] [PubMed]
6. Koster, R.W.; Beenen, L.F.; van der Boom, E.B.; Spijkerboer, A.M.; Tepaske, R.; van der Wal, A.C.; Beesems, S.G.; Tijssen, J.G. Safety of mechanical chest compression devices AutoPulse and LUCAS in cardiac arrest: A randomized clinical trial for non-inferiority. *Eur. Heart J.* **2017**, *38*, 3006–3013. [CrossRef] [PubMed]
7. Milling, L.; Mikkelsen, S.; Astrup, B.S. Characteristics of mechanical CPR-related injuries: A case series. *J. Forensic Leg. Med.* **2020**, *70*, 101918. [CrossRef]
8. Smekal, D.; Lindgren, E.; Sandler, H.; Johansson, J.; Rubertsson, S. CPR-related injuries after manual or mechanical chest compressions with the LUCAS™ device: A multicentre study of victims after unsuccessful resuscitation. *Resuscitation* **2014**, *85*, 1708–1712. [CrossRef] [PubMed]
9. Sinning, C.; Ahrens, I.; Cariou, A.; Beygui, F.; Lamhaut, L.; Halvorsen, S.; Nikolaou, N.; Nolan, J.P.; Price, S.; Monsieurs, K.; et al. The cardiac arrest centre for the treatment of sudden cardiac arrest due to presumed cardiac cause—Aims, function and structure: Position paper of the Association for Acute CardioVascular Care of the European Society of Cardiology (AVCV), European Association of Percutaneous Coronary Interventions (EAPCI), European Heart Rhythm Association (EHRA), European Resuscitation Council (ERC), European Society for Emergency Medicine (EUSEM) and European Society of Intensive Care Medicine (ESICM). *Eur. Heart J. Acute Cardiovasc. Care* **2020**, *9*, S193–S202. [CrossRef] [PubMed]
10. DeVoe, W.B.; Abourezk, M.; Goslin, B.J.; Saraswat, N.; Kiel, B.; Bach, J.A.; Suh, K.I.; Eriksson, E.A. Surgical stabilization of severe chest wall injury following cardiopulmonary resuscitation. *J. Trauma Acute Care Surg.* **2022**, *92*, 98–102. [CrossRef] [PubMed]
11. Drahos, A.; Fitzgerald, M.; Ashley, D.; Christie, D.B., 3rd. Chest wall stabilization with rib plating after cardiopulmonary resuscitation. *J. Thorac. Dis.* **2019**, *11*, S1103–S1105. [CrossRef] [PubMed]
12. Prins, J.T.H.; Van Lieshout, E.M.M.; Van Wijck, S.F.M.; Scholte, N.T.B.; Den Uil, C.A.; Vermeulen, J.; Verhofstad, M.H.J.; Wijffels, M.M.E. Chest wall injuries due to cardiopulmonary resuscitation and the effect on in-hospital outcomes in survivors of out-of-hospital cardiac arrest. *J. Trauma Acute Care Surg.* **2021**, *91*, 966–975. [CrossRef] [PubMed]
13. Edwards, J.G.; Clarke, P.; Pieracci, F.M.; Bemelman, M.; Black, E.A.; Doben, A.; Gasparri, M.; Gross, R.; Jun, W.; Long, W.B.; et al. Chest Wall Injury Society collaborators. Taxonomy of multiple rib fractures: Results of the chest wall injury society international consensus survey. *J. Trauma Acute Care Surg.* **2020**, *88*, e40–e45. [CrossRef]
14. Enarson, D.A.; Didier, E.P.; Gracey, D.R. Flail chest as a complication of cardiopulmonary resuscitation. *Heart Lung J. Crit. Care* **1977**, *6*, 1020–1022.
15. Pieracci, F.M.; Leasia, K.; Bauman, Z.; Eriksson, E.A.; Lottenberg, L.; Majercik, S.; Powell, L.; Sarani, B.; Semon, G.; Thomas, B.; et al. A multicenter, prospective, controlled clinical trial of surgical stabilization of rib fractures in patients with severe, nonflail fracture patterns (Chest Wall Injury Society NONFLAIL). *J. Trauma Acute Care Surg.* **2020**, *88*, 249–257. [CrossRef] [PubMed]
16. Kasotakis, G.; Hasenboehler, E.A.; Streib, E.W.; Patel, N.; Patel, M.B.; Alarcon, L.; Bosarge, P.L.; Love, J.; Haut, E.R.; Como, J.J. Operative fixation of rib fractures after blunt trauma: A practice management guideline from the Eastern Association for the Surgery of Trauma. *J. Trauma Acute Care Surg.* **2017**, *82*, 618–626. [CrossRef] [PubMed]
17. Beks, R.B.; Peek, J.; de Jong, M.B.; Wessem, K.J.P.; Öner, C.F.; Hietbrink, F.; Leenen, L.P.H.; Groenwold, R.H.H.; Houwert, R.M. Fixation of flail chest or multiple rib fractures: Current evidence and how to proceed. A systematic review and meta-analysis. *Eur. J. Trauma Emerg. Surg.* **2019**, *45*, 631–644. [CrossRef] [PubMed]
18. Ingoe, H.M.; Coleman, E.; Eardley, W.; Rangan, A.; Hewitt, C.; McDaid, C. Systematic review of systematic reviews for effectiveness of internal fixation for flail chest and rib fractures in adults. *BMJ Open* **2019**, *9*, e023444. [CrossRef] [PubMed]
19. Peek, J.; Beks, R.B.; Hietbrink, F.; Heng, M.; De Jong, M.B.; Beeres, F.J.P.; Leenen, L.P.H.; Groenwold, R.H.H.; Houwert, R.M. Complications and outcome after rib fracture fixation: A systematic review. *J. Trauma Acute Care Surg.* **2020**, *89*, 411–418. [CrossRef]
20. Kocher, G.J.; Sharafi, S.; Azenha, L.F.; Schmid, R.A. Chest wall stabilization in ventilator-dependent traumatic flail chest patients: Who benefits? *Eur. J. Cardiothorac. Surg.* **2017**, *51*, 696–701. [CrossRef]
21. Awais, M.; Salam, B.; Nadeem, N.; Rehman, A.; Baloch, N.U. Diagnostic Accuracy of Computed Tomography Scout Film and Chest X-ray for Detection of Rib Fractures in Patients with Chest Trauma: A Cross-sectional Study. *Cureus* **2019**, *11*, e3875. [CrossRef]

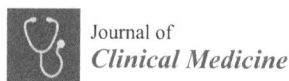

Article

Beneficial Effects of Adjusted Perfusion and Defibrillation Strategies on Rhythm Control within Controlled Automated Reperfusion of the Whole Body (CARL) for Refractory Out-of-Hospital Cardiac Arrest

Sam Joé Brixius [1,*], Jan-Steffen Pooth [1], Jörg Haberstroh [2], Domagoj Damjanovic [1], Christian Scherer [1], Philipp Greiner [1], Christoph Benk [1], Friedhelm Beyersdorf [1] and Georg Trummer [1]

[1] Department of Cardiovascular Surgery, Faculty of Medicine, University Medical Centre Freiburg, University of Freiburg, 79106 Freiburg, Germany; jan-steffen.pooth@uniklinik-freiburg.de (J.-S.P.); domagoj.damjanovic@uniklinik-freiburg.de (D.D.); christian.scherer@uniklinik-freiburg.de (C.S.); greiner-philipp@uniklinik-freiburg.de (P.G.); christoph.benk@uniklinik-freiburg.de (C.B.); friedhelm.beyersdorf@uniklinik-freiburg.de (F.B.); georg.trummer@uniklinik-freiburg.de (G.T.)

[2] Centre for Experimental Models and Transgenic Service, Department of Experimental Surgery, Faculty of Medicine, University Medical Centre Freiburg, University of Freiburg, 79104 Freiburg, Germany; joerg.haberstroh@uniklinik-freiburg.de

* Correspondence: sam.brixius@uniklinik-freiburg.de

Abstract: Survival and neurological outcomes after out-of-hospital cardiac arrest (OHCA) remain low. The further development of prehospital extracorporeal resuscitation (ECPR) towards Controlled Automated Reperfusion of the Whole Body (CARL) has the potential to improve survival and outcome in these patients. In CARL therapy, pulsatile, high blood-flow reperfusion is performed combined with several modified reperfusion parameters and adjusted defibrillation strategies. We aimed to investigate whether pulsatile, high-flow reperfusion is feasible in refractory OHCA and whether the CARL approach improves heart-rhythm control during ECPR. In a reality-based porcine model of refractory OHCA, 20 pigs underwent prehospital CARL or conventional ECPR. Significantly higher pulsatile blood-flow proved to be feasible, and critical hypotension was consistently prevented via CARL. In the CARL group, spontaneous rhythm conversions were observed using a modified priming solution. Applying potassium-induced secondary cardioplegia proved to be a safe and effective method for sustained rhythm conversion. Moreover, significantly fewer defibrillation attempts were needed, and cardiac arrhythmias were reduced during reperfusion via CARL. Prehospital CARL therapy thus not only proved to be feasible after prolonged OHCA, but it turned out to be superior to conventional ECPR regarding rhythm control.

Keywords: cardiopulmonary resuscitation; extracorporeal circulation; post-resuscitation care

1. Introduction

Sudden out-of-hospital cardiac arrest (OHCA) is one of the leading causes of death in Europe and a major health care problem [1,2]. Its survival rate is still reported to be poor, with a significant number of patients suffering from permanent neurological disability [1,3–5]. In recent years, extracorporeal cardiopulmonary resuscitation (ECPR) has shown promising results and consequentially found consideration in the guidelines as a rescue therapy in refractory cardiac arrest (CA) for selected patients [6–8].

However, uncontrolled reperfusion leads to the development of so-called ischaemia-reperfusion injury (IRI), causing further multi-organ damage [9,10]. The pathophysiologic mechanisms of IRI include systemic inflammatory response, oxidative stress and microcirculatory deficits [9,11]. In particular, cardiac IRI often interferes with the aim of re-establishing a regular heart rhythm. As a result, cardiac arrhythmias are frequently detected during

ECPR. Early rhythm conversion and termination of these arrhythmias reduce myocardial oxygen consumption and are essential to unloading the left ventricle [12,13]. As a result, the exacerbation of myocardial ischaemic injury and potential side effects of cardiac standstill during extracorporeal circulation (ECC), such as left ventricle distension or intracardiac thrombus formation, can be prevented [14,15]. Early restoration of a regular cardiac rhythm and preventing further cardiac arrhythmias should therefore be among the highest priorities during ECPR.

To further improve the outcome after CA, a concept based on ECC has been developed, called Controlled Automated Reperfusion of the Whole Body (CARL). CARL enables users to treat and minimise IRI by controlling the initial reperfusion phase and applying basic scientific principles. Its rationale has been reported [9,16–18]. In addition to acquiring and modifying several reperfusion parameters, reperfusion with high, pulsatile blood flow and high reperfusion pressures are key elements of CARL therapy. Based on this, an adapted approach to rhythm conversion using cardiac surgery techniques such as secondary cardioplegia (SC) is followed here [16,19,20].

Our first study aim was to investigate whether a pulsatile, high blood flow approach is feasible despite expected hypovolemia and vasoplegia during refractory cardiopulmonary resuscitation. Second, we wanted to investigate whether modified reperfusion targets when applying CARL therapy have any effects on the rhythm conversion rate and heart rhythm control in comparison to conventional ECPR.

2. Materials and Methods

This animal study protocol was approved by the local animal welfare committee (Regierungspräsidium Freiburg, G-15/148). All experiments were carried out in accordance with the regulations of the German animal protection law and animal care guidelines of the European Community (2010/63/EU).

To create a reality-based porcine model of refractory OHCA, local response times for OHCA were included in our study protocol. For this purpose, the experimental procedure proceeded realistically in individual stages (see Figure 1), starting with a normothermic whole-body ischaemic phase. In this stage, bystanders witness the collapse, CA is observed, and the emergency medical services are dispatched (5 min). In the second stage, basic life support is attempted via high quality chest compression and rescue breaths (8 min). When the specialized rescue forces arrive, additional rescue attempts and advanced life support are started (22 min).

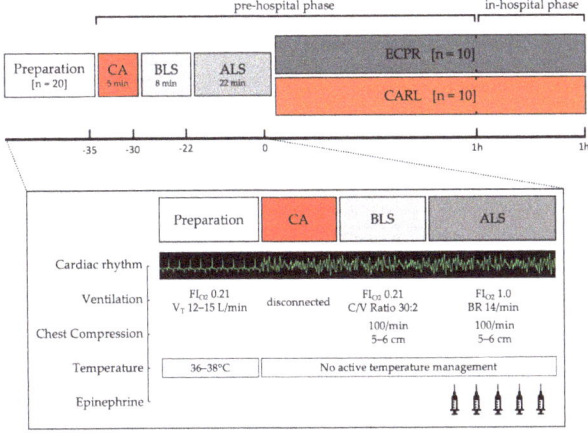

Figure 1. Schematic presentation of the experimental protocol. CA Cardiac arrest, BLS Basic life support, ALS Advanced life support, FiO$_2$ Fraction of inspired oxygen, V$_T$ Tidal volume, C/V Chest compression to ventilation ratio, BR Breathing rate.

A total of 35 min after the CA onset, the therapy is escalated to one of the extracorporeal systems (conventional ECPR versus CARL). The extracorporeal resuscitation phase was further divided into two sections: a pre-hospital and an in-hospital section.

The preparations and realization of each phase according to the group's allocation are explained in detail below.

2.1. Anaesthesia and Surgical Procedures

In our experimental protocol, 20 Landrace-Hybrid pigs of 50–75 kg bodyweight were premedicated with ketamine (20 mg/kg) and midazolam (5 mg/kg) intramuscularly. Anaesthesia was induced by injecting propofol (2–4 mg/kg) through a venous catheter placed in the marginal ear vein. After neuromuscular relaxation with vecuronium (10 mg), endotracheal intubation was performed with an endotracheal tube (size 7.0–8.0 mm). Volume-controlled mechanical ventilation was provided to normalize pH, arterial partial pressure of oxygen (P_{O2}) and arterial partial pressure of carbon dioxide (P_{CO2}). Anaesthesia was maintained with inhaled isoflurane (2% Volume), fentanyl (1–5 µg/kg/h) and vecuronium (0.2 mg/kg/h). Hypokalaemia and hypomagnesemia, as routinely observed in prior experiments, were compensated accordingly with 5 mL potassium chloride 7.45% and 1 g magnesium. An antibiotic prophylaxis was provided with ceftriaxone (2 g). Ringer's solution (10 mL/kg/h) was used as primary fluid substitution to maintain euvolemia. We employed a continuous intraoperative monitoring, which recorded heart rate, pulse strength, oxygen saturation, ECG and blood pressure automatically (Siemens, SC 9000XL, Washington, DC, USA). Body temperature was recorded via a nasopharyngeal temperature probe and kept constant in the physiological range until the experimental protocol was started.

Animals were placed in a horizontal supine position on a specially designed resuscitation board with a built-in connection point for the mechanical resuscitation device [21]. The neck vessels were exposed by chirurgical dissection on the right side of the neck. Two catheters were placed in the right common carotid artery to continuously record the arterial blood pressure and collect arterial blood samples. Another catheter was placed in the external jugular vein for venous blood sampling. Information on pulmonary arterial and central venous pressures as well as cardiac output was obtained via a Swan–Ganz catheter (Swan-Ganz Pacing-TD Catheter, Edwards Lifesciences, Irvine, CA, USA), which was placed in the right subclavian vein. Coronary perfusion pressure was calculated as the difference between the diastolic and central venous pressure [22]. The right femoral artery and right external jugular vein were prepared for later cannulation.

At fixed time points during the experiment, blood samples were taken for arterial and venous blood gas analyses.

2.2. Cardiac Arrest

Cardiac arrest was induced by electrical fibrillation using the pacing electrodes of the Swan–Ganz catheter. The so induced cardiac arrest was kept for the next five minutes. At the same time the animals were disconnected from mechanical ventilation. During this phase, the supply of all drugs was stopped, and no resuscitation of any kind took place.

To prepare for extracorporeal circulation, a 22–24 F cannula was advanced in the exposed right jugular vein for venous drainage, as was a 14–16 F cannula in the right femoral artery for arterial inflow. Each cannula was flushed with saline and 5000 I.U. of heparin to prevent clot formation; they remained clamped during the CA and CPR periods.

2.3. Basic Life Support

Basic life support (BLS) was provided for eight minutes in accordance with the BLS algorithm of the European Resuscitation Council (ERC) [23]. Chest compressions were performed using a mechanical chest compression device (LUCAS 2 Chest Compression Device, Stryker Medical, Portage, MI, USA) at a frequency of 100 compressions per minute and compression depth of 5–6 cm. The time ratio between compression and decompression was 50/50, and active decompression was applied. The animals were manually ventilated with ambient air (21% oxygen) by connecting the endotracheal tube to a ventilation bag. The chest compression to ventilation ratio was 30 to 2.

2.4. Advanced Life Support

In the subsequent advanced life support (ALS) phase, the inspiratory oxygen concentration was raised to 100% and chest compressions were no longer interrupted for ventilation. Ventilation occurred at a rate of 14/min with a tidal volume of 10 mL/kg. In accordance with ERC guidelines, each animal received 1 mg epinephrine (10 mL diluted 1:10 with NaCl 0.9%) every 4 min via intravenous access. Cumulatively, each animal received 5 mg of epinephrine flushed with 20 mL of saline solution. Electrical or chemical defibrillation attempts were not made throughout the duration of conventional CPR to simulate refractory CA and prevent a premature return of spontaneous circulation (ROSC). Anaesthesia was resumed with propofol (10–15 mg/kg/h), fentanyl (1–5 µg/kg/h) and vecuronium (0.2 mg/kg/h) to prevent awareness.

2.5. Animal Groups

Following five minutes of normothermic CA and 30 min of conventional resuscitation, ECC was established for 90 min according to a group-specific protocol. n = 10 pigs were allocated to each group. In both groups, chest compressions were stopped after establishing ECC, and rhythm conversion to a regular heart rhythm was attempted. Any cardiac arrhythmias during reperfusion were treated when hemodynamically relevant.

2.5.1. Conventional Extracorporeal Cardiopulmonary Resuscitation (ECPR)

The selected reperfusion targets and settings in the group receiving conventional ECPR were realized just as they are already practiced in OHCA in many places. ECC was established using a diagonal pump (Deltastream DP3, Medos Medizintechnik AG, Stolberg, Germany) and a commercially available reperfusion set (Medos Medizintechnik AG, Stolberg, Germany). The system was primed with a total of 1.2 L crystalloid solution (Jonosteril Infusion Solution, Fresenius Kabi Deutschland GmbH, Bad Homburg, Germany) at room temperature and 15,000 I.U. heparin. Reperfusion was performed with a blood flow of 50 mL/kg/min and sweep gas flow of 2.5–3.5 L/min with 100% oxygen supply via the membrane oxygenator. The inspiratory oxygen concentration was set to 100% and ventilation was continued with a tidal volume of 10 mL/kg/min.

Persistent shockable cardiac arrhythmias were treated in accordance with the ALS-algorithm [6]. If defibrillation was indicated, up to three shocks were applied at an energy of 200 J followed by an initial dose of amiodarone (10 mg/kg) if unsuccessful. A second dose of amiodarone (5 mg/kg) was administered after the fifth shock, if needed. Persistent shockable arrhythmias beyond that were subjected to subsequent shocks, along with 2 g magnesium and 100 mg lidocaine. All defibrillation attempts were made with the animal in antero-apical pad position.

Due to laminar blood flow induced by conventional ECC and the lack of invasive blood pressure and blood gas measurements, no information regarding blood pressure and blood gases were available in conventional ECPR during the first 60 min (prehospital situation). Consequently, no vasoactive drugs were applied and no active modification of blood gas parameters took place during the pre-hospital ECPR phase. In case of venous-cannula suction events, a bolus of 300–500 mL crystalloid fluid was administered.

In the second, in-hospital section (60–90 min), hypotension was treated with norepinephrine and crystalloid fluid administration to enable a mean arterial blood pressure (MAP) > 65 mmHg [24]. Arterial acidosis was counteracted by injecting sodium bicarbonate in order to achieve a pH greater than 7.2.

2.5.2. Controlled Automated Reperfusion of the Whole Body (CARL)

In the CARL group, the CARL controller (Resuscitec GmbH, Freiburg, Germany) was used for reperfusion, and CARL therapy was applied [16–18]. In accordance with CARL therapy, more than 14 blood parameters and 4 specific reperfusion conditions were modified [16,25]. Before use, the system was primed with 1.0 L specially developed priming solution (CARL Priming Solution, Dr. Franz Köhler Chemie GmbH, Bensheim, Germany) [16]. Initial reperfusion was performed at a high, pulsatile blood flow of 80–100 mL/kg/min, and pulsatility was maintained for 45 min or until the heart regained its own ejection. As provided, a fibreoptic catheter (CARL Arterial Pressure Sensor, Resuscitec GmbH, Freiburg, Germany) was placed in the ascending aorta via the integrated connection site in the arterial line to monitor arterial pressure immediately after initiating reperfusion. A MAP of 80–100 mmHg was targeted by injecting norepinephrine and fluids (priming solution and crystalloid fluid). Immediate hypothermia up to 32 °C was induced in the first 60 min followed by gradual rewarming to normothermic body temperature Mechanical ventilation was performed in a volume-controlled manner with one-third of the tidal volume required before, and the inspiratory oxygen concentration was set to 30% until the heart regained its own ejection. The sweep gas flow and oxygen supply via the membrane oxygenator was adjusted to achieve the target values required in CARL therapy (arterial P_{O2} 100–200 mmHg, arterial P_{CO2} 35–45 mmHg). By injecting sodium bicarbonate, a physiologic pH was targeted form the 45th min onwards.

Shockable cardiac arrhythmias during the reperfusion process were managed by injecting 40 mL potassium (7.45%) to evoke a transient asystole, and allow for a rhythm conversation into an organized hearth rhythm. This form of potassium-induced secondary cardioplegia was repeated once if the arrhythmia persisted before more conversion attempts were made with repeated electrical defibrillations at 200 joules. After the first electrical defibrillation, supportive 10 mg/kg amiodarone was administered via peripheral venous access, followed by another dose of 5 mg/kg after the third shock. If ventricular fibrillation persisted, additional 100 mg lidocaine and 2 g magnesium were applied. To further evaluate the effect of SC beyond the CARL therapy, it was also applied in n = 4 animals in the ECPR group showing refractory ventricular fibrillation (VF) at different time points.

2.6. Statistical Analyses

Statistics were analysed and data were visualised using the statistical software RStudio (version 1.4.11) and R package ggplot2 [26,27]. Data were tested for normal distribution by Shapiro–Wilk test. Means and standard deviation (SD) or medians and ranges were calculated as appropriate. Differences between groups were compared applying Mann–Whitney rank sum test or t-Test as appropriate. The number of defibrillations required was tested in a generalised linear model using Poisson Regression. Analysis of categorical data, such as cardiac arrhythmias, is limited to descriptive analysis due to small subgroup size. Statistical analyses regarding blood pressure and haemoglobin concentration were conducted in a mixed-effects model for each phase of the experiment using the R packages lme4 and lmerTest [28,29]. In this model, bodyweight, time of measurement and group allocation were considered as fixed effects. A group size of n = 10 in each group allowed the discrimination of differences with an effect size greater than 1.2, a power of 0.8 and a one-tailed significance value of 0.05.

3. Results

3.1. Haemoperfusion

In the CARL group, a mean blood flow of 5.26 ± 0.36 L/min was achieved compared to 3.12 ± 0.36 L/min in the ECPR group ($p < 0.001$). This required significantly more fluid administration in the CARL group over the entire reperfusion period than in the ECPR group (Table 1, CARL: 1556 ± 687 mL, ECPR: 430 ± 286 mL, $p < 0.01$).

Table 1. Norepinephrine and fluid use in reperfusion phase.

	n	Mean ± SD	
		Norepinephrine (µg/kg/min)	Fluid (mL)
CARL	8 *	1.15 ± 0.70	1556 ± 687
ECPR	10	1.82 ± 1.33	430 ± 286
p-Value		0.22	0.002

* No information on drug application available for n = 2 pigs (loss of data).

The pulsatile blood flow generated by the CARL controller's second diagonal pump could be tracked in the abdominal aorta as well as in the common carotid artery (Figure 2). As is standard with CARL therapy, we observed an amplitude of 15–20 mmHg in both vessels at a 50/min pulse rate.

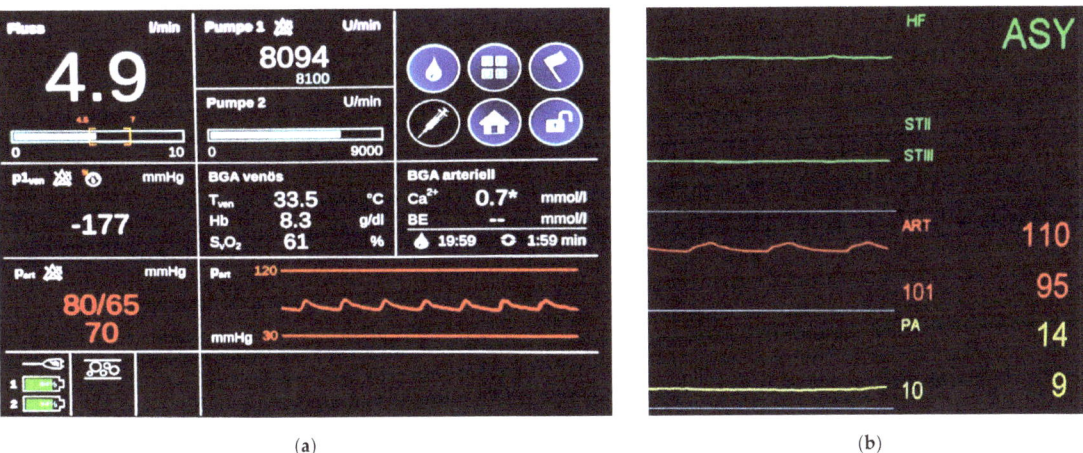

(a)   (b)

Figure 2. Pulsatile blood flow on ECC during CARL therapy: (**a**) Screenshot from real-time measurements on the CARL controller during asystole reperfusion. A pulsatile blood pressure was observed during extracorporeal circulation in the ascending aorta during asystole phase (red curve); (**b**) Screenshot of experimental monitoring during ECC. Despite asystole (green curve), a pulsatile blood flow (red curve) is detected in the common carotid. Pulmonary artery (PA) pressure is displayed in yellow.

We observed no complications in relation to pulsatility or the high flow approach such as aortic valve insufficiency or left ventricle distension.

3.2. Haemodynamics

Neither group differed significantly in MAP during baseline, ischaemia and mechanical resuscitation (see Figure 3a). A trend towards decreasing blood pressure was observed during the BLS and ALS phases, which was interrupted by repetitive peaks in the ALS phase. These peaks corresponded to the repeated application of epinephrine. However, this blood pressure-increasing effect exhibited a visibly decreasing course as the number of applications rose. The effect of the fifth application, two minutes before the start of ECC, coincided with the initial phase of reperfusion and contributed to a further blood pressure peak after extracorporeal reperfusion in both groups.

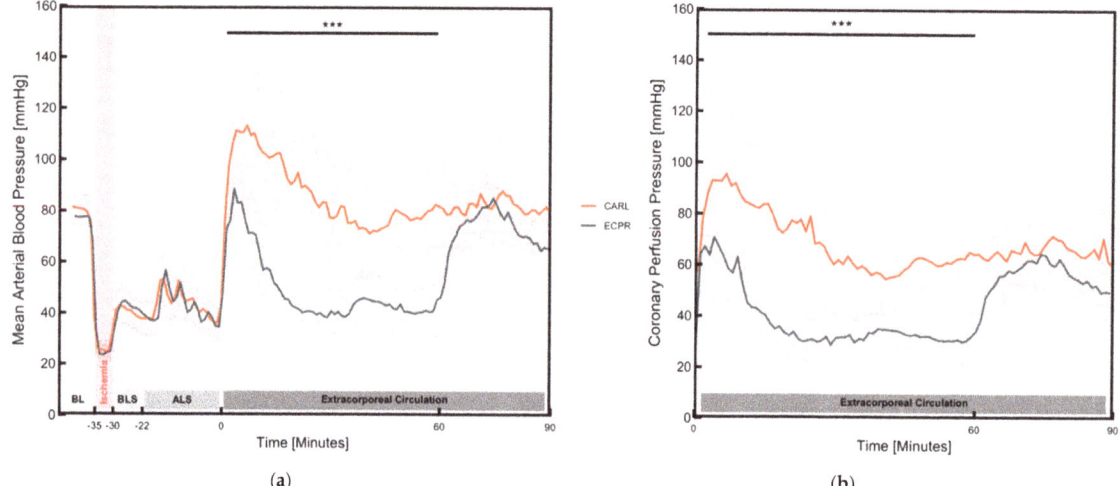

Figure 3. Longitudinal course of haemodynamic parameters: (**a**) Mean arterial blood pressure; (**b**) Coronary perfusion pressure. Data are expressed as mean ± SD. BL Baseline, BLS Basic life support, ALS Advanced life support. (*** $p < 0.001$).

This initial peak revealed a rapid decline in accordance with the half-life of epinephrine (3–10 min) in the ECPR group. Due to the unavailability of prehospital arterial pressure measurements, we could not respond appropriately to this drop, resulting in a critical MAP less than 60 mmHg from the fifteenth minute on in all ten animals. At the beginning of the in-hospital phase after 60 min of ECC, we were able to treat low arterial pressure by injecting norepinephrine and fluids as in Table 1, resulting in a sufficient MAP of 72 ± 7 mmHg in the ECPR group.

The CARL group revealed a significantly higher MAP during the first 60 min of the experiment (pre-hospital phase). The combination of catecholamine and fluid application and the pulsatile, high flow approach resulted in a MAP of 87 ± 13 mmHg.

Concomitant with the CARL group's higher MAP, they also achieved higher coronary perfusion pressures (CPPs) during the first hour of ECC than did the ECPR group (see Figure 3b, CARL: 69.3 ± 14.0 mmHg, ECPR: 36.8 ± 4.6 mmHg, $p < 0.001$). In the second reperfusion phase, CPPs in both groups were similar with the CARL group tending towards higher coronary pressures (CARL: 65.2 ± 12.5 mmHg, ECPR: 54.1 ± 8.7 mmHg, $p = 0.10$). Although both groups required similar numbers of vasopressor applications, the CARL group needed three times as much fluid.

As shown in Figure 4, the haemoglobin concentration rose significantly during chest compressions compared to baseline (13.0 ± 0.7 g/dL vs. 9.3 ± 0.7 g/dL, $p < 0.001$), indicating a relevant haemoconcentration caused by volume shift during cardiac arrest. We detected no differences between the groups until the onset of reperfusion. After starting reperfusion, we noted a complete return to baseline values in the CARL group, but the ECPR group's haemoglobin concentration did not entirely return to baseline values. Even after a prolonged period of reperfusion, they still differed significantly from the CARL group ($p < 0.001$). We found that animal body weight proved to be a significant confounder for haemoglobin concentrations during reperfusion ($p = 0.044$) with higher haemoglobin concentrations in heavier animals.

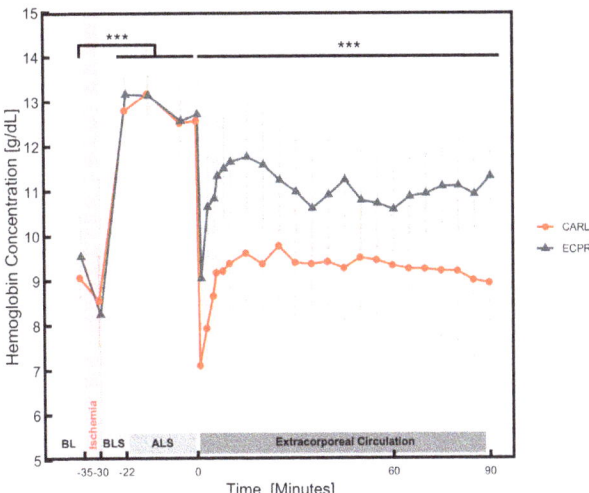

Figure 4. Haemoglobin concentration's longitudinal course in arterial blood. Data are expressed as mean ± SD. BL Baseline, BLS Basic life support, ALS Advanced life support. (*** $p < 0.001$).

3.3. Arterial Blood Gases

Arterial blood gas analysis revealed no differences in baseline values and no differences at the end of the ALS phase between booth groups (see Table 2).

Arterial P_{O2} during ECC was higher in the ECPR group ($p < 0.001$), as well as arterial P_{CO2} ($p < 0.01$) in the pre-hospital phase. No differences were seen in lactate and glucose concentration between booth groups. Arterial pH showed a significant reduction in the ECPR group 30 ($p < 0.05$) and 60 ($p < 0.001$) minutes after the onset of ECC.

Table 2. Arterial blood gas analysis.

	ECPR						CARL					
	BL	ALS	3′	30′	60′	90′	BL	ALS	3′	30′	60′	90′
pH	7.45 ± 0.02	7.09 ± 0.16	7.01 ± 0.09	7.08 * ± 0.06	7.11 *** ± 0.08	7.29 ± 0.05	7.45 ± 0.02	7.07 ± 0.10	7.01 ± 0.05	7.17 * ± 0.08	7.29 *** ± 0.08	7.33 ± 0.06
Base excess, mmol/L	3.6 ± 1.2	−14.4 ± 2.9	−15.1 * ± 3.5	−13.5 ± 1.9	−13.0 * ± 2.4	−5.8 ± 1.2	3.8 ± 1.3	−15.8 ± 3.3	−18.4 * ± 1.6	−14.9 ± 4.1	−9.1 * ± 4.2	−6.2 ± 2.9
Arterial P_{O2}, mmHg	93 ± 17	110 ± 140	207 ± 82	233 *** ± 71	255 *** ± 94	424 *** ± 104	91 ± 7	71 ± 30	224 ± 64	118 *** ± 31	103 *** ± 29	115 *** ± 41
Arterial P_{CO2}, mmHg	40 ± 1	56 ± 24	64 ** ± 9	58 *** ± 10	55 ** ± 10	43 ± 7	41 ± 2	54 ± 25	53 ** ± 6	39 *** ± 7	37 ** ± 8	38 ± 5
Glucose, mg/dL	98 ± 20	276 ± 168	305 ± 164	238 ± 163	201 ± 140	171 ± 141	102 ± 9	381 ± 79	296 ± 76	234 ± 68	226 ± 61	219 ± 52
Lactate, mmol/L	1.6 ± 0.4	10.7 ± 2.5	12.0 ± 2.1	12.0 ± 1.2	12.1 ± 1.6	14.7 ± 1.7	1.5 ± 0.5	10.9 ± 1.6	10.2 ± 1.2	11.4 ± 1.6	13.2 ± 1.7	14.0 ± 1.7

Values are expressed as mean ± SE. BL Baseline, ALS End of advanced life support. (* $p < 0.05$, ** $p < 0.01$, *** $p < 0.001$).

3.4. Effects on Rhythm Conversion and Cardiac Arrhythmias during Reperfusion
3.4.1. Termination of Ventricular Fibrillation

Following ALS, all pigs exhibited persistent VF. With the onset of ECC in the CARL group, the reperfusion solution containing lidocaine and a high concentration of magnesium induced a transient asystole in all animals. Spontaneous rhythm conversion to sinus rhythm was observed in n = 4 animals (see Table 3). In two of those animals (2/4), the sinus rhythm proved to be stable until the end of the observation period. VF in the remaining n = 8 pigs was managed by potassium-induced secondary cardioplegia (SC) as described above. All animals receiving SC showed a transient asystole phase interrupted by either sinus rhythm or further cardiac arrhythmias. Sustained asystole after SC was not observed in any animal. The sinus rhythm achieved in one pig (1/8) after SC appeared to be stable until the end of the observation period. A mean increase in serum potassium concentration of 0.8 ± 0.1 mmol/L per application was observed. The remaining pigs (7/10) with shockable arrhythmias underwent further defibrillation attempts in accordance with the guidelines.

Table 3. Rhythm conversation procedure.

Group	Spontaneous Rhythm Conversion		Secondary Cardioplegia		Electric Defibrillation	
	With Reperfusion (n)	Sustained (n)	Required (n)	Attempts Median (min, max)	Required (n)	No. of Shocks Median (min, max)
CARL	4/10	2/4	8/10	2 (1,2)	7/10	5 (1,8)
ECPR	0/10	0/0	4/10	1 (1,1)	10/10	8 (3,14)

To further evaluate the SC effect beyond CARL therapy, we also evaluated it in n = 4 animals in the ECPR group suffering from refractory VF despite several defibrillations (range 9–13 attempts) at different time points. SC was applied in n = 2 animals during the pre-hospital phase with a MAP of 33 and 36 mmHg, respectively, during administration, another n = 2 animals received SC during the in-hospital phase with a MAP of 58 and 87 mmHg during administration. All animals (4/4) showed a transient asystole followed by persistent sinus rhythm until the end of the observation period. No further cardiac arrhythmias were observed in those animals.

3.4.2. Number of Defibrillations

In the ECPR group, a median of 8 (range 3–14) electrical defibrillation attempts were necessary to achieve sustained rhythm stability, compared to 5 (range 1–8) attempts in the CARL group (see Figure 5). This difference was statistically significant ($p < 0.01$) and remained significant even when considering the treatment attempts with secondary cardioplegia (median CARL 6 (range 1–10), ECPR 8.5 (range 3–15), $p < 0.05$).

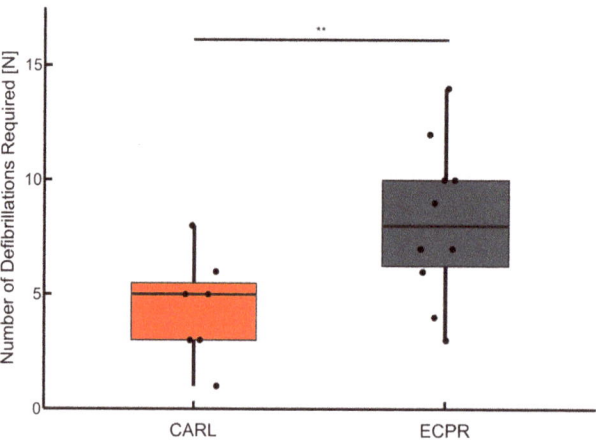

Figure 5. Number of shocks (200 J) delivered. Each point represents the number of electric defibrillations required per animal for sustained rhythm conversion to sinus rhythm (** $p < 0.01$).

3.4.3. Cardiac Arrhythmias

Wide QRS complex bradycardias were observed in both groups after initial VF conversion (see Table 4). All bradycardias required therapeutic interventions, except for one animal in the ECPR group. Internal over-pacing at a rate of 100–120/min via the implanted pacemaker catheter was performed to maintain cardiac output.

Table 4. Cardiac arrhythmias during reperfusion.

Group	Bradyarrhythmia		Tachyarrhythmia	
	n	Therapy-Needed	n	Therapy-Needed
CARL	1/10	1/1	1/10	1/1
ECPR	4*/10	3/4	2*/10	1/2

* One animal exhibited bradyarrhythmia and tachyarrhythmia.

Tachycardiac arrhythmias were documented in two animals, including a bigeminus rhythm in one pig and pulseless ventricular tachycardia (pVT) in two others. Defibrillation was performed for pVT, and the bigeminus rhythm appeared to be self-limiting.

All documented cardiac arrythmias in the ECPR group occurred before the application of secondary cardioplegia. We identified no significant differences in potassium levels between animals with or without cardiac arrhythmias (arrhythmias: 5.22 ± 0.57 mmol/L, no arrhythmias: 5.17 ± 0.93, $p = 0.544$).

4. Discussion

ECPR has been gaining increasing acceptance in the treatment of refractory cardiac arrest. Prolonged low-flow as that accompanying conventional CPR prior to ECPR is known to worsen the neurologic outcome after CA [30]. More and more pre-hospital ECPR programs have been launched to minimise the duration of low-flow. Over the last few decades, a concept specialized in pre-hospital ECPR named CARL was developed. By recording and modifying the most important reperfusion parameters, clinicians aim to achieve the greatest possible reduction in reperfusion damage using CARL [16–18,25].

The purpose of the present study was to investigate whether a pulsatile, high blood-flow approach is feasible when applying CARL therapy, and whether any effects on rhythm control appear in a reality-based porcine model of prolonged CPR. The rationale of this approach and effects on heart rhythm control compared to conventional ECPR are discussed below.

4.1. High Pressure and Pulsatile, High-Flow Reperfusion

It is well known that the cerebral no-reflow phenomenon is exacerbated in proportion to the duration of ischaemia, and that it can be reversed by raising reperfusion pressure [31,32]. Clinical studies have shown that high MAP and CPP are, together with high systolic blood pressure, associated with lower mortality and better neurological outcomes [33–35]. Moreover, dysfunctional cerebral autoregulation is often observed after CA, necessitating higher perfusion pressures to ensure adequate perfusion of all regions in the central nervous system [36]. Due to the unavailability of pre-hospital blood pressure monitoring on ECC, we observed relevant hypotension in the ECPR group. As shown in a systematic review by Bhate et al., the presence of hypotensive phases after ROSC is associated with increased mortality [35]. We detected no hypotensive phases in our CARL group, a finding that again highlights the importance of monitoring key reperfusion parameters including blood pressure as early as possible.

Higher perfusion pressures are also achievable especially on ECC by increasing blood flow. Together with pulsatile blood flow, beneficial effects on survival and neurological outcome have been described in conjunction with CARL therapy before [18]. In the present study we observed that even when using comparatively small cannulas, the pulsatility generated by the CARL controller can be maintained in the vascular system downstream in the smaller blood vessels. Despite the extreme haemoconcentration that occurs after prolonged cardiac arrest, we found this pulsatile, high-flow, high-pressure approach to be feasible.

Haemoconcentration occurs as a result of blood plasma redistributed from the intravascular to the extravascular space due to failure of the energy-dependent sodium–potassium pump combined with enhanced cell permeability and increased intracellular osmolarity [37].

Beyond that, the compression of upper abdominal organs during chest compression contributes to the rise in the haemoglobin concentration. However, haemoconcentration and accompanying increased blood viscosity have been proven to trigger impaired cerebral circulation after ischaemia [32]. As our experiments showed, a haemoconcentrated state raises the fluid demand, which was adequately fulfilled in the CARL group. More research is needed to determine whether additional haemodilution beyond baseline values reveals beneficial effects regarding cerebral blood flow and functional outcome in conjunction with CARL therapy.

4.2. Impact on Rhythm Conversion and Cardiac Arrhythmias

As mentioned above, CARL therapy takes a modified approach for rhythm conversion in shockable arrhythmias via established cardiac surgery techniques [16,19,20]. The combination of lidocaine–magnesium-induced and potassium-induced cardiac standstill led to sustained rhythm conversion in 30% of all animals not requiring any electrical defibrillation, encouraging evidence in light of the potential harmful side effects of defibrillations such as electrical and contractile dysfunction [38–40]. Even when cardioplegia failed, thus requiring defibrillation, we observed that the number of defibrillations required was significantly reduced using CARL. There is ample evidence of the positive effects of high MAP and CPP on the efficacy of defibrillation and survival [33,34]. It is thus likely that the effects we observed can be at least partially attributed to the CARL group's higher CPP. In their study, Lee et al. also demonstrated a decrease in the number of countershocks required after potassium-induced cardiac standstill. Interestingly, their groups' MAP and CPP were similar, suggesting a CPP-independent effect [41]. Furthermore, defibrillation and rhythm stability may be facilitated by a more rapid recovery of the acid–base balance as well as the more physiologic oxygen and carbon dioxide partial pressures during CARL therapy.

As our findings suggest, potassium-induced secondary cardioplegia is effective regardless of CARL therapy, as indicated by its efficacy in four ECPR-group animals. As shown in two animals, SC's anti-arrhythmic effect remains intact even at lower perfusion pressures close to those at the end of the ALS phase, which raises the question of SC's role and effectiveness in conventional CPR. Lee et al. demonstrated beneficial effects of potassium and potassium–lidocaine-induced cardiac standstill even in conventional CPR without employing ECC [41,42]. In their study, animals receiving potassium required fewer countershocks, smaller doses of adrenaline, and their CPR was of shorter duration [41]. However, it is well known that inducing cardiac standstill in the clinical routine, regardless of how it is implemented, should only be performed when stable circulatory support is available via extracorporeal circulation.

It should also be noted that repeated applications of secondary cardioplegia are known to raise the concentration of serum potassium. This may become relevant when considering hyperkalaemia as an accompanying consequence or even possible cause of CA [6]. In this situation, the additional administration of potassium could be associated with an increase in potentially harmful bradyarrhythmias and, thus, worsen CA outcome. We observed no increase in bradyarrhythmias in our study despite repeated applications of potassium-induced cardioplegia. On the contrary, applying CARL therapy, we detected a decrease in cardiac arrhythmias. Moreover, employing a point-of-care blood gas analyser or the CARL controller with its integrated arterial blood gas analyser enables patient-specific therapy due to the immediate availability of electrolyte measurements. This in turn enables diagnosis of pre-existing hyperkalaemia and immediate treatment after the onset of reperfusion. Potassium-induced secondary cardioplegia should be avoided in this case.

4.3. Limitations

Our study has several limitations. In our model, CA was induced electrically and not by any organic pathology. Moreover, to prevent premature ROSC, no amiodarone and no defibrillations were allowed during conventional CPR.

For logistical reasons, as we were unable to extend the observation period, the ECC phase, especially, turned out to be rather short. Longer observation periods are obviously needed to assess long-term cardiac effects. Furthermore, we only investigated myocardial factors in this study, whereas the limitation of neurological damage needs to be investigated in further studies.

Moreover, cardiac IRI occurs as a result of multiple mechanisms impacting rhythm conversion and provoking cardiac arrhythmias. Most of these mechanisms, such as inflammatory response or microcirculatory deficits, were not considered in this study; although, it is well known that they play a crucial role in the development of cardiac IRI.

5. Conclusions

Our results indicate that despite the dramatically excessive haemoconcentration that occurs during cardiac arrest, CARL therapy makes high-pressure, pulsatile, high-flow reperfusion feasible. Life-threatening hypotension can be prevented during the pre-hospital phase of extracorporeal resuscitation by applying CARL. Moreover, controlling the heart rhythm via CARL reperfusion proved to be effective by minimizing defibrillation attempts and cardiac arrhythmias. Even spontaneous rhythm conversions were observed during CARL therapy. This suggests CARL therapy's potential benefit in alleviating refractory OHCA, thus improving the outcomes of patients undergoing ECPR.

Author Contributions: Conceptualization, S.J.B., G.T., J.H., C.S., P.G. and D.D.; methodology, G.T., C.B., S.J.B., J.H., C.S., P.G. and D.D.; formal analysis, S.J.B. and J.-S.P.; investigation S.J.B., J.-S.P., J.H., D.D., C.S., P.G., C.B. and G.T.; writing—original draft preparation, S.J.B.; writing—review and editing, S.J.B., J.-S.P., J.H., D.D., C.S., P.G., C.B., G.T. and F.B.; visualization, S.J.B.; supervision, F.B., G.T. and C.B. All authors have read and agreed to the published version of the manuscript.

Funding: The authors received support in form of material loans for the experiments by Resuscitec GmbH, Germany (CARL System).

Institutional Review Board Statement: The animal study protocol was approved by the local animal welfare committee of the city of Freiburg, Germany, Regierungspräsidium Freiburg (G-15/148 and date of approval: 21 January 2016).

Informed Consent Statement: Not applicable.

Acknowledgments: We thank Patric Diel, Marcia Hohoff, Fabienne Frensch, Rita Fastenau and Tabea Neubert for their technical support during the animal experiments.

Conflicts of Interest: F.B., C.B. and G.T. are shareholders in Resuscitec GmbH, Freiburg, Germany, which is a start-up company of the University Medical Centre Freiburg. J.-S.P., S.J.B., P.G., D.D. and C.S. are part-time employees of Resuscitec GmbH, Freiburg, Germany. The remaining authors have disclosed that they have no conflicts of interest to declare.

References

- Atwood, C.; Eisenberg, M.S.; Herlitz, J.; Rea, T.D. Incidence of EMS-Treated out-of-Hospital Cardiac Arrest in Europe. *Resuscitation* **2005**, *67*, 75–80. [CrossRef] [PubMed]
- Gräsner, J.-T.; Lefering, R.; Koster, R.W.; Masterson, S.; Böttiger, B.W.; Herlitz, J.; Wnent, J.; Tjelmeland, I.B.M.; Ortiz, F.R.; Maurer, H.; et al. EuReCa ONE-27 Nations, ONE Europe, ONE Registry: A Prospective One Month Analysis of out-of-Hospital Cardiac Arrest Outcomes in 27 Countries in Europe. *Resuscitation* **2016**, *105*, 188–195. [CrossRef] [PubMed]
- Fischer, M.; Wnent, J.; Gräsner, J.-T.; Seewald, S.; Brenner, S.; Bein, B.; Ristau, P.; Bohn, A. Die teilnehmenden Rettungsdienste am Deut- schen Reanimationsregister Öffentlicher Jahresbericht 2020 Des Deutschen Reanimationsregisters: Außerklinische Reanimation 2020. 2020. Available online: https://www.reanimationsregister.de/downloads (accessed on 12 January 2022).
- Gräsner, J.-T.; Wnent, J.; Herlitz, J.; Perkins, G.D.; Lefering, R.; Tjelmeland, I.; Koster, R.W.; Masterson, S.; Rossell-Ortiz, F.; Maurer, H.; et al. Survival after Out-of-Hospital Cardiac Arrest in Europe—Results of the EuReCa TWO Study. *Resuscitation* **2020**, *148*, 218–226. [CrossRef] [PubMed]
- Reynolds, J.C.; Frisch, A.; Rittenberger, J.C.; Callaway, C.W. Duration of Resuscitation Efforts and Functional Outcome after Out-of-Hospital Cardiac Arrest: When Should We Change to Novel Therapies? *Circulation* **2013**, *128*, 2488–2494. [CrossRef] [PubMed]

6. Soar, J.; Böttiger, B.W.; Carli, P.; Couper, K.; Deakin, C.D.; Djärv, T.; Lott, C.; Olasveengen, T.; Paal, P.; Pellis, T.; et al. European Resuscitation Council Guidelines 2021: Adult Advanced Life Support. *Resuscitation* **2021**, *161*, 115–151. [CrossRef] [PubMed]
7. Yannopoulos, D.; Bartos, J.; Raveendran, G.; Walser, E.; Connett, J.; Murray, T.A.; Collins, G.; Zhang, L.; Kalra, R.; Kosmopoulos, M.; et al. Advanced Reperfusion Strategies for Patients with Out-of-Hospital Cardiac Arrest and Refractory Ventricular Fibrillation (ARREST): A Phase 2, Single Centre, Open-Label, Randomised Controlled Trial. *Lancet* **2020**, *396*, 1807–1816. [CrossRef]
8. Abrams, D.; MacLaren, G.; Lorusso, R.; Price, S.; Yannopoulos, D.; Vercaemst, L.; Bělohlávek, J.; Taccone, F.S.; Aissaoui, N.; Shekar, K.; et al. Extracorporeal Cardiopulmonary Resuscitation in Adults: Evidence and Implications. *Intensive Care Med.* **2021**, *48*, 1–15. [CrossRef]
9. Daniele, S.G.; Trummer, G.; Hossmann, K.A.; Vrselja, Z.; Benk, C.; Gobeske, K.T.; Damjanovic, D.; Andrijevic, D.; Pooth, J.-S.; Dellal, D.; et al. Brain Vulnerability and Viability after Ischaemia. *Nat. Rev. Neurosci.* **2021**, *22*, 553–572. [CrossRef]
10. Kalogeris, T.; Baines, C.P.; Krenz, M.; Korthuis, R.J. Cell Biology of Ischemia/Reperfusion Injury. In *International Review of Cell and Molecular Biology*; Elsevier: Amsterdam, The Netherlands, 2012; Volume 298, pp. 229–317.
11. Bingol Tanriverdi, T.; Patmano, G.; Bozkurt, F.T.; Kaya, B.C.; Tercan, M. Prognostic Value of C-reactive Protein to Albumin Ratio in Patients Resuscitated from Out-of-hospital Cardiac Arrest. *Int. J. Clin. Pract.* **2021**, *75*, e14227. [CrossRef]
12. Kern, K.B.; Garewal, H.S.; Sanders, A.B.; Janas, W.; Nelson, J.; Sloan, D.; Tacker, W.A.; Ewy, G.A. Depletion of Myocardial Adenosine Triphosphate during Prolonged Untreated Ventricular Fibrillation: Effect on Defibrillation Success. *Resuscitation* **1990**, *20*, 221–229. [CrossRef]
13. Kusuoka, H.; Chacko, V.P.; Marban, E. Myocardial Energetics during Ventricular Fibrillation Investigated by Magnetization Transfer Nuclear Magnetic Resonance Spectroscopy. *Circ. Res.* **1992**, *71*, 1111–1122. [CrossRef] [PubMed]
14. Weber, C.; Deppe, A.-C.; Sabashnikov, A.; Slottosch, I.; Kuhn, E.; Eghbalzadeh, K.; Scherner, M.; Choi, Y.-H.; Madershahian, N.; Wahlers, T. Left Ventricular Thrombus Formation in Patients Undergoing Femoral Veno-Arterial Extracorporeal Membrane Oxygenation. *Perfusion* **2018**, *33*, 283–288. [CrossRef] [PubMed]
15. Reis, R.L.; Cohn, L.H.; Morrow, A.G. Effects of Induced Ventricular Fibrillation on Ventricular Performance and Cardiac Metabolism. *Circulation* **1967**, *35*, I-234. [CrossRef] [PubMed]
16. Beyersdorf, F.; Trummer, G.; Benk, C.; Pooth, J.-S. Application of Cardiac Surgery Techniques to Improve the Results of Cardiopulmonary Resuscitation after Cardiac Arrest: Controlled Automated Reperfusion of the Whole Body. *JTCVS Open* **2021**, S2666273621003569. [CrossRef]
17. Taunyane, I.C.; Benk, C.; Beyersdorf, F.; Foerster, K.; Cristina Schmitz, H.; Wittmann, K.; Mader, I.; Doostkam, S.; Heilmann, C.; Trummer, G. Preserved Brain Morphology after Controlled Automated Reperfusion of the Whole Body Following Normothermic Circulatory Arrest Time of up to 20 Minutes. *Eur. J. Cardiothorac. Surg.* **2016**, *50*, 1025–1034. [CrossRef]
18. Kreibich, M.; Trummer, G.; Beyersdorf, F.; Scherer, C.; Förster, K.; Taunyane, I.; Benk, C. Improved Outcome in an Animal Model of Prolonged Cardiac Arrest Through Pulsatile High Pressure Controlled Automated Reperfusion of the Whole Body: Animal Model of Prolonged Ca through Pulsatile High Pressure Carl. *Artif. Organs* **2018**, *42*, 992–1000. [CrossRef]
19. Watanabe, G.; Yashiki, N.; Tomita, S.; Yamaguchi, S. Potassium-Induced Cardiac Resetting Technique for Persistent Ventricular Tachycardia and Fibrillation After Aortic Declamping. *Ann. Thorac. Surg.* **2011**, *91*, 619–620. [CrossRef]
20. Almdahl, S.M.; Damstuen, J.; Eide, M.; Mølstad, P.; Halvorsen, P.; Veel, T. Potassium-Induced Conversion of Ventricular Fibrillation after Aortic Declamping. *Interact. CardioVascular Thorac. Surg.* **2013**, *16*, 143–150. [CrossRef]
21. Wollborn, J.; Ruetten, E.; Schlueter, B.; Haberstroh, J.; Goebel, U.; Schick, M.A. Standardized Model of Porcine Resuscitation Using a Custom-Made Resuscitation Board Results in Optimal Hemodynamic Management. *Am. J. Emerg. Med.* **2018**, *36*, 1738–1744 [CrossRef]
22. Otlewski, M.P.; Geddes, L.A.; Pargett, M.; Babbs, C.F. Methods for Calculating Coronary Perfusion Pressure During CPR. *Cardiovasc. Eng.* **2009**, *9*, 98–103. [CrossRef]
23. Olasveengen, T.M.; Semeraro, F.; Ristagno, G.; Castren, M.; Handley, A.; Kuzovlev, A.; Monsieurs, K.G.; Raffay, V.; Smyth, M.; Soar, J.; et al. European Resuscitation Council Guidelines 2021: Basic Life Support. *Resuscitation* **2021**, *161*, 98–114. [CrossRef] [PubMed]
24. Nolan, J.P.; Sandroni, C.; Böttiger, B.W.; Cariou, A.; Cronberg, T.; Friberg, H.; Genbrugge, C.; Haywood, K.; Lilja, G.; Moulaert, V.R.M.; et al. European Resuscitation Council and European Society of Intensive Care Medicine Guidelines 2021: Post-Resuscitation Care. *Resuscitation* **2021**, *161*, 220–269. [CrossRef] [PubMed]
25. Trummer, G.; Benk, C.; Beyersdorf, F. Controlled Automated Reperfusion of the Whole Body after Cardiac Arrest. *J. Thorac. Dis.* **2019**, *11*, S1464–S1470. [CrossRef] [PubMed]
26. R Core Team. *R: A Language and Environment for Statistical Computing*; R Foundation for Statistical Computing: Vienna, Austria, 2017.
27. Hadley Wickham. *Ggplot2: Elegant Graphics for Data Analysis*; Springer: New York, NY, USA, 2009; ISBN 978-0-387-98140-6.
28. Bates, D.; Mächler, M.; Bolker, B.; Walker, S. Fitting Linear Mixed-Effects Models Using Lme4. *J. Stat. Soft.* **2015**, *67*, 1–48 [CrossRef]
29. Kuznetsova, A.; Brockhoff, P.B.; Christensen, R.H.B. LmerTest Package: Tests in Linear Mixed Effects Models. *J. Stat. Soft.* **2017**, *82*, 1–26. [CrossRef]
30. Wengenmayer, T.; Rombach, S.; Ramshorn, F.; Biever, P.; Bode, C.; Duerschmied, D.; Staudacher, D.L. Influence of Low-Flow Time on Survival after Extracorporeal Cardiopulmonary Resuscitation (ECPR). *Crit. Care* **2017**, *21*, 157. [CrossRef]

31. Fischer, E.G.; Ames, A.; Lorenzo, A.V. Cerebral Blood Flow Immediately Following Brief Circulatory Stasis. *Stroke* **1979**, *10*, 423–427. [CrossRef]
32. Fischer, E.G.; Ames, A. Studies on Mechanisms of Impairment of Cerebral Circulation Following Ischemia: Effect of Hemodilution and Perfusion Pressure. *Stroke* **1972**, *3*, 538–542. [CrossRef]
33. Reynolds, J.C.; Salcido, D.D.; Menegazzi, J.J. Conceptual Models of Coronary Perfusion Pressure and Their Relationship to Defibrillation Success in a Porcine Model of Prolonged Out-of-Hospital Cardiac Arrest. *Resuscitation* **2012**, *83*, 900–906. [CrossRef]
34. Maryam, Y.; Sutton, R.M.; Friess, S.H.; Bratinov, G.; Bhalala, U.; Kilbaugh, T.J.; Lampe, J.; Nadkarni, V.M.; Becker, L.B.; Berg, R.A. Blood Pressure and Coronary Perfusion Pressure Targeted Cardiopulmonary Resuscitation Improves 24-Hour Survival from Ventricular Fibrillation Cardiac Arrest. *Crit. Care Med.* **2016**, *44*, e1111–e1117.
35. Bhate, T.D.; McDonald, B.; Sekhon, M.S.; Griesdale, D.E.G. Association between Blood Pressure and Outcomes in Patients after Cardiac Arrest: A Systematic Review. *Resuscitation* **2015**, *97*, 1–6. [CrossRef] [PubMed]
36. Sundgreen, C.; Larsen, F.S.; Herzog, T.M.; Knudsen, G.M.; Boesgaard, S.; Aldershvile, J. Autoregulation of Cerebral Blood Flow in Patients Resuscitated From Cardiac Arrest. *Stroke* **2001**, *32*, 128–132. [CrossRef] [PubMed]
37. Jehle, D.; Fiorello, A.B.; Brader, E.; Cottington, E.; Kozak, R.J. Hemoconcentration during Cardiac Arrest and CPR. *Am. J. Emerg. Med.* **1994**, *12*, 524–526. [CrossRef]
38. Kodama, I.; Shibata, N.; Sakuma, I.; Mitsui, K.; Iida, M.; Suzuki, R.; Fukui, Y.; Hosoda, S.; Toyama, J. Aftereffects of High-Intensity DC Stimulation on the Electromechanical Performance of Ventricular Muscle. *Am. J. Physiol. Heart Circ. Physiol.* **1994**, *267*, H248–H258. [CrossRef] [PubMed]
39. Al-Khadra, A.; Nikolski, V.; Efimov, I.R. The Role of Electroporation in Defibrillation. *Circ. Res.* **2000**, *87*, 797–804. [CrossRef]
40. Efimov, I.; Ripplinger, C.M. Virtual Electrode Hypothesis of Defibrillation. *Heart Rhythm.* **2006**, *3*, 1100–1102. [CrossRef]
41. Lee, H.Y.; Lee, B.K.; Jeung, K.W.; Lee, S.M.; Jung, Y.H.; Lee, G.S.; Heo, T.; Min, Y.I. Potassium Induced Cardiac Standstill during Conventional Cardiopulmonary Resuscitation in a Pig Model of Prolonged Ventricular Fibrillation Cardiac Arrest: A Feasibility Study. *Resuscitation* **2013**, *84*, 378–383. [CrossRef]
42. Kook Lee, B.; Joon Lee, S.; Woon Jeung, K.; Youn Lee, H.; Jeong, I.S.; Lim, V.; Hun Jung, Y.; Heo, T.; Il Min, Y. Effects of Potassium/Lidocaine-induced Cardiac Standstill During Cardiopulmonary Resuscitation in a Pig Model of Prolonged Ventricular Fibrillation. *Acad. Emerg. Med.* **2014**, *21*, 392–400. [CrossRef]

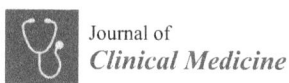

Article

The Impact of Withdrawn vs. Agitated Relatives during Resuscitation on Team Workload: A Single-Center Randomised Simulation-Based Study

Timur Sellmann [1,2,†], Andrea Oendorf [3,4,†], Dietmar Wetzchewald [3], Heidrun Schwager [3], Serge Christian Thal [2,5] and Stephan Marsch [6,*]

1. Department of Anaesthesiology and Intensive Care Medicine, Bethesda Hospital, 47053 Duisburg, Germany; t.sellmann@bethesda.de
2. Department of Anaesthesiology 1, Witten/Herdecke University, 58455 Witten, Germany; serge.thal@uni-wh.de
3. Institute of Emergency Medicine, 59755 Arnsberg, Germany; andrea.oendorf@rub.de (A.O.); d.wetzchewald@aim-arnsberg.de (D.W.); h.schwager@aim-arnsberg.de (H.S.)
4. Department of Internal Medicine, Gertrudis Hospital, 45701 Herten, Germany
5. Department of Anaesthesiology, Helios University Hospital, 42283 Wuppertal, Germany
6. Department of Intensive Care, University Hospital, 4031 Basel, Switzerland
* Correspondence: stephan.marsch@usb.ch; Fax: +41-612-655-300
† These authors contributed equally to this work.

Abstract: Background: Guidelines recommend that relatives be present during cardiopulmonary resuscitation (CPR). This randomised trial investigated the effects of two different behaviour patterns of relatives on rescuers' perceived stress and quality of CPR. Material and methods: Teams of three to four physicians were randomised to perform CPR in the presence of no relatives (control group), a withdrawn relative, or an agitated relative, played by actors according to a scripted role, and to three different models of leadership (randomly determined by the team or tutor or left open). The scenarios were video-recorded. Hands-on time was primary, and the secondary outcomes comprised compliance to CPR algorithms, perceived workload, and the influence of leadership. Results: 1229 physicians randomised to 366 teams took part. The presence of a relative did not affect hands-on time (91% [87–93] vs. 92% [88–94] for "withdrawn" and 92 [88–93] for "agitated" relatives; $p = 0.15$). The teams interacted significantly less with a "withdrawn" than with an "agitated" relative (11 [7–16]% vs. 23 [15–30]% of the time spent for resuscitation, $p < 0.01$). The teams confronted with an "agitated" relative showed more unsafe defibrillations, higher ventilation rates, and a delay in starting CPR (all $p < 0.05$ vs. control). The presence of a relative increased frustration, effort, and perceived temporal demands (all <0.05 compared to control); in addition, an "agitated" relative increased mental demands and total task load (both $p < 0.05$ compared to "withdrawn" and control group). The type of leadership condition did not show any effects. Conclusions: Interaction with a relative accounted for up to 25% of resuscitation time. Whereas the presence of a relative *per se* increased the task load in different domains, only the presence of an "agitated" relative had a marginal detrimental effect on CPR quality (GERMAN study registers number DRKS00024761).

Keywords: cardiopulmonary resuscitation; team performance; randomised controlled trial; family presence; simulation; NASA task load index

Citation: Sellmann, T.; Oendorf, A.; Wetzchewald, D.; Schwager, H.; Thal, S.C.; Marsch, S. The Impact of Withdrawn vs. Agitated Relatives during Resuscitation on Team Workload: A Single-Center Randomised Simulation-Based Study. *J. Clin. Med.* **2022**, *11*, 3163. https://doi.org/10.3390/jcm11113163

Academic Editor: Giorgio Costantino

Received: 19 April 2022
Accepted: 30 May 2022
Published: 2 June 2022

Publisher's Note: MDPI stays neutral with regard to jurisdictional claims in published maps and institutional affiliations.

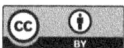

Copyright: © 2022 by the authors. Licensee MDPI, Basel, Switzerland. This article is an open access article distributed under the terms and conditions of the Creative Commons Attribution (CC BY) license (https://creativecommons.org/licenses/by/4.0/).

1. Introduction

Discussing the presence of a relative during cardiopulmonary resuscitation (CPR) dates back to the 1980s and has been a controversial issue since [1–4]. Current guidelines recommend that resuscitation teams should offer family members of cardiac arrest (CA) patients the opportunity to be present during the resuscitation attempt in cases where this opportunity can be provided safely, and a member of the team can be allocated to provide support to the patient's family [5–7]. Data on the effects of the different behaviour patterns of relatives (e.g., from withdrawn to agitated) on the quality of CPR and on the psychological impact on rescuers are sparse [8], and this trial aims at closing this gap.

Resuscitation per se is a stressful task [9]. Studies addressing the additional stress inflicted by family presence showed conflicting results covering an extent of no perceived additional strain to a sensed significant impairment of own activity due to family presence [1,4,10–13]. Regarding the quality of CPR, real-life studies and simulations have repeatedly shown high variability in CPR provision and sub-optimal compliance with guideline algorithms [14–18], but until now, however, no data reporting negative effects on patient outcomes have been published from institutions allowing relatives to be present during resuscitation [19,20]. Moreover, the presence of a "normally" behaving "unobtrusive" relative during simulated CA increased task load and frustration but did not impair the quality of CPR [13]. However, not all relatives can be expected to behave "normally" during the CPR of a loved one. Overtly aggressive or disruptive relatives or relatives who are withdrawn may well have a different impact on rescuers' stress levels and the quality of CPR. It is mostly unknown if leadership (if any) may alleviate any impact of added strain caused by the presence of a relative.

Analysing the effect of a family member's presence on the quality of resuscitation in a randomised controlled trial and under controlled conditions is quite challenging in reality, as the causes of cardiac arrest may vary from case to case. Simulations allow team performance to be studied in a realistic and standardised way [21], both overall and in individual subtasks, and performance metrics in simulation-based trials show a high level of consistency with resuscitation results. The object of our randomised, controlled, and prospective study was, therefore, to analyse the impact of family attendance with a withdrawn or agitated relative on the rescuer's felt task burden as well as to assess leadership designation in this setting on the quality of CPR.

2. Materials and Methods

2.1. Participants

The Working Group on Intensive Care Medicine, Arnsberg, Germany (http://www.aim-arnsberg.de, assessed on 18 April 2022), arranges postgraduate educational, medical courses for physicians from Germany and German-speaking countries, mainly residents in the 2nd to 3rd year in internal medicine, Anaesthesiology, or surgery, who work in emergency and intensive care medicine. Attendees were offered participation in optional simulator-based training and were notified that the simulations would be video-recorded for scientific purposes. Physicians not willing to participate were offered identical workshops, but these were not filmed. The study was conducted according to the rules of the Declaration of Helsinki and authorised by the Ethics Committee of the Medical Association of Westphalia-Lippe (amendment to 2016-558-f-N, dated 6 September 2017), which waived the requirement to provide informed consent. The trial was registered with the German Clinical Trials Registry (www.drks.de, assessed on 18 April 2022; DRKS00024761) and is reported here according to the extensions of the CONSORT statements of the Reporting Guidelines for Health Care Simulation Research [22].

2.2. Study Design

This was a prospective, randomised, single-blind trial. The randomisations were carried out using computer-generated numbers. The participants were randomly assigned to teams of three to five physicians. The teams were then randomly allocated to perform CPR under three conditions: (1) no relative present, (2) "withdrawn" relative present, and (3) agitated relative present. A detailed description of the role can be found in the Appendix. In addition, the teams were randomly assigned so that either no leader was designated (no intervention), the team itself designated a leader (the rescue team received the mission of designating leadership before the scenario began), or the tutor designated a leader (leadership was attributed to a haphazardly selected group member by the tutor before the start of the scenario). The nominated leaders wore a coloured waistcoat and could thus be clearly recognised from the recordings. Aside from the attendance of a relative and allocated leadership, the requirements and conditions were the same for the teams.

2.3. Simulator and Scenario

The Ambu Man Wireless manikin (Ambu GmbH, Bad Nauheim, Germany) was employed. Attendants underwent a standardised implementation of the workshop, the manikin and the available CPR equipment. All members of the team were then briefed that their part during the subsequent setting was either that of an in- or out-of-hospital rescue team called to an unwitnessed cardiac arrest. The patient found (manikin) was pulseless, apnoeic, and had a Glasgow Coma Score of 3 (unresponsive, comatose). Once attached, ventricular fibrillation could be monitored on the defibrillator. The investigation period began when the first participant entered the room and stopped after the third defibrillation. The resuscitation manikins were served by trained tutors who were briefed not to perform any interventions until the investigation period ended.

2.4. Family Member Presence

A total of four actors were instructed to display two types of the patient's relatives following scripted roles (see Appendix A). The attributes included quiet crying, mourning, and quiet observation for the "withdrawn" relative and loud crying or mourning as well as walking around the room worried and upset for the "agitated" relative. In order to ensure consistent quality in the course of the study, the video recordings were repeatedly discussed with all of the actors in the presence of an auditor. The teams assigned to the "relatives" groups met the relative at the scene of the incident beside the patient. The relative reported that the patient had collapsed in his presence and was unresponsive.

2.5. NASA Task Load Index

Subsequent to concluding the simulation, attendants were invited to fill out the NASA Task load index (NASA-TLX). The NASA-TLX was designed to evaluate the workload throughout or after a task. Six areas were rated after being assessed on visual analogue scales (0 to 100): Mental, Physical, and Time Demand, Frustration, Effort, and Own Performance [23]. It has been comprehensively ratified, is easily used and is comprehensively applied in various fields such as driving, teamwork, flying, and medicine [24,25].

2.6. Data Analysis

The data analysis was conducted by A.O., T.S. and S.M. using video recordings that were taken during the simulations. The starting point for the timing of all of the events was the first contact with the patient by one of the attendants.

2.7. Statistical Analysis

The primary outcome measure was the percentage of hands-on time, specified as the time of de facto chest compressions (CC), depicted as a fraction (in percent) of the total time available for CC. A power analysis adapted from pilot experiment data showed that it was necessary to study around 100 teams per study arm to identify a 10% difference between the groups in the primary outcome measure with a significance level of 0.05 (two-sided tested) and a power of 80%. Therefore, we determined to stop the trial once a minimum of 100 videotapes of adequate quality were available for each study arm. Due to organisational causes, the number of accessible video files of satisfactory quality could not be determined until the completion of the respective training course.

The secondary outcome measures involved the level of interaction with the relative, NASA TLX data, and compliance with different aspects of national and international guidelines on CPR. Additionally, the impact of the appointed leader was evaluated as a secondary outcome measure.

The complete data were scored on an intention-to-treat basis. The data are presented as medians [IQR (inter-quartile range)] unless otherwise reported. Statistical analysis was conducted using SPSS (version 25). Non-parametric ANOVA (Kruskal–Wallis test) was used for analysing the numerical data, subsequently followed by Mann–Whitney-U tests for independent samples where necessary. To obtain the estimates for differences between the medians and their approximate confidence intervals, the Hodges–Lehmann estimation was applied. The effect of leadership and the interactive term leadership × relative on outcomes was assessed using SPSS's general linear model procedure with leadership assignment and relative assignment (i.e., study group) as fixed factors. The chi-square test was used for testing categorical data. A $p < 0.05$ (two-tailed) was considered statistically significant.

3. Results

3.1. Participants

After allocation and follow-up, the data of 335 teams (113 control, 117 "agitated", and 105 "withdrawn") were analysed (CONSORT flow chart, Figure 1). The teams consisted of 3 [3–4] physicians with no significant difference ($p = 0.16$) between the study groups. Verbal interactions with the "withdrawn" relative took place during a total of 11 [7–16]% of the study time and with the "agitated" relative in 23 [15–30]% (Difference 11% 95% CI 8–13; $p < 0.01$). Leadership had no influence on the allocation of interaction time ($p = 0.54$).

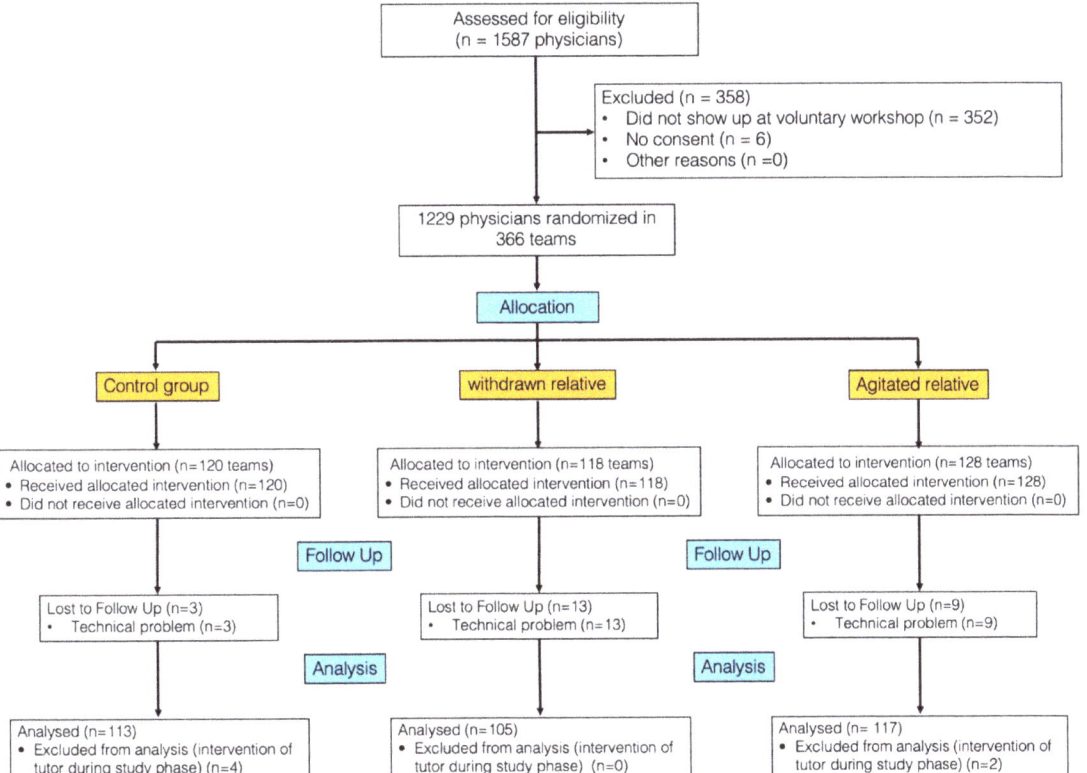

Figure 1. CONSORT flow chart.

3.2. Primary Outcomes

Hands-on time was 91% [87–93] in the control group, 92% [88–94] in the "withdrawn" relative group, and 92% [88–93] in the "agitated" relative group ($p = 0.15$; Figure 2). Assigned leadership positions (p = 0.65) had no effect on hands-on time, and there was no significant relationship between hands-on and absolute (p = 0.64) or percentage of time (p = 0.54) spent verbally interacting with the relative.

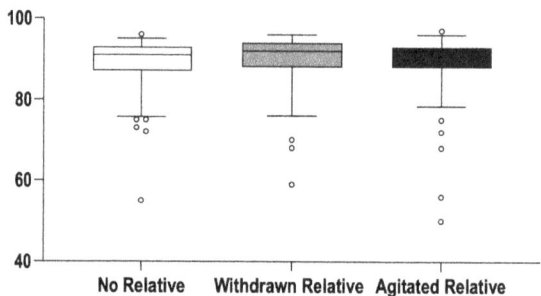

Figure 2. Primary outcome parameter ("Hands-on time"). Box and whisker plot of the percentage hands-on time. Boxes represent medians and interquartile range; whiskers delineate the 10th and 90th percentile, respectively; circles denote values outside the range from 10th to 90th percentile. There was no significant difference between the groups.

3.3. Secondary Outcomes

The secondary outcomes are presented in Table 1. There were no differences between the control group and the withdrawn relative group for any quality marker of CPR. By contrast, compared to the control group, we observed a later start of resuscitation, more unsafe defibrillations, and higher ventilation rates in the agitated relative group. Leadership assignments showed no significant effect on the quality of CPR.

Table 1. Secondary outcome parameters.

	No Relative (Control) (n = 113)	Withdrawn Relative (n = 105)	Agitated Relative (n = 117)
	Chest compression		
Time interval to CPR start (s)	14 [12–19]	17 [13–21]	18 [14–24] *
Start of CPR with CC (teams)	112/113	102/105	114/117
CC rates (strokes/min)	118 [112–125]	121 [112–126]	120 [111–127]
CC < 100/min (teams)	6/113	3/105	4/117
Change-overs per 2 min CPR (n)	1.4 [0.9–1.6]	1.5 [1.0–1.8]	1.3 [0.9–1.7]
	Defibrillation		
Time to 1st defibrillation (s)	75 [55–102]	71 [52–103]	71 [53–106]
Shock with adequate (≥150 J) energy (teams)	113/113	105/105	117/117
VF not recognised ≥ once (teams)	4/113	2/105	4/117
Unsafe defibrillation ≥ once (teams)	30/113	31/105	54/117 *
	Airway Management		
Advanced Airway Management (teams)	111/113	100/105	111/117
Time to Advanced Airway Management (s)	142 [95–194]	140 [111–205]	150 [105–214]
Advance airway position confirmed by capnography (teams)	89/111	85/100	90/111
Ventilation rate (b/min)	12 [4–10]	13 [8–19]	15 [10–20] *

Table 1. Cont.

	No Relative (Control) (n = 113)	Withdrawn Relative (n = 105)	Agitated Relative (n = 117)
	Medication		
Time to i.v. line insertion (s)	112 [77–146]	93 [66–132]	111 [70–163]
Epinephrine administered (teams)	80/113	68/105	71/111
Correct dose (1 mg) administered (teams)	80/80	68/68	71/71
2nd dose after 3–5 min (teams)	2/6	0/6	2/5
Amiodarone administered (teams)	79/113	75/105	79/117
Correct dose (300 mg) administered (teams)	79/79	75/75	79/79
Administered after epinephrine AND 3rd shock (teams)	41/79	41/75	43/117
False ACLS drug administered (teams)	0/113	0/105	0/117

CC = chest compressions; ACLS = advanced cardiac life support; Data are medians [IQR] or proportions. Unsafe defibrillation was defined as not explicitly announcing the release of an electroshock or defibrillating while the patient was touched by a team member or a relative. Incorrect ACLS drugs are all drugs administered other than epinephrine and amiodarone. * = $p < 0.05$ vs. Control group.

The NASA-TLX findings are summarised in Table 2 and Figure 3. Regardless of the relatives' behaviour, the presence of a family member was related to higher scores for the domains temporal demand, effort, and frustration. In addition, "agitated" relatives increased the overall perceived task load and mental demand. The effects of leadership are summarised in Table 3.

Table 2. NASA Task load findings– single components.

	No Relative (Control) (n = 407)	Withdrawn Relative (n = 403)	Agitated Relative (n = 419)
Task Load	63 [54–71]	64 [59–73]	69 [61–73] *,†
Mental demand	70 [50–80]	70 [55–85]	75 [60–85] *,†
Physical demand	50 [30–70]	55 [40–75]	55 [35–70]
Temporal demand	70 [55–80]	75 [60–90] *	80 [65–90] *
Performance	55 [35–70]	55 [35–70]	55 [35–70]
Effort	65 [50–75]	70 [55–75] *	75 [60–85] *,†
Frustration	50 [30–70]	60 [45–75] *	65 [45–80] *,†

Data are medians [IQR]. Ratings are based on visual analogue scales ranging from 0 (minimum) to 100 (maximum). * = $p < 0.05$ vs. Control group; † = $p < 0.05$ vs. Withdrawn family member presence group.

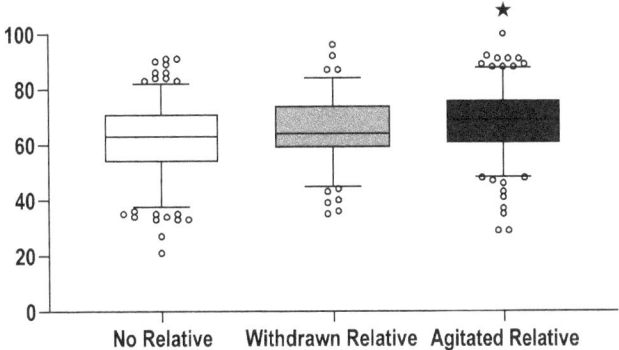

Figure 3. NASA TLX—weight average of components (according to [24]). Box and whisker plot of the perceived overall weighted task load. Boxes depict medians and interquartile range; whiskers outline the 10th and 90th percentile accordingly; circles denote values outside the range from 10th to 90th percentile. Ratings underlying the calculation of the task load are based on visual analogue

scales ranging from 0 (minimum) to 100 (maximum). ★ In the agitated relative group, the task load was significantly higher than in the control group ($p < 0.001$) and the withdrawn relative group ($p = 0.008$). The difference between control and withdrawn relative group was of borderline significance ($p = 0.058$).

Table 3. Effects of leadership assignment.

	Effect of Leadership Assignment	Effect of Relative Assignment	Interactive Term Leadership × Relative
	Chest compression		
Hands-on time	0.65	0.55	0.09
Time interval to start of CPR	0.46	**0.015**	0.92
Start of CPR with massage	0.99	0.99	0.92
Chest compression rates	0.70	0.34	0.83
Compression rates < 100/min	0.92	0.83	0.89
Change-overs per 2 min CPR	0.43	0.08	0.67
	Defibrillation		
Time to 1st defibrillation	0.38	0.52	**0.017**
VF not recognised ≥ once	0.99	0.99	0.98
Unsafe defibrillation ≥ once	0.31	**0.03**	0.62
	Airway Management		
Advanced Airway Management	0.99	0.99	0.82
Time to Advanced Airway Management	0.45	0.59	0.31
Capnography to confirm airway position	0.87	0.67	0.20
Ventilation rate	0.72	0.06	0.16
	Medication		
Time to i.v. line insertion	0.60	0.12	0.31
Time to epinephrine administration	0.46	0.12	0.60
Epinephrine administered	0.15	0.25	0.23
Amiodarone administered	0.46	0.79	0.36
Administered after epinephrine AND 3rd shock	0.25	0.82	0.94
	NASA Taskload		
Task Load	0.98	**0.001**	0.31
Mental demand	0.35	**0.007**	0.29
Physical demand	0.60	0.08	0.74
Temporal demand	0.48	**0.001**	0.30
Performance	0.20	0.65	**0.003**
Effort	0.46	**0.001**	0.30
Frustration	0.09	**0.001**	0.09

Data are p values obtained from SPSS's general linear model procedure with outcomes listed as dependent variables and leadership assignment and relative assignment (i.e., study group) as fixed factors. Unsafe defibrillation was defined as not explicitly announcing the release of an electroshock or defibrillating while the patient was touched by a team member or a relative. The significant interactive term for "time to 1st defibrillation" relates to swifter defibrillation in teams led by a tutor-designated leader in the agitated relative group; the significant interactive term for "performance" relates to higher ratings in teams without a designated leader in the agitated relative group. Bold: highlight the statistical significance.

4. Discussion

The present study demonstrates that regardless of their behaviour, the presence of family members during CPR increased rescuers' perceived task load in several domains. While withdrawn relatives had no impact on the quality of CPR, the presence of an agitated relative was associated with minor effects on the start of CPR and defibrillation patterns.

Although family member presence during CPR is still a discussed and controversial issue [1–4], there is not yet sufficient evidence of the impact of the intervention on the outcome for the patient or family, and concerns about a performance effect exist among professionals and family members [7]. Data for relatives, who are belligerent or hinder CPR activities, are even more scarce [1,10,11]. As far as we know, this is the first study to quantify the burden of a rescue team during CPR dealing with a withdrawn or agitated relative.

4.1. Primary Outcome

By reemphasising the importance of high-quality chest compressions in the current guidelines, we selected hands-on time as the primary outcome variable [5]. We were unable to demonstrate a negative effect on hands-on time, which is in line with prior findings [13]. Interestingly, none of the papers on relatives' presence during CPR quoted here commented on CPR quality itself [1–4,10]. Observational studies of facilities that allow relatives to be present during CPR found no obvious differences in patient outcomes after changing their protocols [20,26,27]. So far, there is only limited moderate to low-quality evidence suggesting that the presence of family members does not affect paediatric or adult CPR outcomes. The generalisation of these results beyond the out-of-hospital and emergency department setting is restricted owing to the lack of studies in alternative areas of health care [28]. A follow-up review appealing for further integration of relatives again describes no effects on CPR quality [29]. Although the controversial discussion regarding the presence of relatives during CPR may not be conclusively resolved, our present results show that at least CPR quality is not hampered and thus not a valid argument against their presence.

4.2. Secondary Outcomes

Honarmand and Crowley recently described a set of ACLS guideline deviations and their impact on outcomes from in-hospital cardiac arrest [30,31]. Selecting these deviations as secondary outcomes for the present trial, we observed no significant effect due to the presence of a "withdrawn" relative. For groups dealing with "agitated" relatives, statistically significant but clinically small effects were found for more unsafe defibrillations and higher ventilation rates as well as delays in starting CPR. These results are consistent with two previous trials where the attendance of a relative led to deferred defibrillation and fewer defibrillation attempts [11,13]. The observable slight delay in the onset of CPR could be a very subtle signal of initial distraction. However, as these findings are of little, if at all, medical relevance, we deduce that the physical attendance of a relative has no relevant negative influence on resuscitation quality.

4.3. NASA TLX

Emergency department personnel were reporting aggravated stress due to the attendance of relatives throughout resuscitation, and six out of twenty interviewees claimed to be hindered in their work [1,4]. In a post-incident survey offering options to answer 'true', 'false', or 'I don't know', no difference in stress scores was found in relation to the attendance of relatives in a large clinical study [10]. Confirming the results of a prior trial with "normally" behaving family presence [13], the present trial found that family presence is associated with increased perceived temporal and mental demands and frustration of the rescuers involved. This effect is even more pronounced if confronted with an "agitated" relative.

In contrast to previous studies [10], our participants were able to provide more specific answers using the Likert scale of the validated NASA TLX [24]. In addition, it is rather uncommon for medical professionals to describe themselves as "stressed" in a dichotomous way, as this admission could give the impression of being weak or not resilient [13].

4.4. Strengths and Limitations

The identical conditions for all teams at all times in a large sample, together with the detailed evaluation of a large number of CPR tasks and subtasks right from the beginning of the scenario, are strengths of our simulation study. In contrast, there are often mentioned limitations in the context of a simulation study, such as the lack of real patients and—in the present study—also real family members. Due to the study centre and location, teams in the trial presented here comprised only physicians, so the results cannot necessarily be transferred to other team compositions.

5. Conclusions

Regardless of their behaviour, relatives present during CPR of a next of kin increase the perceived task load of rescuers involved. The presence of withdrawn relatives has no effect on CPR quality, while the presence of agitated relatives results in minor deviations only. Thus, the CPR quality is not an argument against family presence per se. In the case of massive disruption by agitated family members, teams might consider removing them from the setting to increase patient safety.

Author Contributions: Conceptualization, T.S., A.O. and S.M.; data curation, T.S., A.O. and S.M.; formal analysis, T.S., A.O. and S.M.; funding acquisition, D.W. and H.S.; investigation, T.S. and A.O.; methodology, T.S., A.O. and S.M.; project administration, T.S., D.W., H.S. and S.M.; resources, H.S.; software, S.M.; supervision, T.S., D.W. and S.M.; validation, S.M.; visualization, S.M.; writing—original draft, T.S. and A.O.; writing—review & editing, A.O., S.C.T. and S.M. All authors have read and agreed to the published version of the manuscript.

Funding: This research received no external funding.

Institutional Review Board Statement: The study was conducted in accordance with the Declaration of Helsinki, and approved by the Ethics Committee of Aerztekammer Westfalen-Lippe (Amendment to 2016-558-f-N, dated from 6 September 2017).

Informed Consent Statement: Informed consent was obtained from all subjects involved in the study.

Data Availability Statement: Not applicable.

Conflicts of Interest: The authors declare no conflict of interest.

Appendix A

Scripts for the roles of relatives ("withdrawn" vs. "agitated") Adapted from [12].
Setting:
Emergency team is summoned to an in- or out-of-hospital unobserved cardiac arrest. A relative (actor) is present when the team arrives.
Attributes of the "withdrawn" relative:

- quiet crying/mourning
- quietly observes what is happening
- does not talk directly to the participants; except when asked by the doctors
- does not touch the patient or the participants
- asks to stay with the relative in case the participants want to expel him/her from the room

Attributes of the "agitated" relative:

- loud crying/mourning
- walks around the room worried and upset
- tries to touch the patient once or twice
- During resuscitation, asks the participants questions about the measures performed, the further procedure and the patient's chances of survival
- vehemently insists on staying with his relative in case the participants want to expel him from the room.

No details of the patient's medical history should be given by the actor!

References

1. Doyle, C.J.; Post, H.; Burney, R.E.; Maino, J.; Keefe, M.; Rhee, K.J. Family participation during resuscitation: An option. *Ann. Emerg. Med.* **1987**, *16*, 673–675. [CrossRef]
2. Barreto, M.D.S.; Peruzzo, H.E.; Garcia-Vivar, C.; Marcon, S.S. Family presence during cardiopulmonary resuscitation and invasive procedures: A meta-synthesis. *Rev. Esc. Enferm. USP* **2019**, *53*, e03435. [CrossRef]
3. Downar, J.; Kritek, P.A. Family Presence during Cardiac Resuscitation. *N. Engl. J. Med.* **2013**, *368*, 1060–1062.
4. Fernandes, A.P.; de Souza, C.C.; Geocze, L.; Batista Santos, V.; Guizilini, S.; Lopes Moreira, R.S. Experiences and opinions of health professionals in relation to the presence of the family during in-hospital cardiopulmonary resuscitation: An integrative review. *J. Nurs. Educ. Pract.* **2014**, *4*, 85–94. [CrossRef]
5. Perkins, G.D.; Graesner, J.T.; Semeraro, F.; Olasveengen, T.; Soar, J.; Lott, C.; Van de Voorde, P.; Madar, J.; Zideman, D.; Mentzelopoulos, S.; et al. European Resuscitation Council Guidelines 2021: Executive summary. *Resuscitation* **2021**, *161*, 1–60. [CrossRef]
6. Mentzelopoulos, S.D.; Couper, K.; Voorde, P.V.; Druwé, P.; Blom, M.; Perkins, G.D.; Lulic, I.; Djakow, J.; Raffay, V.; Lilja, G.; et al. European Resuscitation Council Guidelines 2021: Ethics of resuscitation and end of life decisions. *Resuscitation* **2021**, *161*, 408–432. [CrossRef]
7. Madar, J.; Roehr, C.C.; Ainsworth, S.; Ersdal, H.; Morley, C.; Rüdiger, M.; Skåre, C.; Szczapa, T.; Te Pas, A.; Trevisanuto, D.; et al. European Resuscitation Council Guidelines 2021: Newborn resuscitation and support of transition of infants at birth. *Resuscitation* **2021**, *161*, 291–326. [CrossRef]
8. Bjørshol, C.A.; Myklebust, H.; Nilsen, K.L.; Hoff, T.; Bjørkli, C.; Illguth, E.; Søreide, E.; Sunde, K. Effect of socioemotional stress on the quality of cardiopulmonary resuscitation during advanced life support in a randomized manikin study. *Crit. Care Med.* **2011**, *39*, 300–304. [CrossRef]
9. Hunziker, S.; Semmer, N.K.; Tschan, F.; Schuetz, P.; Mueller, B.; Marsch, S. Dynamics and association of different acute stress markers with performance during a simulated resuscitation. *Resuscitation* **2012**, *83*, 572–578. [CrossRef]
10. Jabre, P.; Belpomme, V.; Azoulay, E.; Jacob, L.; Bertrand, L.; Lapostolle, F.; Tazarourte, K.; Bouilleau, G.; Pinaud, V.; Broche, C.; et al. Family Presence during Cardiopulmonary Resuscitation. *N. Engl. J. Med.* **2013**, *368*, 1008–1018. [CrossRef]
11. Fernandez, R.; Compton, S.; Jones, K.A.; Velilla, M.A. The presence of a family witness impacts physician performance during simulated medical codes. *Crit. Care Med.* **2009**, *37*, 1956–1960. [CrossRef]
12. Sak-Dankosky, N.; Andruszkiewicz, P.; Sherwood, P.R.; Kvist, T. Integrative review: Nurses' and physicians' experiences and attitudes towards inpatient-witnessed resuscitation of an adult patient. *J. Adv. Nurs.* **2014**, *70*, 957–974. [CrossRef]
13. Willmes MSellmann, T.; Semmer, N.K.; Tschan, F.; Wetzchewald, D.; Schwager, H.; Russo, S.G.; Marsch, S. The impact of family presence during cardiopulmonary resuscitation on team performance and perceived task load: A prospective randomized simulator-based trial. *BMJ Open* **2022**, *12*, e056798. [CrossRef]
14. Abella, B.S.; Sandbo, N.; Vassilatos, P.; Alvarado, J.P.; O'Hearn, N.; Wigder, H.N.; Hoffman, P.; Tynus, K.; Vanden Hoek, T.L.; Becker, L.B. Chest compression rates during cardiopulmonary resuscitation are suboptimal: A prospective study during in-hospital cardiac arrest. *Circulation* **2005**, *111*, 428–434. [CrossRef]
15. Abella, B.S.; Alvarado, J.P.; Myklebust, H.; Edelson, D.P.; Barry, A.; O'Hearn, N.; Vanden Hoek, T.L.; Becker, L.B. Quality of Cardiopulmonary Resuscitation During In-Hospital Cardiac Arrest. *J. Am. Med. Assoc.* **2005**, *293*, 305–310. [CrossRef]
16. Hunziker, S.; Tschan, F.; Semmer, N.K.; Zobrist, R.; Spychiger, M.; Breuer, M.; Hunziker, P.R.; Marsch, S.C. Hands-on time during cardiopulmonary resuscitation is affected by the process of teambuilding: A prospective randomised simulator-based trial. *BMC Emerg. Med.* **2009**, *9*, 3. [CrossRef]
17. Marsch, S.C.; Muller, C.; Marquardt, K.; Conrad, G.; Tschan, F.; Hunziker, P.R. Human factors affect the quality of cardiopulmonary resuscitation in simulated cardiac arrests. *Resuscitation* **2004**, *60*, 51–56. [CrossRef]
18. Tschan, F.; Vetterli, M.; Semmer, N.K.; Hunziker, S.; Marsch, S.C. Activities during interruptions in cardiopulmonary resuscitation: A simulator study. *Resuscitation* **2011**, *82*, 1419–1423. [CrossRef]
19. Goldberger, Z.D.; Nallamothu, B.K.; Nichol, G.; Chan, P.S.; Curtis, J.R.; Cooke, C.R. Policies Allowing Family Presence During Resuscitation and Patterns of Care During In-Hospital Cardiac Arrest. *Circ. Cardiovasc. Qual. Outcomes* **2015**, *8*, 226–234. [CrossRef]
20. Waldemar, A.; Bremer, A.; Holm, A.; Strömberg, A.; Thylén, I. In-hospital family-witnessed resuscitation with a focus on the prevalence, processes, and outcomes of resuscitation: A retrospective observational cohort study. *Resuscitation* **2021**, *165*, 23–30. [CrossRef]
21. Arriaga, A.F.; Bader, A.M.; Wong, J.M.; Lipsitz, S.R.; Berry, W.R.; Ziewacz, J.E.; Hepner, D.L.; Boorman, D.J.; Pozner, C.N.; Smink, D.S.; et al. Simulation-Based Trial of Surgical-Crisis Checklists. *N. Engl. J. Med.* **2013**, *368*, 246–253. [CrossRef] [PubMed]
22. Cheng, A.; Kessler, D.; Mackinnon, R.; Chang, T.P.; Nadkarni, V.M.; Hunt, E.A.; Duval-Arnould, J.; Lin, Y.; Cook, D.A.; Pusic, M.; et al. Reporting Guidelines for Health Care Simulation Research: Extensions to the CONSORT and STROBE Statements. *Simul. Healthc.* **2016**, *11*, 238–248. [CrossRef]
23. Hart, S.; Staveland, L. Development of NASA-TLX (Task Load Index): Results of Empirical and Theoretical Research. In *Human Mental Workload*; Hancock, P., Meshkati, N., Eds.; North Holland Press: Amsterdam, The Netherlands, 1988; pp. 139–183.
24. Hart, S.G. Nasa-Task Load Index (NASA-TLX); 20 Years Later. *Proc. Hum. Factors Ergon. Soc. Annu. Meet.* **2006**, *50*, 904–908. [CrossRef]

25. Colligan, L.; Potts, H.W.W.; Finn, C.T.; Sinkin, R.A. Cognitive workload changes for nurses transitioning from a legacy system with paper documentation to a commercial electronic health record. *Int. J. Med. Inform.* **2015**, *84*, 469–476. [CrossRef] [PubMed]
26. Jabre, P.; Tazarourte, K.; Azoulay, E.; Borron, S.W.; Belpomme, V.; Jacob, L.; Bertrand, L.; Lapostolle, F.; Combes, X.; Galinski, M.; et al. Offering the opportunity for family to be present during cardiopulmonary resuscitation: 1-year assessment. *Intensive Care Med.* **2014**, *40*, 981–987. [CrossRef] [PubMed]
27. Goldberger, Z.D.; Chan, P.S.; Berg, R.A.; Kronick, S.L.; Cooke, C.R.; Lu, M.; Banerjee, M.; Hayward, R.A.; Krumholz, H.M.; Nallamothu, B.K.; et al. Duration of resuscitation efforts and survival after in-hospital cardiac arrest: An observational study *Lancet* **2012**, *380*, 1473–1481. [CrossRef]
28. Oczkowski, S.J.; Mazzetti, I.; Cupido, C.; Fox-Robichaud, A.E. The offering of family presence during resuscitation: A systematic review and meta-analysis. *J. Intensive Care* **2015**, *3*, 41. [CrossRef]
29. Toronto, C.E.; LaRocco, S.A. Family perception of and experience with family presence during cardiopulmonary resuscitation: An integrative review. *J. Clin. Nurs.* **2019**, *28*, 32–46. [CrossRef]
30. Crowley, C.P.; Salciccioli, J.D.; Kim, E.Y. The association between ACLS guideline deviations and outcomes from in-hospital cardiac arrest. *Resuscitation* **2020**, *153*, 65–70. [CrossRef]
31. Honarmand, K.; Mepham, C.; Ainsworth, C.; Khalid, Z. Adherence to advanced cardiovascular life support (ACLS) guidelines during in-hospital cardiac arrest is associated with improved outcomes. *Resuscitation* **2018**, *129*, 76–81. [CrossRef]

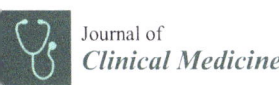

Article

Application of the Team Emergency Assessment Measure for Prehospital Cardiopulmonary Resuscitation

Sangsoo Han [1], Hye Ji Park [2], Won Jung Jeong [3], Gi Woon Kim [1], Han Joo Choi [4], Hyung Jun Moon [5], Kyoungmi Lee [6], Hyuk Joong Choi [7], Yong Jin Park [8], Jin Seong Cho [9] and Choung Ah Lee [2,*]

1. Department of Emergency Medicine, Soonchunhyang University Bucheon Hospital, Bucheon 14584, Korea
2. Department of Emergency Medicine, Hallym University, Dongtan Sacred Heart Hospital, Hwaseong 18450, Korea
3. Department of Emergency Medicine, Catholic University of Korea, St. Vincent's Hospital, Seoul 06591, Korea
4. Department of Emergency Medicine, Dankook University Hospital, Cheonan 31116, Korea
5. Department of Emergency Medicine, College of Medicine, Soonchunhyang University, Cheonan 31151, Korea
6. Department of Emergency Medicine, Myongji Hospital, Goyang 10475, Korea
7. Department of Emergency Medicine, Hanyang University Guri Hospital, Guri 11923, Korea
8. Department of Emergency Medicine, Chosun University Hospital, Gwangju 61453, Korea
9. Department of Emergency Medicine, Gil Medical Center, Gachon University College of Medicine, Incheon 21565, Korea
* Correspondence: cuccum@hanmail.net; Tel.: +82-31-8086-2611

Abstract: Introduction: Communication and teamwork are critical for ensuring patient safety, particularly during prehospital cardiopulmonary resuscitation (CPR). The Team Emergency Assessment Measure (TEAM) is a tool applicable to such situations. This study aimed to validate the TEAM efficiency as a suitable tool even in prehospital CPR. Methods: A multi-centric observational study was conducted using the data of all non-traumatic out-of-hospital cardiac arrest patients aged over 18 years who were treated using video communication-based medical direction in 2018. From the extracted data of 1494 eligible patients, 67 sample cases were randomly selected. Two experienced raters were assigned to each case. Each rater reviewed 13 or 14 videos and scored the TEAM items for each field cardiopulmonary resuscitation performance. The internal consistency, concurrent validity, and inter-rater reliability were measured. Results: The TEAM showed high reliability with a Cronbach's alpha value of 0.939, with a mean interitem correlation of 0.584. The mean item–total correlation was 0.789, indicating significant associations. The mean correlation coefficient between each item and the global score range was 0.682, indicating good concurrent validity. The mean intra-class correlation coefficient was 0.804, indicating excellent agreement. Discussion: The TEAM can be a valid and reliable tool to evaluate the non-technical skills of a team of paramedics performing CPR.

Keywords: Team Emergency Assessment Measure (TEAM); prehospital cardiopulmonary resuscitation (CPR); out-of-hospital cardiac arrest (OHCA)

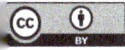

1. Introduction

Teamwork and leadership are known to be important non-technical skills (NTSs) in healthcare [1]. NTS are defined as "the cognitive, social, and personal resource skills that complement technical skills and contribute to safe and efficient task performance" [2]. NTSs include situational awareness, decision making, communication, teamwork, leadership, stress management, and coping with fatigue [3]. These are important for preventing medical errors and ensuring patient safety [4]. Moreover, in many studies, NTSs were correlated with the high clinical performance of the team.

Teamwork plays an important role in the prevention of adverse events [5]. A large-scale survey by the UK National Health Service reported that efficient teams had lower levels of patient mortality and sickness absence [6]. In another study, the implementation of a team training program reduced the surgical mortality rate of inpatients by 18% [7]. Since CPR is performed in a team, there is evidence suggesting that it affects NTS and CPR results [8]. A study showed a clear difference in leadership and task distribution between the team that succeeded in CPR and the team that failed [9]. Hunziker et al. found significant differences in the chest compression start time, the total chest compression time, and the chest compression speed when the technique training group and the leadership training group were compared [10].

Currently, there are no randomized controlled trials in which teamwork is evaluated in association with patient outcomes after a cardiac arrest [11]. Teamwork and leadership are recognized as important aspects of medicine [12]. Resuscitation efforts are delivered using complex, high-risk, and dynamic methods and require efficient interprofessional team coordination and collaboration to deliver safe and high-quality care. Leadership and teamwork training involves building a team of high-performing healthcare professionals from a group of highly skilled clinicians to provide efficient resuscitation to improve patient outcomes. The 2015 European Resuscitation Council guidelines highlighted that NTS training, including training in teamwork, leadership, and structured communication skills, are essential adjuncts to skills training, especially for those expected to perform cardiopulmonary resuscitation (CPR) [13].

Paramedics are responsible for initiating advanced life support during an out-of-hospital cardiac arrest (OHCA), which is a vital link in the chain of survival. Prehospital resuscitation is more difficult than in-hospital resuscitation. During OHCA, personnel with varying degrees of technical skills and NTSs form an improvised team to participate in CPR. In addition, stress, fatigue, and the frequent switching of positions are common factors that may threaten the teamwork of paramedics [14]. Further, the prehospital resuscitation procedure lacks human and material resources, is prone to litigation, and is often criticized by medical institutions and guardians, which puts the paramedics in a mentally vulnerable state [15]. Therefore, strong leadership and teamwork skills are needed, especially during prehospital resuscitations [16].

The standard measures of prehospital team performance are lacking, which makes it difficult to quantitatively assess the team performance of emergency medical services (EMS) [17]. This may be because, in critical, real-life situations, there are not enough resources to treat patients; hence, there are no experts to participate in the objective evaluation. As a result, most prehospital research is based on simulation training [11].

Therefore, this study aimed to evaluate the TEAM [18], which is considered to be the most promising approach in CPR situations among the currently known teamwork evaluation tools [19], to prehospital situations, and confirm its suitability in prehospital CPR performed by the EMS.

2. Materials and Methods

2.1. Patients Selection

This was a multi-centric observational study. Teamwork was evaluated by experts using the video data recorded from the Smart Advanced Life Support (SALS) registry. SALS is a method of advanced resuscitation performed by paramedics under a video communication-based direction for patients older than 18 years with OHCA of non-traumatic causes in South Korea [20]. After arriving at the field, the paramedics used a mobile application to request medical direction from an emergency physician through video call, after which the on-site performance of the paramedics and the doctor's medical guidance were recorded. If using the application was not possible, the medical direction was provided via video or voice calls.

2.2. Intervention

From 1 January 2018 to 31 December 2018, among the 2536 cases that were recorded in the SALS registry, 1725 cases for which the application was used were selected. Further, 1339 of the selected cases were extracted by excluding the cases in which it was difficult to evaluate teamwork due to poor audio and video conditions and short on-site CPR time (<10 min). To ensure the representativeness of the sample, 5% of the population was selected through simple randomization [21]. Finally, 67 cases were analyzed.

Ten experts participated in the video evaluation. The expert group consisted of emergency physicians who conducted direct medical directions. The median age was 41 years, and males accounted for 81.8% of all the experts. They had 15 years of experience as an emergency physician and 48 months as medical directors for SALS (Table 1). Two experts were assigned to evaluate the teamwork for each case according to a predetermined sequence. Each expert reviewed 13 or 14 videos and evaluated the prehospital teamwork of each team (Figure 1).

Table 1. Demographic characteristics of experts (*n* = 10).

Characteristics	n (%) or Median (IQR)
Age	41 (38–43)
Sex, male	9 (81.8)
Career of clinical physician (years)	15 (12–18)
Career of medical director by videophone (months)	48 (24–61)

IQR, interquartile range.

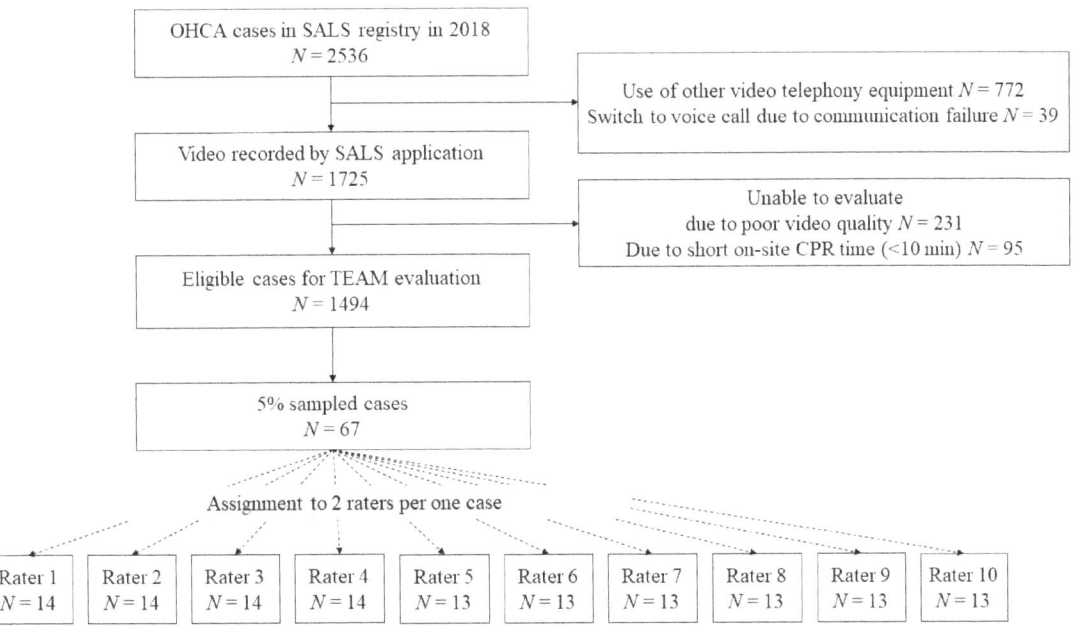

Figure 1. Flowchart of selection of eligible cases and allocation to raters. Abbreviations: OHCA, out-of-hospital cardiac arrest; SALS, Smart Advanced Life Support; CPR, cardiopulmonary resuscitation; TEAM, Team Emergency Assessment Measure.

2.3. Instrument

The TEAM developed by Cooper et al. was used as a tool for prehospital teamwork evaluation [18]. It consists of 11 items in 3 categories: leadership, teamwork, and task management. These items were rated on a 5-point Likert scale ('0' = never to '4' = always) with a total score ranging from 0 to 44. The overall performance was rated on a global rating scale, ranging from 1 to 10. The original English version of the TEAM was translated into Korean according to World Health Organization guidelines [22]. Following forward translation, expert-panel back-translation, pretesting, and cognitive interviewing, the final version was completed, which was approved for use by the developer.

The raters participating in this study were emergency physicians directing medical interventions through video and consisted of advanced life support training managers for paramedics. The training course is based on a scenario in which a video-based medical direction is received during resuscitation. Therefore, the selected raters thoroughly understood the gap between the video performance and the actual situation. All the raters completed a 30-minute theoretical tutorial on the TEAM before evaluation and agreed upon the scoring level through trial evaluations of three sample cases. The evaluations were conducted in separate spaces to prevent the raters from sharing their results with each other.

2.4. Ethical Approval

This study was approved by the relevant Institutional Review Board of the Hallym University Dongtan Sacred Heart Hospital (approval number: HDT 2019-12-011). Written informed consent was obtained from all the participants of this study.

2.5. Statistical Analysis

All analyses were performed using SPSS v. 25 (IBM, New York, NY, USA). The baseline participant and event characteristics of the OHCAs are reported as numbers and percentages for qualitative variables and median and interquartile ranges for continuous variables. The measurement properties of the TEAM were evaluated for internal consistency, concurrent validity, inter-rater reliability, and floor/ceiling effect.

The internal consistency was examined using the mean interitem and item–total correlations and Cronbach's alpha coefficient. An item–total correlation of >0.40 and Cronbach's alpha >0.70 were considered satisfactory [23]. The concurrent validity was evaluated through the correlation of item scores with global ratings. The inter-rater reliability was measured using the intraclass correlation coefficient (ICC) with a 95% confidence interval. An ICC value of less than 0.4 was regarded as poor agreement [24]. The floor effect includes the proportion of observations with the lowest possible scores, whereas the ceiling effect represents observations with the highest possible score. The floor and ceiling effects of less than 15% of the observations were considered adequate [23].

3. Results

3.1. Characteristics of Clinical Cases

Table 2 shows the characteristics of the cardiac arrest cases used for evaluation. The median age of the patients was 61 years. Men accounted for 65.7% of the patients, cardiac arrest was witnessed in 64.2% of the patients, and 31.3% of the cases had an initial shockable rhythm. The median scene time for prehospital management was 21 minutes, and 50.7% of the patients had a prehospital return of spontaneous circulation (ROSC).

Table 2. Characteristics of patients and events ($n = 67$).

Characteristics	n (%)
Age, years, median (IQR)	61 (50–71)
Sex, male	44 (65.7)
Witnessed	43 (64.2)
Initial rhythm	
Shockable	21 (31.3)
Non-shockable	46 (68.7)
Scene time interval, min	21 (19–28)
Prehospital ROSC	34 (50.7)

IQR, interquartile range; ROSC, return of spontaneous circulation.

3.2. Measurement Properties

The TEAM showed high reliability with a Cronbach's alpha value of 0.939, and Cronbach's alpha values for each item of leadership, teamwork, and task management were

0.828, 0.913, and 0.895, respectively. The interitem correlation ranged from 0.463 to 0.811, and the mean interitem correlation was 0.584. The mean item–total correlation was 0.789 (r = 0.708–0.822), which indicates significant item–total score associations (Table 3).

Table 3. The TEAM outcomes (67 clinical cases, 134 observations).

	Median (IQR)	Score Range *	Item–Total Correlation	p-Value
Q1. The team leader let the team know what was expected of them through direction and command.	2 (2–3)	0–4	0.759	<0.001
Q2. The team leader maintained a global perspective	2 (1–3)	0–4	0.807	<0.001
Q3. The team communicated effectively.	2 (1–3)	0–4	0.793	<0.001
Q4. The team worked together to complete tasks in a timely manner.	2 (2–3)	0–4	0.765	<0.001
Q5. The team acted with composure and control.	3 (2–3)	1–4	0.708	<0.001
Q6. The team morale was positive.	2 (2–3)	1–4	0.800	<0.001
Q7. The team adapted to changing situations.	2 (1–3)	0–4	0.814	<0.001
Q8. The team monitored and reassessed the situation.	2 (1–3)	0–4	0.797	<0.001
Q9. The team anticipated potential situations.	2 (1–3)	0–4	0.822	<0.001
Q10. The team prioritized tasks.	2 (2–3)	0–4	0.806	<0.001
Q11. The team followed approved standards/guidelines	2 (2–3)	0–4	0.803	<0.001
Total mean.	25 (18–30)			

TEAM, Team Emergency Assessment Measure; SD, standard deviation. * Score range: 0 = never or hardly ever; 1 = seldom; 2 = about as often as not; 3 = very often; 4 = always/nearly always.

The median score for the single-item global rating was 6 (IQR, 4–7), and the median TEAM was 24.50 (IQR, 17.75–30.25). The mean correlation coefficient between each item and the global score range was 0.682 (r = 0.595 to 0.741, all p < 0.001), indicating good concurrent validity. The mean intraclass correlation coefficient (ICC) was 0.804, with excellent agreement between the raters. However, in 1 of the 67 clinical events, the ICC was 0.323, indicating poor agreement.

The distribution of the lowest and highest scores was within 15% of all the items, which showed no floor or ceiling effects (Figure 2).

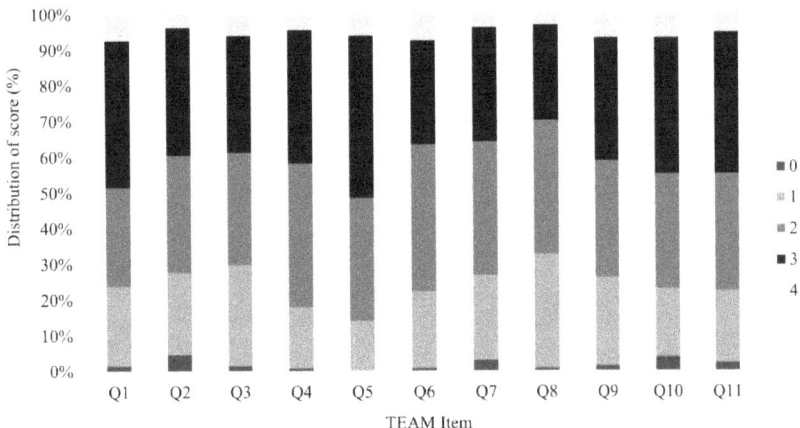

Figure 2. Distribution of the results of the TEAM. Abbreviation: TEAM, Team Emergency Assessment Measure.

4. Discussion

To the best of our knowledge, this is the first study to investigate the validity of a tool that evaluates teamwork during a prehospital cardiac arrest situation rather than a simulation. In this study, the feasibility of the evaluation of teamwork was also suggested even in prehospital OHCA situations.

Although the importance of teamwork in the prehospital stage is sufficiently recognized, only a few studies were conducted due to the lack of data sources. This is because it is challenging to evaluate leadership and communication skills, which are the elements of NTS, only with paper records. Digital technology, such as video records, can be used as a reliable source for situational evaluation in the prehospital stage [25].

To determine the effectiveness of intervention programs to improve team performance, a valid and reliable tool is required. The Clinical Teamwork Scale [26], Observational Skill-based Clinical Assessment Tool for Resuscitation [27], Modified Non-Technical Skills Scale for Trauma [28], and TEAM [18] are well-known tools applicable to critical situations. Among these tools, the TEAM has shown validity in clinical settings and among staff and trainees. It is considered the most promising tool given its measurement of evidence [19]. However, no teamwork evaluation tool, including the TEAM, has been verified in actual prehospital clinical settings. Therefore, this study evaluated whether the TEAM is the most reliable measurement that can be used in prehospital CPR situations.

The mean score for each item in the TEAM was 1.99–2.43, which was lower than that of a previous study (2.69–3.30) in the in-hospital situation. The mean total score was 24.26, which was very different from 34.65 in that previous study [28]. The scores of the leadership category were lower in the in-hospital resuscitation situation [28], but the scores for responding to a changing situation and re-evaluating the situation were low during prehospital resuscitation. These results reflect the characteristics of prehospital situations. Compared with the in-hospital cardiac arrest patients, the OHCA patients were remarkably similar in demographics and most comorbidities, but they had low ROSC and survival rates [29]. In Korea, when a cardiac arrest occurs, a two-tiered EMS system is operated, i.e., two teams are immediately merged to form one team. The EMS that arrives first must respond in an early stage with two or three paramedics. However, during an unrecognized cardiac arrest, the activation of the second EMS team is delayed, making it more difficult to deal with manpower [15]. In addition, there is a lack of facilities and equipment, and it is also affected by the weather and location of the patient. Insufficient human and material resources and several unpredictable factors impede situational adaptation and assessment.

In our study, the internal consistency of prehospital resuscitations was high, with a Cronbach's alpha value of 0.939, which was similar to that in the previous study (Cronbach's alpha = 0.94) that evaluated in-hospital resuscitation situations [30]. In addition, the mean interitem and item–total correlations in our study were strongly significant at 0.584 and 0.789, respectively, which were similar to those of the in-hospital resuscitations (mean interitem correlation, $(r = 0.60)$; mean item–total correlation $(r = 0.795)$) [30].

In the concurrent validity evaluation, the item ratings were significantly associated with the global ratings $(r = 0.682)$; however, this correlation was low compared with that of the evaluation conducted using video records of simulations $(r = 0.80$ to $0.94)$ [31] and the French version of the simulation study $(r = 0.78)$ [32]. The mean ICC of the 11 TEAM items showed a high agreement rate of 0.804, with the exception of one case that showed poor agreement. The video of this case was reviewed by the authors, and it was observed that the performance of the paramedics was very poor; therefore, both raters gave 0 or 1 point for all the items. The ICC should be interpreted with caution, as it is affected by the range of measurements in the study population. For example, if the measured values of the study group were all high, and the range was small, the interindividual variation would be smaller than the intraindividual variation, and the ICC would be low.

This study has several limitations. First, we did not conduct evaluations in real time during the resuscitation. We analyzed and evaluated video records. Moreover, it was difficult to evaluate the leader's situational awareness, decision-making ability, or skills by simply observing their behavior. To reduce the error caused by this, only the expert group of video-guided medical directors were designated as the raters in this study. Second, we could not calculate the test–retest reliability. The videos used for analysis were stored on a secure server to protect patient privacy and could only be reviewed on a designated computer after prior approval. Due to this, it was difficult to perform retesting. Hence, for the various case reviews in this study, two raters were assigned to each case to calculate the inter-rater reliability. Third, because the video data could not be processed, the raters could not check whether the patient had an on-site ROSC. It is possible that the patient's outcome, along with the performance of the paramedics, may have affected the TEAM score.

5. Conclusions

NTSs in the prehospital stage should be appropriately evaluated for patient safety. The TEAM can be a valid and reliable tool to evaluate the efficiency of a team of healthcare workers during real-life CPR situations.

Author Contributions: Conceptualization, C.A.L.; method, S.H. and C.A.L.; software, S.H. and C.A.L.; validation, C.A.L.; formal analysis, C.A.L., H.J.P. and S.H.; investigation, W.J.J., G.W.K., H.J.C. (Han Joo Choi), H.J.M., K.L., H.J.C. (Hyuk Joong Choi), Y.J.P. and J.S.C.; resources, H.J.P. and S.H.; data curation, H.J.P. and S.H.; writing—original draft preparation, S.H. and C.A.L.; writing—review and editing, C.A.L.; visualization, S.H. and C.A.L.; supervision, C.A.L.; project administration, C.A.L. All authors have read and agreed to the published version of the manuscript.

Funding: This study received honoraria from the Soonchunhyang University Research Fund (grant no. 10210064).

Institutional Review Board Statement: This study was approved by the relevant Institutional Review Board. Written informed consent was obtained from all the participants of this study.

Informed Consent Statement: Informed consent was obtained from all the subjects involved in this study.

Data Availability Statement: The data used to support the findings of this study are available from the corresponding author upon request. The original video data used in this study cannot be disclosed to protect personal information.

Conflicts of Interest: The authors of this work have no conflict of interest to disclose.

References

1. Flin, R.; Maran, N. Identifying and training non-technical skills for teams in acute medicine. *Qual. Saf. Health Care* **2004**, *13* (Suppl. 1), i80–i84. [CrossRef] [PubMed]
2. Flin, R.; Martin, L.; Goeters, K.M.; Hörmann, H.J. Development of the NOTECHS (nontechnical skills) system for assessing pilots' CRM skills. In *Human Factors and Aerospace Safety*, 1st ed.; Harris, D., Muir, H.C., Eds.; Routledge: London, UK, 2018; pp. 95–117.
3. Mitchell, L.; Flin, R. Non-technical skills of the operating theatre scrub nurse: Literature review. *J. Adv. Nurs.* **2008**, *63*, 15–24. [CrossRef] [PubMed]
4. Katzenbach, J.R.; Smith, D.K. The discipline of teams. *Harv. Bus Rev.* **1993**, *71*, 111–120.
5. Manser, T. Teamwork and patient safety in dynamic domains of healthcare: A review of the literature. *Acta Anaesthesiol. Scand.* **2009**, *53*, 143–151. [CrossRef] [PubMed]
6. Lyubovnikova, J.; West, M.A.; Dawson, J.F.; Carter, M.R. 24-Karat or fool's gold? Consequences of real team and co-acting group membership in healthcare organizations. *Eur. J. Work Organ Psychol.* **2015**, *24*, 929–950. [CrossRef]
7. Neily, J.; Mills, P.D.; Young-Xu, Y.; Carney, B.T.; West, P.; Berger, D.H.; Mazzia, L.M.; Paull, D.E.; Bagian, J.P. Association between implementation of a medical team training program and surgical mortality. *JAMA* **2010**, *304*, 1693–1700. [CrossRef]
8. Hunziker, S.; Johansson, A.C.; Tschan, F.; Semmer, N.K.; Rock, L.; Howell, M.D.; Marsch, S. Teamwork and leadership in cardiopulmonary resuscitation. *J. Am. Coll Cardiol.* **2011**, *57*, 2381–2388. [CrossRef]
9. Marsch, S.C.U.; Müller, C.; Marquardt, K.; Conrad, G.; Tschan, F.; Hunziker, P.R. Human factors affect the quality of cardiopulmonary resuscitation in simulated cardiac arrests. *Resuscitation* **2004**, *60*, 51–56. [CrossRef]
10. Hunziker, S.; Bühlmann, C.; Tschan, F.; Balestra, G.; Legeret, C.; Schumacher, C.; Semmer, N.K.; Hunziker, P.; Marsch, S. Brief leadership instructions improve cardiopulmonary resuscitation in a high-fidelity simulation: A randomized controlled trial. *Crit. Care Med.* **2010**, *38*, 1086–1091. [CrossRef]
11. Kuzovlev, A.; Monsieurs, K.G.; Gilfoyle, E.; Finn, J.; Greif, R.; Education Implementation and Teams Task Force of the International Liaison Committee on Resuscitation. The effect of team and leadership training of advanced life support providers on patient outcomes: A systematic review. *Resuscitation* **2021**, *160*, 126–139. [CrossRef]
12. Rosen, M.A.; DiazGranados, D.; Dietz, A.S.; Benishek, L.E.; Thompson, D.; Pronovost, P.J.; Weaver, S.J. Teamwork in healthcare: Key discoveries enabling safer, high-quality care. *Am. Psychol.* **2018**, *73*, 433–450. [CrossRef] [PubMed]

13. Soar, J.; Nolan, J.P.; Böttiger, B.W.; Perkins, G.D.; Lott, C.; Carli, P.; Pellis, T.; Sandroni, C.; Skrifvars, M.B.; Smith, G.B.; et al. European Resuscitation Council Guidelines for resuscitation 2015: Section 3. Adult advanced life support. *Resuscitation* **2015**, *95*, 100–147. [CrossRef] [PubMed]
14. Patterson, P.D.; Arnold, R.M.; Abebe, K.; Lave, J.R.; Krackhardt, D.; Carr, M.; Weaver, M.D.; Yealy, D.M. Variation in emergency medical technician partner familiarity. *Health Serv. Res.* **2011**, *46*, 1319–1331. [CrossRef]
15. Patterson, P.D.; Huang, D.T.; Fairbanks, R.J.; Simeone, S.; Weaver, M.; Wang, H.E. Variation in emergency medical services workplace safety culture. *Prehosp. Emerg. Care* **2010**, *14*, 448–460. [CrossRef] [PubMed]
16. Atack, L.; Maher, J. Emergency medical and health providers' perceptions of key issues in prehospital patient safety. *Prehosp. Emerg. Care* **2010**, *14*, 95–102. [CrossRef] [PubMed]
17. Patterson, P.D.; Weaver, M.D. Teams and teamwork in emergency Medical Services. In *Human Factors and Ergonomics of Prehospital Emergency Care: Critical Essays in Human Geography*, 1st ed.; Keebler, J.R., Lazzara, E.H., Misasi, P., Eds.; CRC Press: Boca Raton, FL, USA, 2017; p. 14.
18. Cooper, S.; Cant, R.; Porter, J.; Sellick, K.; Somers, G.; Kinsman, L.; Nestel, D. Rating medical emergency teamwork performance: Development of the Team Emergency Assessment Measure (TEAM). *Resuscitation* **2010**, *81*, 446–452. [CrossRef]
19. Boet, S.; Etherington, N.; Larrigan, S.; Yin, L.; Khan, H.; Sullivan, K.; Jung, J.J.; Grantcharov, T.P. Measuring the teamwork performance of teams in crisis situations: A systematic review of assessment tools and their measurement properties. *BMJ Qual. Saf.* **2019**, *28*, 327–337. [CrossRef]
20. Kim, C.; Choi, H.J.; Moon, H.; Kim, G.; Lee, C.; Cho, J.S.; Kim, S.; Lee, K.; Choi, H.; Jeong, W. Prehospital advanced cardiac life support by EMT with a smartphone-based direct medical control for nursing home cardiac arrest. *Am. J. Emerg. Med.* **2019**, *37*, 585–589. [CrossRef]
21. Park, W.; Son, S.; Park, H.; Park, H. A proposal on determining appropriate sample size considering statistical conclusion validity. *Seoul J. Ind. Relat.* **2010**, *21*, 51–85.
22. World Health Organization. Process of Translation and Adaptation of Instruments, Course Hero. 2013. Available online: https://www.coursehero.com/file/30372721/WHO-Process-of-translation-and-adaptation-of-instrumentspdf/;2013 (accessed on 13 September 2022).
23. Terwee, C.B.; Bot, S.D.M.; de Boer, M.R.; van der Windt, D.A.; Knol, D.L.; Dekker, J.; Bouter, L.M.; de Vet, H.C. Quality criteria were proposed for measurement properties of health status questionnaires. *J. Clin. Epidemiol.* **2007**, *60*, 34–42. [CrossRef]
24. Cicchetti, D.V. Guidelines, criteria, and rules of thumb for evaluating normed and standardized assessment instruments in psychology. *Psychol. Assess.* **1994**, *6*, 284–290. [CrossRef]
25. Vicente, V.; Johansson, A.; Selling, M.; Johansson, J.; Möller, S.; Todorova, L. Experience of using video support by prehospital emergency care physician in ambulance care—An interview study with prehospital emergency nurses in Sweden. *BMC Emerg. Med.* **2021**, *21*, 44. [CrossRef] [PubMed]
26. Guise, J.M.; Deering, S.H.; Kanki, B.G.; Osterweil, P.; Li, H.; Mori, M.; Lowe, N.K. Validation of a tool to measure and promote clinical teamwork. *Simul. Healthc.* **2008**, *3*, 217–223. [CrossRef] [PubMed]
27. Walker, S.; Brett, S.; McKay, A.; Lambden, C.; Vincent, C.; Sevdalis, N. Observational skill-based clinical assessment tool for resuscitation (OSCAR): Development and validation. *Resuscitation* **2011**, *82*, 835–844. [CrossRef]
28. Steinemann, S.; Berg, B.; DiTullio, A.; Skinner, A.; Terada, K.; Anzelon, K.; Ho, H.C. Assessing teamwork in the trauma bay: Introduction of a modified 'NOTECHS' scale for trauma. *Am. J. Surg.* **2012**, *203*, 69–75. [CrossRef]
29. Høybye, M.; Stankovic, N.; Holmberg, M.; Christensen, H.C.; Granfeldt, A.; Andersen, L.W. In-hospital vs. out-of-hospital cardiac arrest: Patient characteristics and survival. *Resuscitation* **2021**, *158*, 157–165. [CrossRef]
30. Cooper, S.; Cant, R.; Connell, C.; Sims, L.; Porter, J.E.; Symmons, M.; Nestel, D.; Liaw, S.Y. Measuring teamwork performance: Validity testing of the Team Emergency Assessment Measure (TEAM) with clinical resuscitation teams. *Resuscitation* **2016**, *101*, 97–101. [CrossRef]
31. Cooper, S.J.; Cant, R.P. Measuring non-technical skills of medical emergency teams: An update on the validity and reliability of the Team Emergency Assessment Measure (TEAM). *Resuscitation* **2014**, *85*, 31–33. [CrossRef]
32. Maignan, M.; Koch, F.X.; Chaix, J.; Phellouzat, P.; Binauld, G.; Collomb Muret, R.; Cooper, S.J.; Labarère, J.; Danel, V.; Viglino, D.; et al. Team Emergency Assessment Measure (TEAM) for the assessment of non-technical skills during resuscitation: Validation of the French version. *Resuscitation* **2016**, *101*, 115–120. [CrossRef]

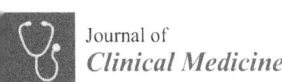

Article

COVID-19 CPR—Impact of Personal Protective Equipment during a Simulated Cardiac Arrest in Times of the COVID-19 Pandemic: A Prospective Comparative Trial

Timur Sellmann [1,2,†], Maria Nur [3,†,‡], Dietmar Wetzchewald [3], Heidrun Schwager [3], Corvin Cleff [4], Serge C. Thal [2] and Stephan Marsch [5,*]

1. Department of Anaesthesiology and Intensive Care Medicine, Bethesda Hospital, 47053 Duisburg, Germany
2. Department of Anaesthesiology 1, Witten/Herdecke University, 58455 Witten, Germany
3. Institution for Emergency Medicine, 59755 Arnsberg, Germany
4. Department of Anaesthesiology and Intensive Care Medicine, Faculty of Medicine and University Hospital Cologne, University of Cologne, 50937 Cologne, Germany
5. Department of Intensive Care, University Hospital, 4031 Basel, Switzerland
* Correspondence: stephan.marsch@usb.ch; Fax: +41-61-265-53-00
† These authors contributed equally to this work.
‡ This work is part of Maria Nur's doctoral thesis.

Abstract: *Background:* Guidelines of cardiopulmonary resuscitation (CPR) recommend the use of personal protective equipment (PPE) during the resuscitation of COVID-19 patients. Data on the effects of PPE on rescuers' stress level and quality of CPR are sparse and conflicting. This trial investigated the effects of PPE on team performance in simulated cardiac arrests. *Methods:* During the pandemic period, 198 teams (689 participants) performed CPR with PPE in simulated cardiac arrests (PPE group) and were compared with 423 (1451 participants) performing in identical scenarios in the pre-pandemic period (control group). Video recordings were used for data analysis. The primary endpoint was hands-on time. Secondary endpoints included a further performance of CPR and the perceived task load assessed by the NASA task-load index. *Results:* Hands-on times were lower in PPE teams than in the control group (86% (83–89) vs. 90% (87–93); difference 3, 95% CI for difference 3–4, $p < 0.0001$). Moreover, PPE teams made fewer change-overs and delayed defibrillation and administration of drugs. PPE teams perceived higher task loads (57 (44–67) vs. 63 (53–71); difference 6, 95% CI for difference 5–8, $p < 0.0001$) and scored higher in the domains physical and temporal demand, performance, and effort. Leadership allocation had no effect on primary and secondary endpoints. *Conclusions:* Having to wear PPE during CPR is an additional burden in an already demanding task. PPE is associated with an increase in perceived task load, lower hands-on times, fewer change-overs, and delays in defibrillation and the administration of drugs. (German study register number DRKS00023184).

Keywords: COVID-19; personal protective equipment; cardiopulmonary resuscitation; simulation; controlled trial

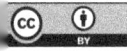

1. Introduction

The current European Resuscitation Council COVID-19 guidelines recommend the use of personal protective equipment (PPE) during the cardiopulmonary resuscitation (CPR) of a suspected COVID-19 victim [1,2]. These recommendations are based on considerations of potential droplet and airborne transmission from the victim to the rescuer during CPR. In addition, international and national recommendations regarding a hygienic faultless dressing ("donning") and removal ("doffing") of PPE have also been published in order to further minimise the risk of contagion [3]. Data concerning CPR during COVID-19 is still limited and the outcome seems worse in comparison to non-COVID-19 patients [4,5]. Two large studies including over 6300 COVID-19 patients reported no survival [6] and 3%

survival in patients aged > 79 years, respectively [7]. The authors of both studies advocate the need for further studies of CPR in COVID-19 and claim that strategies are needed to further optimize CPR for COVID-19, including the use of PPE [6,7]. Current data on the impact of PPE on CPR mostly relate to small studies investigating the quality of chest compressions of single rescuers' in simulated arrests [8–15]. Results are conflicting with studies reporting no effect of PPE [11,12] or negative effects [8,13–16].

The beneficial effects of PPE include counteracting aerosol or droplet transmission-induced infection rates [1–3]. Delays by "donning" PPE in COVID-19 CPR has been discussed [2], but published data preferentially did not show any relevant delay during life-saving procedures in various populations [11,17]. CPR is a stressful task in itself [18] and the need to wear PPE may add supplementary cognitive and emotional demands. Finally, there are no data, though important in CPR teams [19,20], on whether leadership is able to mitigate the effects of additional stress, as may be caused by PPE.

Investigating the impact of PPE on the quality of CPR in COVID-19 patients in large randomized trials would be difficult in real cases for a variety of reasons. Simulation allows the investigation of team performance both globally and in specific subtasks in a realistic and standardized manner [21]. A particular advantage of simulation is the possibility of recording data right from the start. Accordingly, the aim of this trial was to investigate the effects of PPE on rescuers' perceived task load and the quality of CPR, and the mitigating effects of team leadership, if any, in simulated cardiac arrests.

2. Material and Methods

2.1. Participants

The Working Group on Intensive Care Medicine, Arnsberg, Germany (http://www.aim-arnsberg.de; assessed on 19 August 2022), organizes educational courses for physicians, mainly residents in their 2nd to 3rd year of postgraduate medical education in internal medicine, anaesthesia, or surgery, from Germany and German-speaking countries working in intensive care and emergency medicine. Participants of the courses were offered to attend voluntary simulator-based CPR workshops and were informed that simulations were video-taped for scientific reasons. Identical workshops were offered to physicians wishing to participate without being filmed. To capture the actual level of training of the course participants, a specific theoretical instruction on their knowledge of CPR was omitted. The updates in international CPR guidelines (AHA in 2020; ERC in 2021) did not affect the primary and secondary outcomes of the present trial. The trial was carried out following the rules of the Declaration of Helsinki and was approved by the Ethics Committee of "Aerztekammer Westfalen-Lippe" (2020-602-f-S) that waived the obligation to obtain consent. The study is registered at the German Clinical Trial Registry (www.drks.de; assessed on 19 August 2022; DRKS-ID: DRKS00023184) and reported herein according to the extensions to the CONSORT statements of the Reporting Guidelines for Health Care Simulation Research [22].

2.2. Study Design

This is a prospective comparative trial of two cohorts: during the pandemic years 2020 and 2021, all participants of our workshops performed CPR with PPE (PPE group), while a cohort of participants of pre-pandemic workshops of 2016 to 2019 [23–25] served as the control group. Apart from the need to wear PPE, the conditions and settings for both cohorts were identical.

Using computer-generated numbers, participants from single workshops were randomly assigned to teams of three to five physicians. Teams were randomly allocated 1:1:1 to no designated leadership (no intervention), designated leadership by the team (team was given the task to designate a leader prior to the start of the scenario), or designated leadership by a tutor (leader was assigned to a randomly chosen team member by the tutor prior to the start of the scenario). The designated leaders wore a coloured scrub cap and could thus be identified on video-recordings.

2.3. Simulator and Scenario

The mannequin Ambu Man Wireless (Ambu GmbH, Bad Nauheim, Germany) was used. All participants received a standardized introduction to the workshop, the mannequins, and the resuscitation equipment available. Subsequently, all team members were informed that their role during the following scenario was that of a resuscitation team summoned to an unwitnessed cardiac arrest. The victim of the arrest (mannequin) was handed over to the team. Ventricular fibrillation was displayed on the manual defibrillator simulator (ALSI isimulate, iSimulate, LLC, Albany, NY, USA) once the patches were attached. The study period started with the first touch of the patient by one of the participants and ended after the third defibrillation with the return of spontaneous circulation during the following two minutes of CPR. After handing over the victim, tutors, who were instructed to refrain from any intervention until the end of the study period, operated the resuscitation mannequins. The further course of the scenario was at the discretion of the tutor who, after the simulated scenario, gave educational feedback to the teams.

2.4. Personal Protective Equipment (PPE)

The teams were instructed that, like in the real world, they had to put on complete PPE prior to any patient contact. Due to a strict hygiene protocol, N95 masks had to be worn all the time throughout the course. Further PPE consisting of gloves, glasses, gowns, and scrub caps was displayed in sufficient number and different sizes on a table in the scenario room. This made sure that participants were aware that, after "donning", they had to deal with a medical emergency. The time needed for "donning" was defined as the interval between the first touch of PPE equipment by any team member and the first touch of the patient by any team member.

2.5. NASA Task Load Index

Immediately after the completion of their simulation, participants were asked to fill in the NASA task load index (NASA-TLX) questionnaire. The NASA-TLX assesses six domains on visual analogue scales (which range from 0 to 100): mental demand, physical demand, temporal demand, own performance, effort, and frustration [26]. The NASA-TLX has been extensively validated, is easy to administer, and widely used in different domains like flying, driving, teamwork, and medicine [26,27]. Using the unweighted (or "raw") NASA-TLX, values reach from "0" (minimum) to "100" (maximum), with higher values indicating a higher workload.

2.6. Data Analysis

Data analysis was performed using the video recordings obtained during the simulations. The study period started with the first touch of the patient by one of the participants and ended after the third defibrillation. The first touch of the patient by one of the participants was defined to be the starting point for the timing of all events.

2.7. Statistical Analysis

The primary endpoint was the percentage of hands-on time, defined as the time of actual chest compressions divided by the total time interval of the study period. Secondary outcomes included the time of "donning" PPE, adherence to the CPR guidelines, and the NASA-TLX data. The effect of designated leadership was assessed as a secondary outcome for all outcomes analysed.

Data are expressed as medians [IQR], unless otherwise stated. Statistical analysis was performed using SPSS (version 28). Numerical data were analysed by a non-parametric ANOVA, followed by a Mann–Whitney test, if appropriate. The estimates for differences between the medians and their approximate confidence intervals were obtained by the Hodges–Lehmann estimation. Categorical data were analysed using the chi-square test. A $p < 0.05$ (two-tailed) was considered to represent a statistical significance.

3. Results

3.1. Participants

One hundred and ninety-eight PPE teams (689 participants, 354 male) were compared with 423 control teams (1451 participants). The gender of the leaders was equally distributed between the control groups and the PPE teams ($p = 0.31$). The PPE teams needed 62 (50–78) s for "donning".

3.2. Primary Outcome

The hands-on times were lower in the PPE group than in the control group (86% (83–89) vs. 90% (87–93); difference 3, 95% CI for difference 3–4, $p < 0.0001$). Leadership allocation had no effect on the hands-on times ($p = 0.77$). For more information, please see Figure 1.

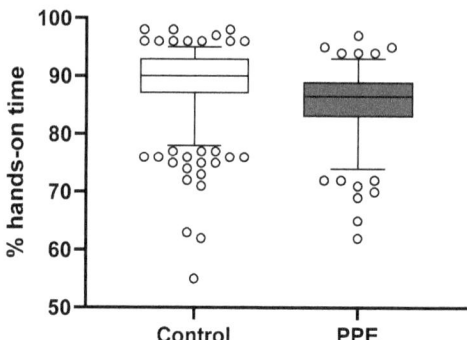

Figure 1. Box and whisker plot of the percentage hands-on time. Boxes represent medians and interquartile range; whiskers delineate the 5th and 95th percentile respectively. Outlier markers indicate teams performing outside the 5th and 95th percentile. White box = control group (no PPE); grey box = group performing CPR with PPE. Hands-on times differed significantly between the groups ($p < 0.0001$).

3.3. Secondary Outcomes

The performance metrics of CPR are displayed in Table 1. The PPE teams made fewer change-overs and delayed defibrillation and the administration of drugs. Leadership allocation had no effect on any performance marker (Table 2).

Table 1. Performance metrics of CPR.

	Control Group (n = 423)	PPE Group (n = 198)	Difference (95% CI)	p
Start cardiac massage (s)	12 (8–16)	12 (8–16)	0 (−1–1)	0.49
Chest compression rate (strokes/min)	118 (108–127)	119 (112–124)	1 (−3–1)	0.46
Change-overs per 2 min (n)	1.3 (1.3–1.7)	0.4 (0.3–0.6)	0.9 (0.9–1.0)	0.0001
AAM completed (CPR cycle)	2 (1–2)	2 (2–2)	0 (0–0)	0.30
Ventilatory rate (breaths/min)	20 (13–28)	18 (12–25)	2 (0–4)	0.28
Time to 1st defibrillation (s)	67 (48–102)	86 (67–119)	19 (13–25)	0.001
Time to epinephrine administration (s)	268 (190–312)	319 (282–371)	66 (48–86)	0.001
Time to amiodarone administration (s)	302 (270–340)	423 (388–465)	121 (109–131)	0.0001

Data are medians [IQR]. Estimates for differences between medians and their approximate confidence intervals were obtained by the Hodges–Lehmann estimation. PPE = personal protective equipment; change over = change of the person performing chest compressions (as CPR guidelines recommend a change over every two minutes a value of 1.0 represents perfect adherence); and AAM = advanced airway management.

Table 2. Effects of leadership on primary and secondary outcomes.

		No Designated Leadership	Designated Leadership by Team	Designated Leadership by Tutor	p
Hands-on time (%)	Control	90 (86–93)	90 (87–92)	90 (87–92)	0.77
	PPE	87 (82–91)	87 (84–89)	85 (82–89)	
Start cardiac massage (s)	Control	13 (7–16)	12 (7–16)	12 (9–16)	0.84
	PPE	12 (8–16)	12 (9–16)	11 (7–14)	
Chest compression rate (strokes/min)	Control	118 (108–129)	118 (106–126)	117 (110–129)	0.38
	PPE	121 (115–121)	119 (112–125)	116 (111–122)	
Change-overs per 2 min (n)	Control	1.3 (1.3–1.7)	1.4 (1.2–1.7)	1.3 (1.3–1.7)	0.31
	PPE	0.5 (0.3–0.6)	0.4 (0.3–0.6)	0.4 (0.3–0.6)	
AAM completed (CPR cycle)	Control	2 (2–2)	2 (1–2)	2 (2–3)	0.14
	PPE	2 (1–2)	2 (2–2)	2 (2–2)	
Ventilatory rate (breaths/min)	Control	19 (13–29)	20 (12–29)	20 (15–27)	0.88
	PPE	20 (12–29)	19 (13–27)	17 (9–21)	
Time to 1st defibrillation (s)	Control	66 (50–101)	68 (48–99)	67 (47–107)	0.16
	PPE	86 (65–119)	80 (67–116)	96 (74–121)	
Time to epinephrine administration (s)	Control	264 (201–312)	263 (185–307)	276 (190–317)	0.82
	PPE	324 (283–348)	326 (277–392)	299 (284–373)	
Time to amiodarone administration (s)	Control	298 (262–339)	301 (276–324)	306 (276–359)	0.42
	PPE	418 (380–448)	430 (392–476)	419 (385–465)	
Total task load	Control	56 (46–70)	58 (45–69)	58 (46–68)	0.63
	PPE	63 (56–71)	62 (51–72)	63 (52–69)	
Mental demand	Control	75 (60–85)	70 (55–85)	70 (55–80)	0.30
	PPE	73 (55–85)	70 (50–85)	70 (55–85)	
Physical demand	Control	60 (40–75)	55 (35–75)	60 (35–75)	0.55
	PPE	60 (35–85)	65 (45–75)	60 (30–75)	
Temporal demand	Control	70 (55–85)	70 (50–85)	70 (50–80)	0.41
	PPE	75 (55–85)	70 (50–85)	75 (55–85)	
Performance	Control	60 (35–75)	55 (35–75)	60 (40–80)	0.35
	PPE	68 (45–85)	65 (45–75)	65 (45–75)	
Effort	Control	65 (50–80)	65 (50–80)	65 (50–80)	0.64
	PPE	70 (55–80)	70 (50–80)	65 (50–75)	
Frustration	Control	55 (30–75)	55 (35–75)	55 (30–70)	0.53
	PPE	48 (25–70)	50 (25–70)	50 (35–70)	

Data are medians [IQR] and were analysed using 2-factor ANOVA with group (control or PPE) and leadership allocation as independent between-subject factors. The P-value indicates the effect of the factor leadership. For all outcomes the interactive term group leadership was statistically not significant. PPE = personal protective equipment.

The PPE teams perceived higher task loads than the control group teams (57 (44–67) vs. 63 (53–71); difference 6, 95% CI for difference 5–8, $p < 0.0001$) and scored higher in the domains physical and temporal demand, performance, and effort (Table 3). Leadership allocation had no effect on the overall task load ($p = 0.63$) nor on any of the six domains (Table 2).

Table 3. NASA task load index questionnaire data.

	Control Group ($n = 1451$)	PPE Group ($n = 689$)	Difference (95% CI)	p
Total task load	57 (44–67)	63 (53–71)	6 (5–8)	0.0001
Mental demand	70 (50–80)	70 (55–85)	0 (0–5)	0.073
Physical demand	55 (35–75)	60 (35–80)	5 (0–5)	0.005
Temporal demand	65 (50–80)	70 (50–85)	5 (5–10)	0.001
Performance	60 (35–75)	65 (45–80)	5 (5–10)	0.001
Effort	60 (50–75)	65 (50–80)	5 (0–5)	0.001
Frustration	50 (30–70)	50 (25–70)	0 (0–5)	0.87

Data are medians [IQR]. Estimates for differences between medians and their approximate confidence intervals were obtained by the Hodges–Lehmann estimation.

4. Discussion

This prospective comparative trial demonstrates that wearing PPE while performing CPR increased the rescuers' task-load and resulted in lower hands-on times, too few change-overs, and delays in defibrillation and the administration of drugs. Designated leadership did not mitigate the additional burden imposed by PPE.

To the best of our knowledge, this is the first large-scale trial on the effects of PPE in CPR teams. Simulator-based cross-over studies from the pre-COVID-19 area reported a significant deterioration in chest compression performance in participants wearing level-C PPE [8,13,14]. Studies conducted during the COVID-19 pandemic show conflicting results: in a simulator-based randomized study involving 36 residents, no significant effect of PPE on both depth and rate of chest compressions, and time for drugs preparation and administration was detected [11]; likewise, a simulator-based randomized cross-over study involving 32 BLS providers reported no negative effect of PPE on the quality of chest compressions [12]; as well as in another randomized controlled non-inferiority triple-crossover study with a total of 48 participants, in which no negative influence of PPE (specifically N95 +/− expiration valve) was found [28]. By contrast, a simulator-based randomized study involving 80 participants (23 physicians, 57 nurses) reported that compared to wearing a surgical mask, wearing an N95 mask increases a rescuer's fatigue and decreases the chest compression quality during CPR [15]. In simulator-based randomized cross-over studisssses with participants dressed in full PPE during the pandemic, an automated chest compression device proved to be superior over manual chest compressions in both 35 students after the successful completion of an ACLS course [10] and 67 paramedics [9]. Of note, all above mentioned studies assessed the quality of performance of single rescuers only and only one [15] included data on hands-on time, the primary outcome of our trial.

In keeping with our findings of increased physical demand, performance, and effort in PPE teams, Chen et al. reported that rescuers' increases in heart rate, mean arterial pressure, and subjective fatigue scores were significantly more obvious with the use of PPE, which was associated with a significant decrease in effective chest compressions [8]. By contrast, Kienbacher et al. were able to demonstrate increased attention when performing basic life support while attention and dexterity were not inferior when wearing PPE, including N95 masks [29]. However, in light of a PPE-related gradual decrease in effective chest compressions resulting from increased rescuers' fatigue, our finding of too few change-overs in PPE teams is worrisome.

As far as we know, this is the first trial investigating leadership in the context of CPR teams equipped with PPE. Our results indicate that designated leadership is not able to mitigate the additional burden imposed by PPE.

Strengths of this trial include the large sample size and the perfectly identical conditions for all teams. Limitations include the non-randomized design and the absence of real patients. However, randomized trials on PPE in real COVID-19 cases are difficult to conduct. Moreover, simulation is increasingly regarded as an accepted tool for evaluation [21] and performance markers in simulator-based studies show a high agreement with findings in real cases.

Our study population consisted of physicians in their 2nd to 3rd year of residency that, at the time of the study, acted as potential first responders for cardiac arrests in their hospitals. In addition, we refrained from using special teaching, special PPE protocols, or habituation with repetitive exposure prior to testing our participants in the simulated scenario. As such, our results reflect the actual state of our participants' knowledge and skills and can be extrapolated to real-world settings. Unfortunately, chest compression depth, a benchmark for fatigue during CPR described in previous studies, could not be assessed with our mannequin due to technical limitations.

Clinical studies have established that deviations from CPR algorithms are associated with decreased rates of return of spontaneous circulation and survival to discharge [30,31]. The present experiment observed several shortcomings and deviations from CPR algorithms associated with PPE. While the negative impact of PPE on any single CPR performance marker may be regarded as small, their aggregated effect in combination with the initial delay of CPR due to "donning" may well be of clinical relevance and contribute to poor outcomes of CPR in COVID-19 patients [5–7].

Our results indicate that training CPR under the conditions which require PPE is warranted and may be a suitable countermeasure against shortcomings and delays. As first responders have to potentially act under various circumstances requiring PPE, PPE sessions should be integrated in regular teaching and training regardless of the current pandemic situation. The participants should be made aware of potential PPE-related increases in rescuers' fatigue and advised to frequently change-over.

5. Conclusions

Having to wear PPE during CPR is an additional burden for rescuers involved in an already demanding task. PPE is associated with an increase in perceived task load and lower hands-on times, fewer change-overs, and delays in defibrillation and the administration of drugs. These findings should be considered in future resuscitation training.

Author Contributions: Conceptualization, M.N., T.S. and S.M.; Data curation, M.N., T.S. and C.C.; Formal analysis, M.N., T.S., S.C.T. and S.M.; Funding acquisition, T.S., D.W. and H.S.; Investigation, M.N., T.S., C.C. and S.M.; Methodology, T.S. and S.M.; Project administration, T.S., S.C.T. and S.M.; Resources, T.S., D.W. and H.S.; Software, S.M.; Supervision, T.S., D.W., H.S. and S.M.; Validation, T.S.; Visualization, S.M.; Writing—Original draft, M.N. and T.S.; Writing—Review & editing, T.S., C.C., S.C.T. and S.M. All authors have read and agreed to the published version of the manuscript.

Funding: This research received no external funding.

Institutional Review Board Statement: The study was conducted according to the guidelines of the Declaration of Helsinki, and approved by the Ethics Committee of Aerztekammer Westfalen-Lippe (2020-602-f-S) that waived the obligation to obtain consent. The study is registered at the German Clinical Trial Registry (www.drks.de (accessed on 7 October 2020); DRKS-ID: DRKS00023184).

Informed Consent Statement: Participants consent was waived due to the anonymity of the compiled data.

Data Availability Statement: The data presented in this study are available on request from the corresponding author.

Conflicts of Interest: The authors declare no conflict of interest.

References

1. Kundra, P.; Vinayagam, S. COVID-19 cardiopulmonary resuscitation: Guidelines and modifications. *J. Anaesthesiol. Clin. Pharm.* **2020**, *36*, S39–S44. [CrossRef]
2. Nolan, J.P.; Monsieurs, K.G.; Bossaert, L.; Bottiger, B.W.; Greif, R.; Lott, C.; Madar, J.; Olasveengen, T.M.; Roehr, C.C.; Semeraro, F.; et al. European Resuscitation Council COVID-19 guidelines executive summary. *Resuscitation* **2020**, *153*, 45–55. [CrossRef]
3. World Health Organization. *Rational Use of Personal Protective Equipment for Coronavirus Disease (COVID-19) and Considerations during Severe Shortages: Interim Guidance, 6 April 2020*; WHO/2019-nCov/IPC_PPE_use/2020.3; World Health Organization: Geneva, Switzerland, 2020.
4. Couper, K.; Taylor-Phillips, S.; Grove, A.; Freeman, K.; Osokogu, O.; Court, R.; Mehrabian, A.; Morley, P.T.; Nolan, J.P.; Soar, J.; et al. COVID-19 in cardiac arrest and infection risk to rescuers: A systematic review. *Resuscitation* **2020**, *151*, 59–66. [CrossRef]
5. Lim, Z.J.; Ponnapa Reddy, M.; Afroz, A.; Billah, B.; Shekar, K.; Subramaniam, A. Incidence and outcome of out-of-hospital cardiac arrests in the COVID-19 era: A systematic review and meta-analysis. *Resuscitation* **2020**, *157*, 248–258. [CrossRef]
6. Thapa, S.B.; Kakar, T.S.; Mayer, C.; Khanal, D. Clinical Outcomes of In-Hospital Cardiac Arrest in COVID-19. *JAMA Intern. Med.* **2021**, *181*, 279–281. [CrossRef] [PubMed]
7. Hayek, S.S.; Brenner, S.K.; Azam, T.U.; Shadid, H.R.; Anderson, H.; Berlin, H.; Pan, M.; Meloche, C.; Feroz, R.; OGÇÖHayer, P.; et al. In-hospital cardiac arrest in critically ill patients with COVID-19: Multicenter cohort study. *BMJ* **2020**, *371*, m3513. [CrossRef] [PubMed]
8. Chen, J.; Lu, K.Z.; Yi, B.; Chen, Y. Chest Compression With Personal Protective Equipment During Cardiopulmonary Resuscitation: A Randomized Crossover Simulation Study. *Medicine (Baltimore)* **2016**, *95*, e3262. [CrossRef]
9. Malysz, M.; Smereka, J.; Jaguszewski, M.; Dabrowski, M.; Nadolny, K.; Ruetzler, K.; Ladny, J.; Sterlinski, M.; Filipiak, K.; Szarpak, L. An optimal chest compression technique using personal protective equipment during resuscitation in the COVID-19 pandemic: A randomized crossover simulation study. *Kardiol. Pol. (Pol. Heart J.)* **2020**, *78*, 1254–1261. [CrossRef] [PubMed]
10. Malysz, M.; Dabrowski, M.; Böttiger, B.W.; Smereka, J.; Kulak, K.; Szarpak, A.; Jaguszewski, M.; Filipiak, K.J.; Ladny, J.R.; Ruetzler, K.; et al. Resuscitation of the patient with suspected/confirmed COVID-19 when wearing personal protective equipment: A randomized multicenter crossover simulation trial. *Cardiol. J.* **2020**, *27*, 497–506.
11. Mormando, G.; Paganini, M.; Alexopoulos, C.; Savino, S.; Bortoli, N.; Pomiato, D.; Graziano, A.; Navalesi, P.; Fabris, F. Life-Saving Procedures Performed While Wearing CBRNe Personal Protective Equipment: A Mannequin Randomized Trial. *Simul. Healthc.* **2021**, *16*, e200–e205. [CrossRef]
12. Rauch, S.; van Veelen, M.J.; Oberhammer, R.; Dal Cappello, T.; Roveri, G.; Gruber, E.; Strapazzon, G. Effect of Wearing Personal Protective Equipment (PPE) on CPR Quality in Times of the COVID-19 Pandemic-A Simulation, Randomised Crossover Trial. *J. Clin. Med.* **2021**, *10*, 1728. [CrossRef] [PubMed]
13. Kim, T.H.; Kim, C.H.; Shin, S.D.; Haam, S. Influence of personal protective equipment on the performance of life-saving interventions by emergency medical service personnel. *Simulation* **2016**, *92*, 893–898. [CrossRef]
14. Shin, D.M.; Kim, S.Y.; Shin, S.D.; Kim, C.H.; Kim, T.H.; Kim, K.Y.; Kim, J.H.; Hong, E.J. Effect of wearing personal protective equipment on cardiopulmonary resuscitation: Focusing on 119 emergency medical technicians. *Korean J. Emerg. Med. Serv.* **2015**, *19*, 19–32. [CrossRef]
15. Tian, Y.; Tu, X.; Zhou, X.; Yu, J.; Luo, S.; Ma, L.; Liu, C.; Zhao, Y.; Jin, X. Wearing a N95 mask increases rescuer's fatigue and decreases chest compression quality in simulated cardiopulmonary resuscitation. *Am. J. Emerg. Med.* **2021**, *44*, 434–438. [CrossRef] [PubMed]
16. Sahu, A.K.; Suresh, S.; Mathew, R.; Aggarwal, P.; Nayer, J. Impact of personal protective equipment on the effectiveness of chest compression—A systematic review and meta-analysis. *Am. J. Emerg. Med.* **2021**, *39*, 190–196. [CrossRef]
17. Doukas, D.; Arquilla, B.; Halpern, P.; Silverberg, M.; Sinert, R. The Impact of Personal Protection Equipment on Intubation Times. *Prehosp. Disaster Med.* **2021**, *36*, 375–379. [CrossRef] [PubMed]
18. Hunziker, S.; Semmer, N.K.; Tschan, F.; Schuetz, P.; Mueller, B.; Marsch, S. Dynamics and association of different acute stress markers with performance during a simulated resuscitation. *Resuscitation* **2012**, *83*, 572–578. [CrossRef]
19. Cooper, S.; Wakelam, A. Leadership of resuscitation teams: "Lighthouse Leadership". *Resuscitation* **1999**, *42*, 27–45. [CrossRef]
20. Hunziker, S.; Johansson, A.C.; Tschan, F.; Semmer, N.K.; Rock, L.; Howell, M.D.; Marsch, S. Teamwork and leadership in cardiopulmonary resuscitation. *J. Am. Coll. Cardiol.* **2011**, *57*, 2381–2388. [CrossRef]
21. Arriaga, A.F.; Bader, A.M.; Wong, J.M.; Lipsitz, S.R.; Berry, W.R.; Ziewacz, J.E.; Hepner, D.L.; Boorman, D.J.; Pozner, C.N.; Smink, D.S.; et al. Simulation-Based Trial of Surgical-Crisis Checklists. *N. Engl. J. Med.* **2013**, *368*, 246–253. [CrossRef]
22. Cheng, A.; Kessler, D.; Mackinnon, R.; Chang, T.P.; Nadkarni, V.M.; Hunt, E.A.; Duval-Arnould, J.; Lin, Y.; Cook, D.A.; Pusic, M.; et al. Reporting Guidelines for Health Care Simulation Research: Extensions to the CONSORT and STROBE Statements. *Simul. Healthc.* **2016**, *1*, 1–13. [CrossRef] [PubMed]
23. Sellmann, T.; Oendorf, A.; Wetzchewald, D.; Schwager, H.; Thal, S.C.; Marsch, S. The Impact of Withdrawn vs. Agitated Relatives during Resuscitation on Team Workload: A Single-Center Randomised Simulation-Based Study. *J. Clin. Med.* **2022**, *11*, 3163. [CrossRef] [PubMed]

24. Willmes, M.; Sellmann, T.; Semmer, N.; Tschan, F.; Wetzchewald, D.; Schwager, H.; Russo, S.G.; Marsch, S. Impact of family presence during cardiopulmonary resuscitation on team performance and perceived task load: A prospective randomised simulator-based trial. *BMJ Open* **2022**, *12*, e056798. [CrossRef] [PubMed]
25. Zöllner, K.; Sellmann, T.; Wetzchewald, D.; Schwager, H.; Cleff, C.; Thal, S.C.; Marsch, S. U SO CARE—The Impact of Cardiac Ultrasound during Cardiopulmonary Resuscitation: A Prospective Randomized Simulator-Based Trial. *J. Clin. Med.* **2021**, *10*, 5218. [CrossRef]
26. Hart, S.G. Nasa-Task Load Index (NASA-TLX); 20 Years Later. *Proc. Hum. Factors Ergon. Soc. Annu. Meet.* **2006**, *50*, 904–908. [CrossRef]
27. Colligan, L.; Potts, H.W.W.; Finn, C.T.; Sinkin, R.A. Cognitive workload changes for nurses transitioning from a legacy system with paper documentation to a commercial electronic health record. *Int. J. Med. Inform.* **2015**, *84*, 469–476. [CrossRef]
28. Kienbacher, C.L.; Grafeneder, J.; Tscherny, K.; Krammel, M.; Fuhrmann, V.; Niederer, M.; Neudorfsky, S.; Herbich, K.; Schreiber, W.; Herkner, H.; et al. The use of personal protection equipment does not impair the quality of cardiopulmonary resuscitation: A prospective triple-cross over randomised controlled non-inferiority trial. *Resuscitation* **2021**, *160*, 79–83. [CrossRef]
29. Kienbacher, C.L.; Grafeneder, J.; Tscherny, K.; Krammel, M.; Fuhrmann, V.; Niederer, M.; Neudorfsky, S.; Herbich, K.; Schreiber, W.; Herkner, H.; et al. The use of personal protection equipment does not negatively affect paramedics' attention and dexterity: A prospective triple-cross over randomized controlled non-inferiority trial. *Scand. J. Trauma Resusc. Emerg. Med.* **2022**, *30*, 2. [CrossRef]
30. Crowley, C.P.; Salciccioli, J.D.; Kim, E.Y. The association between ACLS guideline deviations and outcomes from in-hospital cardiac arrest. *Resuscitation* **2020**, *153*, 65–70. [CrossRef]
31. Honarmand, K.; Mepham, C.; Ainsworth, C.; Khalid, Z. Adherence to advanced cardiovascular life support (ACLS) guidelines during in-hospital cardiac arrest is associated with improved outcomes. *Resuscitation* **2018**, *129*, 76–81. [CrossRef]

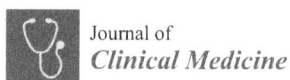

Review

Developments in Post-Resuscitation Care for Out-of-Hospital Cardiac Arrests in Adults—A Narrative Review

Stephan Katzenschlager [1,*], Erik Popp [1], Jan Wnent [2,3,4], Markus A. Weigand [1] and Jan-Thorsten Gräsner [2,3]

1. Department of Anesthesiology, Heidelberg University Hospital, 69120 Heidelberg, Germany; erik.popp@med.uni-heidelberg.de (E.P.); markus.weigand@med.uni-heidelberg.de (M.A.W.)
2. Institute for Emergency Medicine, University Hospital Schleswig-Holstein, 24105 Kiel, Germany; jan.wnent@uksh.de (J.W.); jan-thorsten.graesner@uksh.de (J.-T.G.)
3. Department of Anesthesiology and Intensive Care Medicine, University Hospital Schleswig-Holstein, Campus Kiel, 24105 Kiel, Germany
4. School of Medicine, University of Namibia, Windhoek 9000, Namibia
* Correspondence: stephan.katzenschlager@med.uni-heidelberg.de; Tel.: +49-6221-56-39683

Abstract: This review focuses on current developments in post-resuscitation care for adults with an out-of-hospital cardiac arrest (OHCA). As the incidence of OHCA is high and with a low percentage of survival, it remains a challenge to treat those who survive the initial phase and regain spontaneous circulation. Early titration of oxygen in the out-of-hospital phase is not associated with increased survival and should be avoided. Once the patient is admitted, the oxygen fraction can be reduced. To maintain an adequate blood pressure and urine output, noradrenaline is the preferred agent over adrenaline. A higher blood pressure target is not associated with higher rates of good neurological survival. Early neuro-prognostication remains a challenge, and prognostication bundles should be used. Established bundles could be extended by novel biomarkers and methods in the upcoming years. Whole blood transcriptome analysis has shown to reliably predict neurological survival in two feasibility studies. This needs further investigation in larger cohorts.

Keywords: post-resuscitation care; out-of-hospital cardiac arrest; resuscitation; intensive care

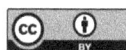

1. Introduction

Out-of-hospital cardiac arrest (OHCA) remains a high burden for society and caregivers, with an annual incidence between 67 and 170 per 100,000 inhabitants in Europe, whereas the percentage of survival is reported to be 8% [1,2]. Studies focusing on specific treatments and populations achieve higher survival rates, which might not reflect the true rates in these countries. Rates of good neurological outcome vary between 3% and 8% for national registries [3,4].

Post-resuscitation care for OHCA has been continually improved over the last few years, with the aim of improving survival with favorable neurological outcomes, according to the cerebral performance category (CPC) or modified ranking scale (mRS). The return of spontaneous circulation (ROSC) is dependent on known factors, such as: shockable rhythm [5,6], preexisting conditions [7], bystander cardiopulmonary resuscitation (CPR) [8,9] and early defibrillation [10]. Early recognition and call for help in patients with typical chest pain is still the main link in the chain of survival [11]. This is easier said than done, as it takes education to recognize a critically ill person and a system to receive the emergency call, send adequate help, give first aid advice and perform telephone-CPR if necessary [12]. If this link is missing, the chances of survival diminish.

Early restoration of circulation, whether spontaneous or assisted via extracorporeal cardiopulmonary resuscitation (eCPR), is one cornerstone to initiate post-resuscitation care in OHCA [13]. Prediction scores for ROSC [14] can help determine which patients might be suitable for eCPR strategies if conventional measures fail at a certain timepoint. A recent evaluation of a prediction score for good neurological outcomes after OHCA identified variables to be of relevance only until admission of the patient [15], indicating that initial circumstances and prehospital therapy are the main drivers of good neurological outcomes.

This review highlights important studies assessing the treatment strategies for post-resuscitation care in patients with OHCA.

Narrative Review

We selected articles cited by recent guidelines on post-resuscitation care [16] and used backwards and forwards reference searching to identify relevant articles. No systematic review was conducted. Articles were considered eligible if they were published within the last couple of years, without applying a strict cut off. No restrictions regarding language, country or type of study (e.g., observational vs. randomized) were made. Studies assessing only in-hospital cardiac arrest were not considered to be eligible for this review.

2. Post-Resuscitation Care—Changes from 2015 to 2021

In 2021, the current joint guideline from the European Resuscitation Council (ERC) and European Society of Intensive Care Medicine (ESICM) for post-resuscitation care in an intensive care unit (ICU) was released [16]. Several changes and novelties were introduced; these are herein summarized and put into context with the current literature.

For the first time, ERC and ESICM are emphasizing on the admission of patients with non-traumatic OHCA to a dedicated cardiac arrest center (CAC) [17]. This is expected to ultimately reduce morbidity and mortality. Due to the logistics of CAC, early percutaneous coronary intervention (PCI), temperature management and computer tomography should be achieved.

In 2015, the guideline recommended a mean arterial pressure (MAP) to achieve a urine output of 1 mL/kg/h and normal or decreasing lactate levels. This changed to the avoidance of hypotension (MAP < 65 mm Hg), urine output of >0.5 mL/kg/h and normal or decreasing lactate levels in the 2021 guidelines. Further, individualized MAP targets should be considered to enable adequate organ perfusion.

Temperature control between 32 °C and 36 °C was specified to be constant for at least 24 h. In addition, avoidance of fever for at least 72 h was explicitly recommended. A routine use of prophylactic antibiotics was not recommended. As for prognostication, neuron-specific enolase (NSE) was further specified with a predefined cut-off value of >60 µg/L at 48 h and 72 h, indicating a poor neurological outcome.

2.1. Oxygenation/Ventilation

After ROSC, it is recommended that patients maintain normoxaemia with an SpO_2 of 94–98% or PaO_2 of 75 to 100 mm Hg [16]. Early titration of oxygen saturation was investigated in patients with prehospital ROSC transported by paramedics [18]. Herein, 425 patients were randomized to the intervention group, which targeted a SpO_2 of 90% to 94%. Patients in the control group were targeted to a SpO_2 of 98% to 100%. The primary outcome was survival to hospital discharge, and there were nine secondary outcomes such as hypoxia or survival with a CPC score of 1–2. Out of 647 eligible patients, 425 were included in the final analysis. The main proportion of patients were male with a median age of 66 and 64 years in the intervention and control groups, respectively.

Both groups had high rates of bystander-witnessed arrests, bystander CPR and shockable rhythm. Survival to hospital discharge was lower in the intervention group, touching the level of significance (odds ratio (OR) 0.68 [95% confidence interval [CI] 0.46 to 1.00]; $p = 0.05$). Secondary analysis showed a significantly higher odds ratio (OR) of hypoxic ($SpO_2 < 90\%$) episodes prior to ICU admission in the interventions group (OR 2.37 [95%CI 1.49 to 3.79]); however, the rates of rearrests and good neurological outcomes were similar. This study indicates that an SpO_2 between 90% and 94% in patients with OHCA and ROSC can decrease survival rates.

In a different study, investigating how different oxygenation strategies in adults with OHCA and ROSC admitted to the ICU can have an impact, Schmidt et al. conducted a randomized controlled trial (RCT) [19]. These patients were randomized to receive either a restrictive (68 to 75 mm Hg) or liberal (98 to 105 mm Hg) oxygenation strategy for up to 5 days. A total of 789 patients were included in the final analysis. Baseline characteristics did not differ between the two groups. A higher proportion of men were included, with a mean age of 62 years, and with high rates of shockable rhythm (85%) and bystander CPR (89%). The primary outcome was death at 90 days or hospital discharge with a CPC score of 3–5, where no differences between both groups were found. Survival rates were 70% across both groups with a median CPC score of 1, indicating an a priori selected group of patients with a good probability of favorable neurological survival. Hypoxic events were not reported.

Early titration with lower targeted SpO_2 values may decrease the chances of survival with good neurological outcomes, whereas in an ICU setting, a restrictive oxygenation strategy can be chosen without compromising the chances of survival. Mortality in correlation to PaO_2 levels in critical ill patients have a U-shaped distribution [20]. Robba et al. performed a secondary analysis of the TTM_2 trial, investigating the effects of hypo- and hyperoxemia within the first 72 h of admission on mortality and neurological status at 6 months. This multivariate Cox regression also showed a U-shaped distribution for PaO_2 with an increased risk for mortality below 69 mm Hg (hypoxemia) and above 195 mm Hg (hyperoxemia); however, it found no correlation for poor neurological outcomes [21]. PaO_2 was significantly lower in non-survivors for up to 32 h after ICU admission. In a different trial, the presence of hyperoxemia ($PaO_2 > 300$ mm Hg) for a 1 h period increased the risk of poor neurological outcomes by 3% (relative risk 1.03 [95% CI 1.02 to 1.05]) [22].

Clinical trials investigating different oxygen levels in OHCA were conducted within the "safe" range of the curve, thus questioning if this U-shaped curve is still of relevance [23]. Several observational studies investigated the association between severe hyperoxemia ($PaO_2 > 300$ mm Hg) and mortality or neurological outcomes. La Via et al. performed a meta-analysis across 13 observational studies and found that severe hyperoxemia is associated with a poor neurological outcome (OR 1.37 [95% CI 1.01 to 1.86]) and higher mortality (OR 1.32 [95% CI 1.11 to 1.57]) [24]. Furthermore, hyperoxemia during the first 36 h of ICU admission showed higher OR for poor neurological outcomes and mortality with 1.52 (95% CI 1.12 to 2.08) and 1.40 (95% CI 1.18 to 1.66), respectively.

Carbon dioxide is recommended to be kept from 35 to 45 mm Hg in patients requiring mechanical ventilation after ROSC. In a retrospective cohort study in Japan, normocapnia (35 to 45 mm Hg) and mild hypercapnia (45 to 55 mm Hg) during the first 24 h after ROSC were associated with a better neurological outcome [25]. This analysis was adjusted for multiple covariates which are known to influence outcomes in patients with OHCA. This study is in line with the guideline recommendations and further emphasizes the avoidance of hypocapnia in patients with ROSC. However, mechanical ventilation during CPR has shown to be unreliable as the overall deviation of the predetermined tidal volume was −21% [26]. This can result in higher $PaCO_2$ levels after ROSC and should be closely monitored. Further, tidal volumes during chest compressions should be assessed if mechanical ventilation is used. An increase in the respiratory rate during OHCA does not seem to have an effect on PCO_2, pH and ROSC rates [27]. Patients suffering from OHCA which achieved sustained ROSC and ICU admission receiving TTM were assessed for impacts of ventilator settings in the initial 72 h on mortality and neurological outcomes [28]. Analyzing ventilator parameters in 1848 patients, a higher respiratory rate was identified as being associated with a higher mortality rate and worse neurological outcomes.

2.2. Circulation/Vasopressors

As per the guideline recommendation, hypotension (MAP < 65 mm Hg) should be avoided. However, there is no clear definition on a MAP target above 65 mm Hg. To test the hypothesis of whether a higher MAP impacts the rate of all-cause mortality or

CPC score 3–4, Kjaergaard et al. conducted a randomized controlled trial comparing two different MAP targets, 63 vs. 77 mm Hg in comatose adults after OHCA [29]. The baseline characteristics are described above in the study by Schmidt et al. To maintain the study's specific MAP target, volume resuscitation, noradrenaline and dobutamine were used. No difference in mortality or unfavorable neurological outcomes between these two groups (32% vs. 34%, p = 0.56) was found. Secondary endpoints also showed no differences between the two groups, indicating that a higher MAP target does not improve overall survival and good neurological outcomes until 90 days.

To achieve and maintain this target, different medications can be used. In a multicenter observational study, 766 patients were included with post-ROSC shock. Of those, 481 received noradrenaline and 285 adrenaline to maintain an adequate MAP. Both groups had high rates of witnessed arrests (90%) and bystander CPR before EMS arrival (71%), with half of the patients having initial shockable rhythm.

Propensity score analysis and adjusted logistic regression found higher OR for all-cause mortality with 2.1 (95% CI 1.1 to 4) and 2.6 (95% CI 1.4 to 4.7), respectively. Unfavorable neurological outcomes (CPC 3-5) at discharge for patients receiving adrenaline had ORs of 4.3 (95% CI 2.2 to 8.3) and 5.5 (95% CI 3 to 10.3), respectively [30]. Although observational trials have certain biases, this finding impacts the further treatment of patients with hypotension after ROSC and supports the guideline recommendations on the usage of noradrenaline.

2.3. Glucose

As hyperglycemia is often observed after OHCA [31], the American Diabetes Association recommended a range from 140 to 180 mg/dL for critically ill patients, respectively, such as those admitted to an ICU after OHCA [32]. In order manage hyperglycemia, a continuous insulin infusion is favored over repetitive applications [16]. As hypoglycemia (<70 mg/dL) is harmful, blood glucose levels should be monitored closely [33].

2.4. Percutaneous Coronary Intervention

After stabilization of the patient, PCI should be performed in all patients with presumed or obvious cardiac causes of cardiac arrest [16]. This has shown to be beneficial in all patients with ECG changes in line with occlusion myocardial infarction (OMI). In patients with ROSC after OHCA without ST-segment elevation, Desch et al. investigated if an immediate PCI strategy would provide a benefit over a delayed PCI strategy [34]. This study investigated death from any cause at 30 days as the primary outcome and survival with severe neurological deficit as a secondary endpoint. In total, 554 patients were randomized to either an immediate or delayed angiography. With similar baseline characteristics, angiography was performed 2.9 h or 46.9 h after OHCA, respectively. This study found no benefit for an immediate angiography, as the primary endpoint was reached in 54% of the immediate group and 46% of the delayed group (hazard ratio [HR] 1.28 [95% CI 1.00 to 1.63]). This finding corroborates other trials that have failed to show survival benefits for an early coronary angiography strategy in patients after OHCA without ST-segment elevation [35–37]. In contrast to these RCTs, observational studies showed results in favor of early angiography [38].

Therefore, the current guidelines recommend early angiography to patients with hemodynamic instability or those of high suspicion for a cardiac cause [39,40].

2.5. Temperature Management/Fever Prevention

Temperature control has been discussed over the last two decades. The initial trials have shown a benefit when patients are initially cooled between 32 °C and 34 °C [41]; however, recent trials have found no difference in survival [42]. This is further corroborated by two meta-analyses from Aneman et al. and Sanfilippo et al. [43,44]. Aneman et al. conducted a Bayesian meta-analysis across seven RCTs, which identified no significant risk ratio (RR) for mortality (RR 0.96 [95%CI 0.82 to 1.04]) and unfavorable neurological outcomes (RR 0.93 [95%CI 0.84 to 1.02]) [43]. Sanfilippo et al. included eight RCTs which compared TTM to either actively controlled or uncontrolled hypothermia [44]. In the overall study group and actively controlled subgroup, no significant differences for mortality were found, with RRs of 1.06 (95% CI 0.94 to 1.20) and 0.97 (95% CI 0.90 to 1.04), respectively. In the passively controlled normothermia subgroup, a significant difference for mortality was observed (RR 1.31 [95% CI 1.07 to 1.59]). Temperature control to 32–34 °C did not influence neurological outcomes, with an overall RR of 1.17 (95% CI 0.97 to 1.41).

While there is a constant debate about patient selection and the time until hypothermia was initiated in those studies, current guidelines recommend the temperature control to be between 32 °C and 36 °C for at least 24 h, and further prevention of fever for 72 h. To understand if a longer TTM strategy after the initial 24 h is beneficial, Hassager et al. conducted a randomized controlled trial. In this study, patients after OHCA who remained comatose were randomized to receive TTM either 12 or 48 h after the initial 24 h. No difference was found in the composite outcome of death or CPC score 3–4 at 90 days (HR 0.99 [95% CI 0.77 to 1.26], $p = 0.70$) [45].

2.6. Antibiotics/Further Medications

Many patients aspirate during cardiac arrest and undergo mechanical ventilation during the initial course of ICU therapy. Due to temperature management and prevention of fever, clinical signs of infection can be missed. Current guidelines do not support the routine administration of antibiotics in patients with ROSC. If clinical signs of an infection persist after OHCA, these patients benefit from an antibiotic treatment. Patients requiring mechanical ventilation after OHCA are at risk of ventilator-associated pneumonia (VAP). Therefore, a preventive strategy with short-term antibiotic therapy was assessed by Francois et al. [46]. Patients with initial shockable rhythm receiving temperature management between 32 °C and 34 °C were randomized to either amoxicillin-clavulanate or placebo. This trial included 194 patients in both groups and resulted in a lower incidence of early VAP in the intervention group (19% vs. 34%). These results were mirrored in the significant reduction in VAP at any timepoint (23% vs. 39%). However, due to the small sample size, this did not impact mortality rates at day 28 (41% vs. 37%) or ICU length of stay. Even if this trial included only patients with shockable rhythm, these findings can be generalized to patients with non-shockable rhythm, as post-resuscitation care is similar between those groups.

A meta-analysis on prophylactic antibiotic use after OHCA did not show a significant increase in overall survival (OR 1.16 [95% CI 0.97 to 1.40]) or survival with good neurological outcomes (OR 2.25 [95% CI 0.93 to 5.45]) [47].

The usage of stress ulcer prophylaxis is recommended, even if it does not reduce mortality in ICU patients [48]. As patients after OHCA often are treated with antiplatelet and anticoagulant medication [49], they are at a higher risk of gastrointestinal (GI) bleeding. The usage of ulcer prophylaxis has shown to reduce the rates of GI bleeding in high-risk ICU patients [50].

2.7. Prognostication

Prognostication can already be started during advanced life support (ALS) using near-infrared spectroscopy (NIRS) to assess cerebral oximetry (rSO_2). During CPR, increasing rSO_2 values might be indicative of ROSC [51]. In an analysis of 52 patients with OHCA, initial rSO_2 values were undetectable (<15%) and increased rapidly with near-normalization in patients who achieved ROSC. Patients with ROSC had a higher maximum value at 47% vs. 31% in those without ROSC [52]. Patients undergoing eCPR with a pre-cannulation rSO_2 between 41% and 60% had the highest chance of good neurological survival (CPC 1 to 2) with almost 40% [53], while patients with a pre-cannulation rSO_2 between 17% and 40% and above 60% had just over 20% good neurological survival. Besides rSO_2, a rise in $etCO_2$ was also found to be of prognostic value. Keeping in mind that $etCO_2$ is prone to confounders such as respiratory rate, tidal volume and the type of airway device, the major limitation is that that an advanced airway must be applied.

After initial ICU treatment, the prognostication of neurological outcomes is one cornerstone in the early post-resuscitation care phase. This remains a challenge in post-resuscitation care as the false positive rate for the prediction of poor neurological outcomes should be 0%. Consequently, the reliable identification of patients who will not benefit from early invasive treatment strategies can be the main consequence of those tests. An inappropriate withdraw of life support must be avoided; this occurs due to a self-fulfilling prophecy bias [54,55]. Therefore, current guidelines recommend the investigation of prognostic biomarkers to be blinded. Withholding results from blood samples can be cumbersome and unethical in daily practice. To minimize these biases, an assessment of neurological outcomes is recommended to be performed at three-to-six months after OHCA [16].

Regarding biomarkers, NSE in combination with other tests is recommended to be the biomarker for neurological prognostication. A sole biomarker has substantial limitations for predictions, failing to safely identify patients with unfavorable neurological outcomes.

NSE is reported to decrease after 24 h in patients with good neurological outcomes and increase in those with unfavorable neurological outcomes between 48 and 96 h. This highlights that a single NSE value should be interpreted with caution; rather, its trend over the first few days is important. Further, hemolysis must be measured in order to detect false high NSE values [56]. Hemolysis was observed in more than half of the patients in up to 4 h after eCPR initiation; this rate decreased to approximately 10% after 24 h. In a retrospective cohort study of patients with OHCA and prehospital eCPR undergoing temperature management, there was a significant difference in NSE at 4 h between those with favorable neurological outcomes and those who died [57]. At 48 h, NSE could reliably distinguish between those with favorable and unfavorable neurological survival; this is while extracorporeal membrane oxygenation was still ongoing. The early withdraw of life support solely based on biomarkers is not recommended and should be avoided.

As a multi-modal approach, electroencephalogram (EEG) and cranial computed tomography (cCT)—besides others—are recommended. EEG has been thoroughly studied to predict brain function and prognosis after cardiac arrest [58]. It is described that EEG is suppressed immediately after OHCA and returns to normal voltage within 24 h in patients with good neurological outcomes [59]. CCT is used to evaluate the ratio between grey and white matter densities (grey–white ratio; GWR); this quantifies the degree of cerebral oedema. It is reported that a 100% specificity for unfavorable neurological outcomes was achieved between 1 h [60] and up to 72 h [61–63] after ROSC.

This bundle of prognostication can be extended by other biomarkers that are currently not recommended such as tau protein, neurofilament light chain, glial fibrillary acidic protein and ubiquitin C-terminal hydrolase-L1, which have recently been described to discriminate between favorable and unfavorable neurological outcomes [64].

In addition to the above-mentioned known and established neurological prognostic options, there is the possibility of whole blood transcriptome analysis [65,66]. One study was able to identify three biomarkers associated with poor neurological outcomes: MAPK3, BCL2 and AKT1 [65]. MAPK3 was significantly up-regulated in patients with poor neurological outcomes. This was further corroborated by multivariate logistic regression, where MAPK3 was the strongest independent predictor for poor neurological outcomes (OR 1.2 [95% CI 1.1 to 16.7]).

Tissier et al. found that HLA family genes were decreased in the group with poor neurological survival [66]. Here, logistic regression was able to predict clinical survival better compared to known person- and setting-specific factors with an area under the curve of 0.94 vs. 0.83, respectively [15]. Organ-specific damage can be assessed using cell-free DNA. This method enables the possibility to assess the potential damage to vital organs such as the brain, heart and lungs. Even if there are no trials in patients with OHCA to date, this method can be used in the future. A limitation can be the availability of expertise to carry out such tests; centralizing these analyses to specialized centers can help overcome this limitation.

These promising first results of additional biomarkers should be studied in future trials, investigating the early prediction of functional neurological outcomes and identifying patients that can benefit from early invasive strategies.

3. Discussion

This review assesses the current literature in post-resuscitation care in patients with OHCA. Herein, novel therapy strategies are highlighted and put into the perspective of current guidelines. Different strategies on oxygen and blood pressure levels did not improve survival. Oxygen titration in the initial ROSC phase can be harmful and should be avoided. Beside recent RCTs, observational trials and secondary analyses have shown that hyperoxemia is harmful and associated with an increased mortality rate, especially if PaO$_2$ exceeds 300 mm Hg. In patients with reliable pulse oximeter values, the titration of oxygen can be safe if SpO$_2$ is >99%, keeping in mind that these patients might deteriorate faster compared to other ventilated patients. Prehospital blood gas analysis can be beneficial in the early phase of ROSC, starting preliminary goal-directed treatment. With the prehospital availability of diagnostic tools, one must not forget that the overarching goal is still to admit the patient to an ICU or emergency department as soon as possible after OHCA. Different aspects of ventilation strategies have been discussed, where a secondary analysis found significantly higher OR for mortality in patients with a higher respiratory rate. Although emerging from a large cohort, these findings should still be interpreted with caution as these data are observational and the original trial focused on TTM [28,42]. Ventilation during OHCA needs further research, especially with respect to different respirators, airway devices and chest compression devices available. These possibilities also include manual chest compression and bag mask ventilation. Whether mild hypercapnia (PaCO$_2$ 50–55 mm Hg) within the first 24 h after OHCA is associated with a favorable neurological survival after six months is currently being investigated in the Targeted Therapeutic Mild Hypercapnia after Resuscitated Cardiac Arrest (TAME) trial [67]. These findings can impact future initial ICU treatment and are awaited to be published in June 2023.

The usage of noradrenaline in post-ROSC shock is corroborated, as a matched cohort study showed worse outcomes in patients receiving adrenaline infusion. As this study was not randomized or blinded, whether these results would change in a randomized study must be critically assessed. Further trials might not be impactful. The guidelines currently do not cover the aspect of return of circulation (ROC). As eCPR programs, in-hospital or pre-hospital are currently established around the globe, this challenge must be faced and recommendations for immediate post-ROC treatment are needed. Future studies can address a targeted MAP in the early phase of patients with eCPR.

PCI remains the primary strategy for patients with ST elevation myocardial infarction and in those with hemodynamic instability despite the lack of ST elevations. These recommendations are based on RCTs and have a good certainty of evidence (CoE).

Fever prevention remains critical and is one of the cornerstones in post-resuscitation care, whereas prophylactic antibiotic use does not increase favorable neurological outcomes Temperature management between 32 and 34 °C was not associated with an increase in favorable neurological outcomes.

Neuroprognostication is made at the patient's peril, as conformation bias affects our judgement. Therefore, the limitations of current methods should be considered when interpretating biomarkers and rSO$_2$. Most of the studies were either retrospective studies, observational trials or secondary analyses, limiting the CoE. Although it may be tempting to start prognosis as early as during the prehospital phase, this underlies certain limitations. RSO$_2$ is independent from motion artefacts, making it valid during CPR; however, cerebral blood flow is controlled by PaCO$_2$ in patients after OHCA [51].

Novel biomarkers and methods will emerge in the upcoming years and should be considered if feasibility is given outside of clinical studies. Further, a better understanding of their predictive value is needed.

4. Conclusions

"*Normo, normo, normo*" is the main goal in post-resuscitation care. Being above the normal ranges has been shown to be harmful in recent studies, especially regarding oxygenation, ventilation and temperature. Strategies to reduce early harm in the treatment of patients with ROSC have yet to be found. Prognostication is still a multi-modal approach, using both technical resources and biomarkers combined.

Author Contributions: Conceptualization, S.K. and J.-T.G.; writing—original draft preparation, S.K.; writing—review and editing, E.P., J.W., M.A.W. and J.-T.G.; supervision E.P. and J.-T.G. All authors have read and agreed to the published version of the manuscript.

Funding: This research received no external funding.

Institutional Review Board Statement: Not applicable.

Informed Consent Statement: Not applicable.

Data Availability Statement: Not applicable.

Conflicts of Interest: The authors declare no conflict of interest.

References

1. Gräsner, J.-T.; Herlitz, J.; Tjelmeland, I.B.; Wnent, J.; Masterson, S.; Lilja, G.; Bein, B.; Böttiger, B.W.; Rosell-Ortiz, F.; Nolan, J.P.; et al. European Resuscitation Council Guidelines 2021: Epidemiology of cardiac arrest in Europe. *Resuscitation* **2021**, *161*, 61–79. [CrossRef] [PubMed]
2. Gräsner, J.-T.; Wnent, J.; Herlitz, J.; Perkins, G.D.; Lefering, R.; Tjelmeland, I.; Koster, R.W.; Masterson, S.; Rossell-Ortiz, F.; Maurer, H.; et al. Survival after out-of-hospital cardiac arrest in Europe—Results of the EuReCa TWO study. *Resuscitation* **2020**, *148*, 218–226. [CrossRef] [PubMed]
3. Benjamin, E.J.; Virani, S.S.; Callaway, C.W.; Chamberlain, A.M.; Chang, A.R.; Cheng, S.; Chiuve, S.E.; Cushman, M.; Delling, F.N.; Deo, R.; et al. Heart Disease and Stroke Statistics-2018 Update: A Report From the American Heart Association. *Circulation* **2018**, *137*, e67–e492. [CrossRef] [PubMed]
4. Ong, M.E.H.; Shin, S.D.; De Souza, N.N.A.; Tanaka, H.; Nishiuchi, T.; Song, K.J.; Ko, P.C.-I.; Leong, B.S.-H.; Khunkhlai, N.; Naroo, G.Y.; et al. Outcomes for out-of-hospital cardiac arrests across 7 countries in Asia: The Pan Asian Resuscitation Outcomes Study (PAROS). *Resuscitation* **2015**, *96*, 100–108. [CrossRef] [PubMed]
5. Andrew, E.; Nehme, Z.; Lijovic, M.; Bernard, S.; Smith, K. Outcomes following out-of-hospital cardiac arrest with an initial cardiac rhythm of asystole or pulseless electrical activity in Victoria, Australia. *Resuscitation* **2014**, *85*, 1633–1639. [CrossRef]
6. Czapla, M.; Zielińska, M.; Kubica-Cielińska, A.; Diakowska, D.; Quinn, T.; Karniej, P. Factors associated with return of spontaneous circulation after out-of-hospital cardiac arrest in Poland: A one-year retrospective study. *BMC Cardiovasc. Disord.* **2020**, *20*, 288. [CrossRef] [PubMed]
7. Hirlekar, G.; Jonsson, M.; Karlsson, T.; Hollenberg, J.; Albertsson, P.; Herlitz, J. Comorbidity and survival in out-of-hospital cardiac arrest. *Resuscitation* **2018**, *133*, 118–123. [CrossRef]
8. Wnent, J.; Tjelmeland, I.; Lefering, R.; Koster, R.W.; Maurer, H.; Masterson, S.; Herlitz, J.; Böttiger, B.W.; Ortiz, F.R.; Perkins, G.D.; et al. To ventilate or not to ventilate during bystander CPR—A EuReCa TWO analysis. *Resuscitation* **2021**, *166*, 101–109. [CrossRef] [PubMed]
9. Dainty, K.N.; Colquitt, B.; Bhanji, F.; Hunt, E.A.; Jefkins, T.; Leary, M.; Ornato, J.P.; Swor, R.A.; Panchal, A.; on behalf of the Science Subcommittee of the American Heart Association Emergency Cardiovascular Care Committee. Understanding the Importance of the Lay Responder Experience in Out-of-Hospital Cardiac Arrest: A Scientific Statement From the American Heart Association. *Circulation* **2022**, *145*, e852–e867. [CrossRef]
10. Krammel, M.; Lobmeyr, E.; Sulzgruber, P.; Winnisch, M.; Weidenauer, D.; Poppe, M.; Datler, P.; Zeiner, S.; Keferboeck, M.; Eichelter, J.; et al. The impact of a high-quality basic life support police-based first responder system on outcome after out-of-hospital cardiac arrest. *PLoS ONE* **2020**, *15*, e0233966. [CrossRef]
11. Deakin, C.D. The chain of survival: Not all links are equal. *Resuscitation* **2018**, *126*, 80–82. [CrossRef] [PubMed]
12. Schnaubelt, S.; Greif, R.; Monsieurs, K. The chainmail of survival: A modern concept of an adaptive approach towards cardiopulmonary resuscitation. *Resuscitation* **2023**, *184*. [CrossRef] [PubMed]
13. Scquizzato, T.; Bonaccorso, A.; Swol, J.; Gamberini, L.; Scandroglio, A.M.; Landoni, G.; Zangrillo, A. Refractory out-of-hospital cardiac arrest and extracorporeal cardiopulmonary resuscitation: A meta-analysis of randomized trials. *Artif. Organs* **2023**. [CrossRef]
14. Gräsner, J.-T.; Meybohm, P.; Lefering, R.; Wnent, J.; Bahr, J.; Messelken, M.; Jantzen, T.; Franz, R.; Scholz, J.; Schleppers, A.; et al. ROSC after cardiac arrest—The RACA score to predict outcome after out-of-hospital cardiac arrest. *Eur. Heart J.* **2011**, *32*, 1649–1656. [CrossRef]

15. Seewald, S.; Wnent, J.; Lefering, R.; Fischer, M.; Bohn, A.; Jantzen, T.; Brenner, S.; Masterson, S.; Bein, B.; Scholz, J.; et al. CaRdiac Arrest Survival Score (CRASS)—A tool to predict good neurological outcome after out-of-hospital cardiac arrest. *Resuscitation* **2020**, *146*, 66–73. [CrossRef]
16. Nolan, J.P.; Soar, J.; Cariou, A.; Cronberg, T.; Moulaert, V.R.M.; Deakin, C.D.; Bottiger, B.W.; Friberg, H.; Sunde, K.; Sandroni, C. European Resuscitation Council and European Society of Intensive Care Medicine guidelines 2021 for post-resuscitation care. *Intensiv. Care Med.* **2021**, *161*, 220–269. [CrossRef]
17. Yeung, J.; Matsuyama, T.; Bray, J.; Reynolds, J.; Skrifvars, M.B. Does care at a cardiac arrest centre improve outcome after out-of-hospital cardiac arrest?—A systematic review. *Resuscitation* **2019**, *137*, 102–115. [CrossRef]
18. Bernard, S.A.; Bray, J.E.; Smith, K.; Stephenson, M.; Finn, J.; Grantham, H.; Hein, C.; Masters, S.; Stub, D.; Perkins, G.D.; et al. Effect of Lower vs Higher Oxygen Saturation Targets on Survival to Hospital Discharge Among Patients Resuscitated After Out-of-Hospital Cardiac Arrest: The EXACT Randomized Clinical Trial. *JAMA* **2022**, *328*, 1818–1826. [CrossRef]
19. Schmidt, H.; Kjaergaard, J.; Hassager, C.; Mølstrøm, S.; Grand, J.; Borregaard, B.; Obling, L.E.R.; Venø, S.; Sarkisian, L.; Mamaev, D.; et al. Oxygen Targets in Comatose Survivors of Cardiac Arrest. *N. Engl. J. Med.* **2022**, *387*, 1467–1476. [CrossRef]
20. Helmerhorst, H.J.F.; Arts, D.; Schultz, M.J.; Van Der Voort, P.H.J.; Abu-Hanna, A.; De Jonge, E.; Van Westerloo, D.J. Metrics of Arterial Hyperoxia and Associated Outcomes in Critical Care. *Crit. Care Med.* **2017**, *45*, 187–195. [CrossRef]
21. Robba, C.; Badenes, R.; Battaglini, D.; Ball, L.; Sanfilippo, F.; Brunetti, I.; Jakobsen, J.C.; Lilja, G.; Friberg, H.; Wendel-Garcia, P.D.; et al. Oxygen targets and 6-month outcome after out of hospital cardiac arrest: A pre-planned sub-analysis of the targeted hypothermia versus targeted normothermia after Out-of-Hospital Cardiac Arrest (TTM2) trial. *Crit. Care* **2022**, *26*, 323. [CrossRef]
22. Roberts, B.W.; Kilgannon, J.H.; Hunter, B.R.; Puskarich, M.A.; Pierce, L.; Donnino, M.; Leary, M.; Kline, J.A.; Jones, A.E.; Shapiro, N.I.; et al. Association Between Early Hyperoxia Exposure After Resuscitation From Cardiac Arrest and Neurological Disability: Prospective multicenter protocol-directed cohort study. *Circulation* **2018**, *137*, 2114–2124. [CrossRef] [PubMed]
23. Martin, D.; de Jong, A.; Radermacher, P. Is the U-shaped curve still of relevance to oxygenation of critically ill patients? *Intensiv. Care Med.* **2023**, 1–3. [CrossRef]
24. LA Via, L.; Astuto, M.; Bignami, E.G.; Busalacchi, D.; Dezio, V.; Girardis, M.; Lanzafame, B.; Ristagno, G.; Pelosi, P.; Sanfilippo, F. The effects of exposure to severe hyperoxemia on neurological outcome and mortality after cardiac arrest. *Minerva Anestesiol.* **2022**, *88*, 853–863. [CrossRef]
25. Okada, N.; Matsuyama, T.; Okada, Y.; Okada, A.; Kandori, K.; Nakajima, S.; Kitamura, T.; Ohta, B. Post-Resuscitation Partial Pressure of Arterial Carbon Dioxide and Outcome in Patients with Out-of-Hospital Cardiac Arrest: A Multicenter Retrospective Cohort Study. *J. Clin. Med.* **2022**, *11*, 1523. [CrossRef]
26. Orlob, S.; Wittig, J.; Hobisch, C.; Auinger, D.; Honnef, G.; Fellinger, T.; Ristl, R.; Schindler, O.; Metnitz, P.; Feigl, G.; et al. Reliability of mechanical ventilation during continuous chest compressions: A crossover study of transport ventilators in a human cadaver model of CPR. *Scand. J. Trauma Resusc. Emerg. Med.* **2021**, *29*, 102. [CrossRef]
27. Prause, G.; Zoidl, P.; Eichinger, M.; Eichlseder, M.; Orlob, S.; Ruhdorfer, F.; Honnef, G.; Metnitz, P.G.; Zajic, P. Mechanical ventilation with ten versus twenty breaths per minute during cardio-pulmonary resuscitation for out-of-hospital cardiac arrest: A randomised controlled trial. *Resuscitation* **2023**, 109765. [CrossRef]
28. Robba, C.; Badenes, R.; Battaglini, D.; Ball, L.; Brunetti, I.; Jakobsen, J.C.; Lilja, G.; Friberg, H.; Wendel-Garcia, P.D.; Young, P.J.; et al. Ventilatory settings in the initial 72 h and their association with outcome in out-of-hospital cardiac arrest patients: A preplanned secondary analysis of the targeted hypothermia versus targeted normothermia after out-of-hospital cardiac arrest (TTM2) trial. *Intensive Care Med.* **2022**, *48*, 1024–1038. [CrossRef]
29. Kjaergaard, J.; Møller, J.E.; Schmidt, H.; Grand, J.; Mølstrøm, S.; Borregaard, B.; Venø, S.; Sarkisian, L.; Mamaev, D.; Jensen, L.O.; et al. Blood-Pressure Targets in Comatose Survivors of Cardiac Arrest. *N. Engl. J. Med.* **2022**, *387*, 1456–1466. [CrossRef]
30. Bougouin, W.; Slimani, K.; Renaudier, M.; Binois, Y.; Paul, M.; Dumas, F.; Lamhaut, L.; Loeb, T.; Ortuno, S.; Deye, N.; et al. Epinephrine versus norepinephrine in cardiac arrest patients with post-resuscitation shock. *Intensive Care Med.* **2022**, *48*, 300–310. [CrossRef]
31. Skrifvars, M.B.; Pettilä, V.; Rosenberg, P.H.; Castrén, M. A multiple logistic regression analysis of in-hospital factors related to survival at six months in patients resuscitated from out-of-hospital ventricular fibrillation. *Resuscitation* **2003**, *59*, 319–328. [CrossRef] [PubMed]
32. American Diabetes Association. 15. Diabetes Care in the Hospital: Standards of Medical Care in Diabetes—2021. 2021. Available online: https://riu.austral.edu.ar/handle/123456789/1617 (accessed on 30 March 2023).
33. The NICE-SUGAR Study Investigators. Hypoglycemia and Risk of Death in Critically Ill Patients. *N. Engl. J. Med.* **2012**, *367*, 1108–1118. [CrossRef] [PubMed]
34. Desch, S.; Freund, A.; Akin, I.; Behnes, M.; Preusch, M.R.; Zelniker, T.A.; Skurk, C.; Landmesser, U.; Graf, T.; Eitel, I.; et al. Angiography after Out-of-Hospital Cardiac Arrest without ST-Segment Elevation. *N. Engl. J. Med.* **2021**, *385*, 2544–2553. [CrossRef]
35. Lemkes, J.S.; Janssens, G.N.; van der Hoeven, N.W.; Jewbali, L.S.; Dubois, E.A.; Meuwissen, M.; Rijpstra, T.A.; Bosker, H.A.; Blans, M.J.; Bleeker, G.B.; et al. Coronary Angiography after Cardiac Arrest without ST-Segment Elevation. *N. Engl. J. Med.* **2019**, *380*, 1397–1407. [CrossRef] [PubMed]

6. Kern, K.B.; Radsel, P.; Jentzer, J.C.; Seder, D.B.; Lee, K.S.; Lotun, K.; Janardhanan, R.; Stub, D.; Hsu, C.-H.; Noc, M. Randomized Pilot Clinical Trial of Early Coronary Angiography Versus No Early Coronary Angiography After Cardiac Arrest Without ST-Segment Elevation: The PEARL Study. *Circulation* 2020, *142*, 2002–2012. [CrossRef]
7. Hauw-Berlemont, C.; Lamhaut, L.; Diehl, J.-L.; Andreotti, C.; Varenne, O.; Leroux, P.; Lascarrou, J.-B.; Guerin, P.; Loeb, T.; Roupie, E.; et al. Emergency vs Delayed Coronary Angiogram in Survivors of Out-of-Hospital Cardiac Arrest: Results of the Randomized, Multicentric EMERGE Trial. *JAMA Cardiol.* 2022, *7*, 700–707. [CrossRef]
8. Kumar, S.; Abdelghaffar, B.; Iyer, M.; Shamaileh, G.; Nair, R.; Zheng, W.; Verma, B.; Menon, V.; Kapadia, S.R.; Reed, G.W. Coronary Angiography in Patients With Out-of-Hospital Cardiac Arrest Without ST-Segment Elevation on Electrocardiograms: A Comprehensive Review. *J. Soc. Cardiovasc. Angiogr. Interv.* 2023, *2*, 100536. [CrossRef]
9. Panchal, A.R.; Bartos, J.A.; Cabañas, J.G.; Donnino, M.W.; Drennan, I.R.; Hirsch, K.G.; Kudenchuk, P.J.; Kurz, M.C.; Lavonas, E.J.; Morley, P.T.; et al. Part 3: Adult Basic and Advanced Life Support: 2020 American Heart Association Guidelines for Cardiopulmonary Resuscitation and Emergency Cardiovascular Care. *Circulation* 2020, *142*, S366–S468. [CrossRef]
10. Ibanez, B.; James, S.; Agewall, S.; Antunes, M.J.; Bucciarelli-Ducci, C.; Bueno, H.; Caforio, A.L.P.; Crea, F.; Goudevenos, J.A.; Halvorsen, S.; et al. 2017 ESC Guidelines for the management of acute myocardial infarction in patients presenting with ST-segment elevation. *Eur. Heart J.* 2018, *39*, 119–177. [CrossRef]
11. Hypothermia after Cardiac Arrest Study Group. Mild Therapeutic Hypothermia to Improve the Neurologic Outcome after Cardiac Arrest. *N. Engl. J. Med.* 2002, *346*, 549–556. [CrossRef]
12. Dankiewicz, J.; Cronberg, T.; Lilja, G.; Jakobsen, J.C.; Levin, H.; Ullén, S.; Rylander, C.; Wise, M.P.; Oddo, M.; Cariou, A.; et al. Hypothermia versus Normothermia after Out-of-Hospital Cardiac Arrest. *N. Engl. J. Med.* 2021, *384*, 2283–2294. [CrossRef] [PubMed]
13. Aneman, A.; Frost, S.; Parr, M.; Skrifvars, M.B. Target temperature management following cardiac arrest: A systematic review and Bayesian meta-analysis. *Crit. Care* 2022, *26*, 58. [CrossRef] [PubMed]
14. Sanfilippo, F.; La Via, L.; Lanzafame, B.; Dezio, V.; Busalacchi, D.; Messina, A.; Ristagno, G.; Pelosi, P.; Astuto, M. Targeted Temperature Management after Cardiac Arrest: A Systematic Review and Meta-Analysis with Trial Sequential Analysis. *J. Clin. Med.* 2021, *10*, 3943. [CrossRef] [PubMed]
15. Hassager, C.; Schmidt, H.; Møller, J.E.; Grand, J.; Mølstrøm, S.; Beske, R.P.; Boesgaard, S.; Borregaard, B.; Bekker-Jensen, D.; Dahl, J.S.; et al. Duration of Device-Based Fever Prevention after Cardiac Arrest. *N. Engl. J. Med.* 2022, *388*, 888–897. [CrossRef] [PubMed]
16. François, B.; Cariou, A.; Clere-Jehl, R.; Dequin, P.-F.; Renon-Carron, F.; Daix, T.; Guitton, C.; Deye, N.; Legriel, S.; Plantefève, G.; et al. Prevention of Early Ventilator-Associated Pneumonia after Cardiac Arrest. *N. Engl. J. Med.* 2019, *381*, 1831–1842. [CrossRef]
17. Couper, K.; Laloo, R.; Field, R.; Perkins, G.D.; Thomas, M.; Yeung, J. Prophylactic antibiotic use following cardiac arrest: A systematic review and meta-analysis. *Resuscitation* 2019, *141*, 166–173. [CrossRef]
18. Krag, M.; Marker, S.; Perner, A.; Wetterslev, J.; Wise, M.P.; Schefold, J.C.; Keus, F.; Guttormsen, A.B.; Bendel, S.; Borthwick, M.; et al. Pantoprazole in Patients at Risk for Gastrointestinal Bleeding in the ICU. *N. Engl. J. Med.* 2018, *379*, 2199–2208. [CrossRef]
19. Gianforcaro, A.; Kurz, M.; Guyette, F.; Callaway, C.W.; Rittenberger, J.C.; Elmer, J. Association of antiplatelet therapy with patient outcomes after out-of-hospital cardiac arrest. *Resuscitation* 2017, *121*, 98–103. [CrossRef]
20. Wang, Y.; Ye, Z.; Ge, L.; Siemieniuk, R.A.C.; Wang, X.; Wang, Y.; Hou, L.; Ma, Z.; Agoritsas, T.; Vandvik, P.O.; et al. Efficacy and safety of gastrointestinal bleeding prophylaxis in critically ill patients: Systematic review and network meta-analysis. *BMJ* 2020, *368*, l6744. [CrossRef]
21. Sandroni, C.; Parnia, S.; Nolan, J.P. Cerebral oximetry in cardiac arrest: A potential role but with limitations. *Intensive Care Med.* 2019, *45*, 904–906. [CrossRef]
22. Prosen, G.; Strnad, M.; Doniger, S.J.; Markota, A.; Stožer, A.; Borovnik-Lesjak, V.; Mekiš, D. Cerebral tissue oximetry levels during prehospital management of cardiac arrest—A prospective observational study. *Resuscitation* 2018, *129*, 141–145. [CrossRef] [PubMed]
23. Bertini, P.; Marabotti, A.; Paternoster, G.; Landoni, G.; Sangalli, F.; Peris, A.; Bonizzoli, M.; Scolletta, S.; Franchi, F.; Rubino, A.; et al. Regional Cerebral Oxygen Saturation to Predict Favorable Outcome in Extracorporeal Cardiopulmonary Resuscitation: A Systematic Review and Meta-Analysis. *J. Cardiothorac. Vasc. Anesthesia* 2023, 1–8. [CrossRef] [PubMed]
24. Sandroni, C.; Cavallaro, F.; Callaway, C.W.; Sanna, T.; D'Arrigo, S.; Kuiper, M.; Della Marca, G.; Nolan, J.P. Predictors of poor neurological outcome in adult comatose survivors of cardiac arrest: A systematic review and meta-analysis. Part 1: Patients not treated with therapeutic hypothermia. *Resuscitation* 2015, *84*, 1310–1323. [CrossRef] [PubMed]
25. Sandroni, C.; Cavallaro, F.; Callaway, C.W.; D'arrigo, S.; Sanna, T.; Kuiper, M.A.; Biancone, M.; Della Marca, G.; Farcomeni, A.; Nolan, J.P. Predictors of poor neurological outcome in adult comatose survivors of cardiac arrest: A systematic review and meta-analysis. Part 2: Patients treated with therapeutic hypothermia. *Resuscitation* 2013, *84*, 1324–1338. [CrossRef]
26. Rundgren, M.; Cronberg, T.; Friberg, H.; Isaksson, A. Serum neuron specific enolase—Impact of storage and measuring method. *BMC Res. Notes* 2014, *7*, 726. [CrossRef]
27. Petermichl, W.; Philipp, A.; Hiller, K.-A.; Foltan, M.; Floerchinger, B.; Graf, B.; Lunz, D. Reliability of prognostic biomarkers after prehospital extracorporeal cardiopulmonary resuscitation with target temperature management. *Scand. J. Trauma Resusc. Emerg. Med.* 2021, *29*, 147. [CrossRef]

58. Friberg, H.; Cronberg, T.; Dünser, M.W.; Duranteau, J.; Horn, J.; Oddo, M. Survey on current practices for neurological prognostication after cardiac arrest. *Resuscitation* **2015**, *90*, 158–162. [CrossRef]
59. Cloostermans, M.C.; Van Meulen, F.B.; Eertman, C.J.; Hom, H.W.; van Putten, M. Continuous electroencephalography monitoring for early prediction of neurological outcome in postanoxic patients after cardiac arrest: A prospective cohort study. *Crit. Care Med.* **2012**, *40*, 2867–2875. [CrossRef]
60. Sandroni, C.; D'arrigo, S.; Cacciola, S.; Hoedemaekers, C.W.E.; Kamps, M.J.A.; Oddo, M.; Taccone, F.S.; Di Rocco, A.; Meijer, F.J.A.; Westhall, E.; et al. Prediction of poor neurological outcome in comatose survivors of cardiac arrest: A systematic review. *Intensive Care Med.* **2020**, *46*, 1803–1851. [CrossRef]
61. Scarpino, M.; Lanzo, G.; Lolli, F.; Carrai, R.; Moretti, M.; Spalletti, M.; Cozzolino, M.; Peris, A.; Amantini, A.; Grippo, A. Neurophysiological and neuroradiological multimodal approach for early poor outcome prediction after cardiac arrest. *Resuscitation* **2018**, *129*, 114–120. [CrossRef]
62. Lee, D.H.; Lee, B.K.; Jeung, K.W.; Jung, Y.H.; Cho, Y.S.; Cho, I.S.; Youn, C.S.; Kim, J.W.; Park, J.S.; Min, Y.I. Relationship between ventricular characteristics on brain computed tomography and 6-month neurologic outcome in cardiac arrest survivors who underwent targeted temperature management. *Resuscitation* **2018**, *129*, 37–42. [CrossRef] [PubMed]
63. Scarpino, M.; Lolli, F.; Lanzo, G.; Carrai, R.; Spalletti, M.; Valzania, F.; Lombardi, M.; Audenino, D.; Celani, M.G.; Marrelli, A.; et al. Neurophysiology and neuroimaging accurately predict poor neurological outcome within 24 hours after cardiac arrest: The ProNeCA prospective multicentre prognostication study. *Resuscitation* **2019**, *143*, 115–123. [CrossRef] [PubMed]
64. Song, H.; Bang, H.J.; You, Y.; Park, J.S.; Kang, C.; Kim, H.J.; Park, K.N.; Oh, S.H.; Youn, C.S. Novel serum biomarkers for predicting neurological outcomes in postcardiac arrest patients treated with targeted temperature management. *Crit. Care* **2023**, *27*, 113 [CrossRef]
65. Eun, J.W.; Yang, H.D.; Kim, S.H.; Hong, S.; Park, K.N.; Nam, S.W.; Jeong, S. Identification of novel biomarkers for prediction of neurological prognosis following cardiac arrest. *Oncotarget* **2017**, *8*, 16144–16157. [CrossRef] [PubMed]
66. Tissier, R.; Hocini, H.; Tchitchek, N.; Deye, N.; Legriel, S.; Pichon, N.; Daubin, C.; Hermine, O.; Carli, P.; Vivien, B.; et al. Early blood transcriptomic signature predicts patients' outcome after out-of-hospital cardiac arrest. *Resuscitation* **2019**, *138*, 222–232 [CrossRef]
67. Nichol, A.; Bellomo, R.; Ady, B.; Nielsen, N.; Hodgson, C.; Parke, R.; McGuinness, S.; Skrifvars, M.; Stub, D.; Barnard, S.; et al. Protocol summary and statistical analysis plan for the Targeted Therapeutic Mild Hypercapnia after Resuscitated Cardiac Arrest (TAME) trial. *Crit. Care Resusc.* **2021**, *23*, 374–385. [CrossRef]

Disclaimer/Publisher's Note: The statements, opinions and data contained in all publications are solely those of the individual author(s) and contributor(s) and not of MDPI and/or the editor(s). MDPI and/or the editor(s) disclaim responsibility for any injury to people or property resulting from any ideas, methods, instructions or products referred to in the content.

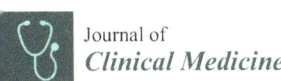

Article

Outcome of Out-of-Hospital Cardiac Arrest Patients Stratified by Pre-Clinical Loading with Aspirin and Heparin: A Retrospective Cohort Analysis

Sascha Macherey-Meyer *, Sebastian Heyne, Max M. Meertens, Simon Braumann, Stephan F. Niessen, Stephan Baldus, Samuel Lee † and Christoph Adler †

Clinic III for Internal Medicine, Faculty of Medicine and University Hospital Cologne, University of Cologne, 50931 Cologne, Germany; sebastian.heyne@uk-koeln.de (S.H.); max.meertens@uk-koeln.de (M.M.M.); simon.braumann@uk-koeln.de (S.B.); franz.niessen@uk-koeln.de (S.F.N.); stephan.baldus@uk-koeln.de (S.B.); samuel.lee@uk-koeln.de (S.L.); christoph.adler@uk-koeln.de (C.A.)
* Correspondence: sascha.macherey-meyer@uk-koeln.de; Tel.: +49-221-478-77753
† These authors contributed equally to this work.

Abstract: Background: Out-of-hospital cardiac arrest (OHCA) has a high prevalence of obstructive coronary artery disease and total coronary occlusion. Consequently, these patients are frequently loaded with antiplatelets and anticoagulants before hospital arrival. However, OHCA patients have multiple non-cardiac causes and high susceptibility for bleeding. In brief, there is a gap in the evidence for loading in OHCA patients. **Objective:** The current analysis stratified the outcome of patients with OHCA according to pre-clinical loading. **Material and Methods:** In a retrospective analysis of an all-comer OHCA registry, patients were stratified by loading with aspirin (ASA) and unfractionated heparin (UFH). Bleeding rate, survival to hospital discharge and favorable neurological outcomes were measured. **Results:** Overall, 272 patients were included, of whom 142 were loaded. Acute coronary syndrome was diagnosed in 103 patients. One-third of STEMIs were not loaded. Conversely, 54% with OHCA from non-ischemic causes were pretreated. Loading was associated with increased survival to hospital discharge (56.3 vs. 40.3%, $p = 0.008$) and a more favorable neurological outcome (80.7 vs. 62.6% $p = 0.003$). Prevalence of bleeding was comparable (26.8 vs. 31.5%, $p = 0.740$). **Conclusions:** Pre-clinical loading did not increase bleeding rates and was associated with favorable survival. Overtreatment of OHCA with non-ischemic origin, but also undertreatment of STEMI-OHCA were documented. Loading without definite diagnosis of sustained ischemia is debatable in the absence of reliable randomized controlled data.

Keywords: OHCA; aspirin; heparin; NSTE-ACS; STEMI

1. Introduction

Out-of-hospital cardiac arrest (OHCA) affects 67 to 170 per 100,000 Europeans per year [1–3]. It is the third leading cause of death in Europe, and prognosis remains poor despite continual efforts to improve treatment algorithms [1,4]. Only 7–11% of patients in all-comer cohorts survive until hospital discharge, and of these, only few have a favorable neurological outcome [1,2,5,6]. Sudden cardiac death remains the main cause of OHCA and is predominantly driven by atherosclerotic coronary artery disease (CAD) [7]. Recent analyses demonstrated that early coronary angiography in all-comer OHCA cohorts without ST-segment elevation is not superior to a delayed strategy [8–10]. However, obstructive CAD is a common finding in OHCA patients, and approximately 20% have acute total coronary artery occlusion [11]. In patients with presumed ongoing ischemia, immediate coronary angiography is still recommended [12–14], but identification of ischemia in these comatose patients might be challenging in pre-clinical settings. In cases of return of spontaneous circulation (ROSC) and ST-segment elevation myocardial infarction

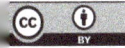

(STEMI), ischemia detection is feasible with high confidence and diagnostic certainty using electrocardiogram (ECG). In acute coronary syndrome without ST-segment elevation (NSTE-ACS), specific clinical criteria are missing. Chest pain is a suggestive symptom, but is non-specific with multiple non-cardiac causes [11,15,16]. Pre-hospital measurement of troponin is technically feasible but not routinely established yet [17,18]. Consequently, pre-clinical suspected diagnosis of NSTE-ACS is often false positive, and patients are at risk for overtreatment [19,20]. In Germany, patients with suspected NSTE-ACS are frequently pretreated by pre-hospital application of aspirin (ASA) and/or unfractionated heparin (UFH)—so called "loading" [19–21]. There is a gap in the evidence for loading in OHCA patients with high prevalence of obstructive CAD, but also other potential causes of cardiac arrest, with high susceptibility for bleeding.

The current analysis aimed to stratify the outcome of patients with OHCA from a single cardiac arrest center according to pre-clinical loading decision.

2. Material and Methods

This retrospective, single-center study is based on a registry of consecutive OHCA patients treated at our cardiac arrest center located in the department of cardiology in a tertiary hospital. The registry generally included all-cause OHCA patients treated at our cardiac arrest center between January 2014 and November 2021, and the vast majority was treated at the department of cardiology. Of these, the majority suffer from OHCA of cardiac origin, as emergency medical services frequently allocate these patients to our hospital to provide extracorporeal cardiopulmonary resuscitation (eCPR). Patients with pre-hospital ROSC, but also under ongoing manual or mechanical CPR, were considered. Adult patients with non-traumatic cardiac arrest and complete information on pre-clinical loading and in-hospital course were eligible for this analysis.

2.1. Treatment Algorithm

Our cardiac arrest center is located in a metropolitan area with approximately 1.1 million inhabitants. The contributing emergency medical service (EMS) covers a 400 km^2 area. In case of pre-hospital cardiac arrest, EMS personnel will be supported by a specialized and trained German emergency physician (EP) leading resuscitation. During ongoing resuscitation, the EP decides whether to stay on scene and continuing pre-clinical treatment until ROSC or termination of cardiopulmonary resuscitation (CPR), or to transport the patient using mechanical CPR (mCPR) devices. According to our local protocol [22], patients with non-traumatic OHCA from presumed cardiac origin are immediately transferred to the catheterization laboratory. Adjudication of cardiac origin is at the discretion of the treating EP after consultation of a cardiologist by phone. In patients with ROSC, the need for urgent coronary angiography is evaluated versus direct transfer to an intensive care unit (ICU). In refractory cardiac arrest or intermittent ROSC, patients will be evaluated by an interdisciplinary heart team for implementation of eCPR or mechanical circulatory support (MCS). Patients with non-cardiac OHCA (e.g., hypothermia, drowning, intoxication) are transferred to the emergency department for further evaluation and are subsequently treated at the ICU. Loading with ASA and UFH, and dosage were at treating EP's discretion.

2.2. Measured Data and Investigated Outcomes

Baseline characteristics were extracted from patient records, including age and gender, data on pre-emergency status, detailed information on resuscitation and pre-hospital treatment, in-hospital outcome data and reasons for cardiac arrest. Arterial blood gas measurements and partial thromboplastin time (PTT) were also extracted. Patients were then stratified according to pre-clinical treatment with ASA and UFH. Additionally, subgroup analysis of STEMI patients was performed, as STEMI guidelines recommend immediate use of antithrombotics and anticoagulants at the time of diagnosis even in pre-clinical settings [13]. Measured outcomes were survival at hospital discharge and favorable neurological outcome at hospital discharge (defined by the Glasgow–Pittsburgh cerebral performance categories (CPC) Score ≤ 2), bleeding complications (defined as a composite of need for red blood cell [RBC] transfusion and intracranial bleeding), ICU and hospital stay. Ethical approval was not necessary in this retrospective, non-interventional analysis of the local OHCA registry.

2.3. Statistical Analysis

Data were described using mean values (±standard deviation), or frequencies and percentages. Student's *t*-test, Fisher's exact test and chi-squared test were used for statistical analyses according to metric or categorial variables. All reported *p*-values were two-sided, and *p*-values less than 0.05 were considered statistically significant. Statistical analyses were performed using SPSS Statistics Version 27.0.0 (IBM Corp., Armonk, NY, USA).

3. Results

3.1. Overall Analysis

Overall, 272 patients were included in the registry analysis (Figure 1). Patients had a mean age of 62.7 years and were more frequently male (*n* = 196) (Table 1). Cardiac arrest was witnessed in 211 (77.6%) patients, and 170 (62.5%) received prompt bystander CPR. Shockable rhythm was present in 174 (64%) patients, and they required a mean of 3 shocks. ROSC could be achieved in 245 (90%) patients, and mean time until ROSC was 26.7 min. mCPR was implemented on-scene or during transport in 75 (27.6%) patients. Immediate coronary angiography was performed in 229 (84.2%) patients, and 48 (17.6%) patients required MCS.

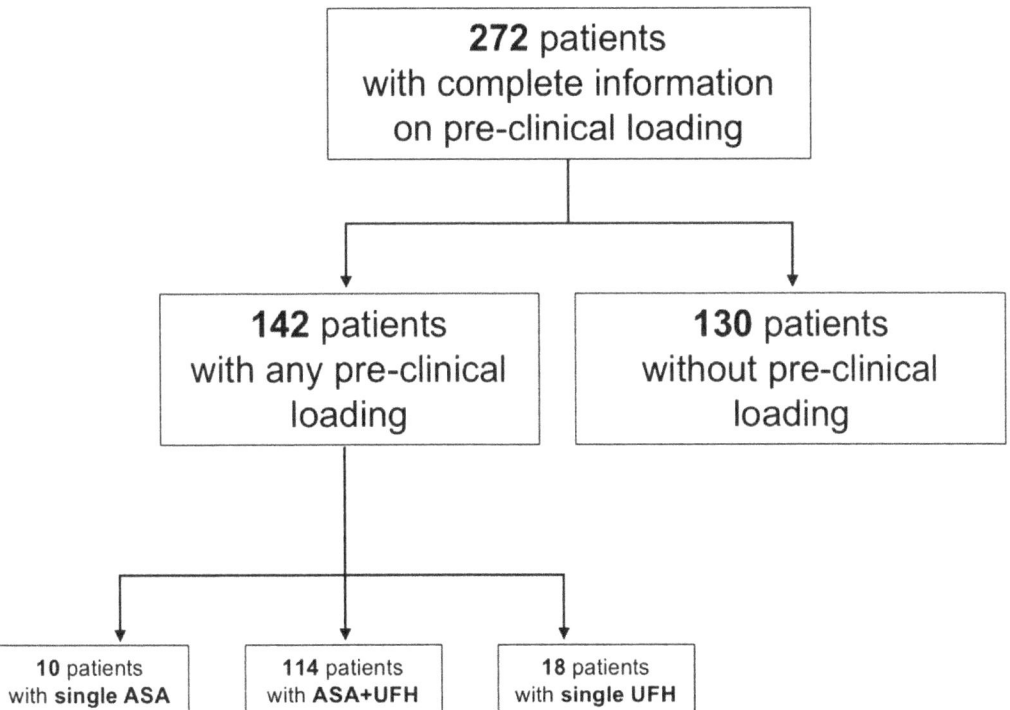

Figure 1. Patient cohort. Abbreviations: ASA: aspirin, UFH: unfractionated heparin.

Table 1. Patient characteristics total cohort.

	Total Cohort N = 272	Pre-Clinical Loading N = 142	No Loading N = 130	p-Value *
Age, mean [SD]	62.7 [±15.5]	61.5 [±14.9]	64.1 [±16.4]	0.168
Gender male (%)	196 (72.1)	108 (76)	88 (67.7)	0.125
Pre-emergency status (%)				0.255
No prior diseases	50 (18.4)	31 (21.8)	19 (14.6)	
Diseases without limitations in daily living	134 (49.3)	72 (50.7)	62 (47.7)	
Diseases with limitation in daily living	41 (15.1)	17 (12)	24 (18.5)	
No independent daily living	4 (1.5)	1 (0.7)	3 (2.3)	
Unknown status	43 (15.8)	21 (14.8)	22 (16.9)	
Pre-hospital characteristics				
Witnessed arrest	211	116	95	**0.037**
Bystander CPR	170 (62.5)	97 (68.3)	73 (56.2)	**0.039**
No-flow time, min	2.2 [±4]	2.1 [±4.1]	2.4 [±4]	0.624
Shockable rhythm	174	99	75	0.114
Shocks, n	2.99 [±3.5]	3.1 [±3.7]	2.9 [±3.3]	0.649
Epinephrine use, n	214	109	105	0.460
Amiodarone use, n	108	49	59	**0.008**
Achieving ROSC before hospital arrival [§]	190	100	90	
Achieving ROSC after hospital arrival [§]	55	28	27	0.914
Never ROSC achieved [§]	25	14	11	
Time until ROSC, min	26.7 [±22.9]	26.4 [±25.5]	27.2 [±19.8]	0.795
EMS transport with mechanical cardiopulmonary resuscitation device	75	40	35	0.854
Presenting arterial blood gases, means				
Initial arterial O_2, mm Hg	182.5 [±106.5]	176 [±88.3]	190.4 [±125.7]	0.419
Initial arterial CO_2, mm Hg	59.8 [±27.9]	58.7 [±25.2]	60.6 [±88.3]	0.829
Initial lactate, mmol/L	7.98 [±6]	7.36 [±5.9]	8.67 [±6.0]	0.073
Initial pH	7.15 [±0.2]	7.17 [±0.2]	7.12 [±0.2]	0.166
Initial hemoglobin g/dL	14.3 [±2.9]	15.1 [±2.3]	13.5 [±3.3]	0.135
In-hospital treatment				
Coronary angiography performed (%)	229 (84.2)	129 (90.8)	100 (76.9)	**0.002**
Mechanical circulatory support implantation (%)				
ECMO	33 (12.1)	16 (11.3)	17 (13.1)	0.631
Axial flow pump (Impella©)	8 (2.9)	6 (4.2)	2 (1.5)	0.286
IABP	7 (2.6)	4 (2.8)	3 (2.3)	1.000
Target temperature management	89 (32.7)	48 (33.8)	41 (31.5)	0.691
PTT, s	50.2 [±31.7]	57 [±31.4]	45.1 [±31.1]	**0.014**
Aspiration pneumonia, n	110	55	55	0.565
Hypoxic ischemic encephalopathy (%)	64 (23.5)	24 (16.9)	40 (30.8)	**0.007**
Ejection fraction, EF (%)				0.101

Table 1. Cont.

	Total Cohort N = 272	Pre-Clinical Loading N = 142	No Loading N = 130	p-Value *
Preserved EF (≥50%)	83 (30.5)	42 (29.6)	41 (31.5)	
Mildly reduced EF (41 to 49%)	42 (15.4)	27 (19)	15 (11.5)	
Reduced EF (≤40%)	86 (31.7)	48 (33.8)	38 (29.2)	
Not estimated	61 (22.5)	25 (17.6)	36 (27.7)	
Cause of non-traumatic cardiac arrest (%)				0.019
Acute coronary syndrome	103 (37.9)	65 (45.8) #	38 (29.2) #	0.005 #
- STEMI	60	40	20	
- NSTE-ACS	43	25	18	
Arrhythmia	76 (27.9)	32 (22.5)	44 (33.8)	
Asphyxia	28 (10.3)	11 (7.7)	17 (13.1)	
Other	65 (23.9)	34 (23.9)	31 (23.9)	

* Chi-square test/Fisher's exact test in categorical variables and t-test in metric variables. [] Standard deviation, () Percentages. # ACS vs. non-ACS. § missing Data: n = 2. Abbreviations: ACS: acute coronary syndrome; CPR: cardiopulmonary resuscitation; ECMO: extracorporeal membrane oxygenation; EF: ejection fraction; EMS: emergency medical service; IABP: intra-aortic balloon pump; NSTE-ACS: non-ST-segment elevation acute coronary syndrome; PTT: partial thromboplastin time; ROSC: return of spontaneous circulation, STEMI: ST-segment elevation myocardial infarction.

Cardiac etiology was the main reason for OHCA. In detail, 103 (37.9%)) patients were classified as having acute coronary syndrome (ACS), 60 presented with STEMI and 43 with NSTE-ACS. Arrhythmia (n = 76, 27.9%) was the second leading cause of OHCA, followed by asphyxia (n = 28, 10.3%). The remaining 65 (23.9%) patients represented a heterogeneous group mainly suffering from distributive, hypovolemic or obstructive shock.

3.2. Loading Status

ASA and/or UFH was used in 142 patients, and 130 did not receive loading before hospital admission (Figure 1). Dosage of aspirin varied between 125 mg and 725 mg. UFH was administered at 5000 or 10,000 units, except in one case in which the EP used 24,000 units.

Patients in the loading group more often had witnessed arrest, were more often treated with bystander CPR, more frequently had ACS and subsequently had a higher proportion of coronary angiography (Table 1). Amiodarone use was more often documented in patients without pre-hospital loading. All other characteristics were distributed evenly between the groups.

Safety analysis showed comparable incidence of bleeding events (26.8 vs. 31.5%, $p = 0.740$) between the groups. This event rate was mainly driven by RBC transfusion (25.4 vs. 28.5%, Table 2). Intracranial bleeding was detected in 2.8% and 5.4% patients by computed tomography ($p = 0.553$).

Both groups had comparable duration of ICU stay, but patients in the loading group showed a trend towards longer overall hospital stay (14.0 vs. 11.1 days, $p = 0.07$).

Patients in the loading group had a significantly higher rate of survival to hospital discharge (56.3 vs. 40.3%, $p = 0.008$). They additionally had a more favorable neurological outcome (80.7 vs. 62.6% $p = 0.003$) compared to patients without loading.

Table 2. Outcome of patients stratified by loading.

	Pre-Clinical Loading N = 142	No Loading N = 130	p-Value *
Patients with bleeding complication, n (%)	38 (26.8)	41 (31.5)	0.740
RBC transfusion, n patients (%)	36 (25.4)	37 (28.5)	0.587
Mean number of RBC transfusion	2.4 [±7]	2.7 [±7]	0.722
Intracranial bleeding, n	4	7	0.553
ICU stay, mean	6.3 [±5.5]	7 [±5.8]	0.557
Hospital stay, mean	14 [±14.5]	11.1 [±10.8]	0.07
Survival to hospital discharge, % total group	56.3	40.3	**0.008**
Favorable neurological outcome at hospital discharge, % of survivors	80.7	62.6	**0.003**

Abbreviations: RBC: red blood cell; ICU: intensive care unit. * Chi-square test/Fisher's exact test in categorical variables and *t*-test in metric variables.

3.3. STEMI Subgroup Analysis

Grouping of STEMI patients according to loading status resulted in 40 patients with pre-clinical loading and 20 patients without pretreatment. Patients in the loading group had numerically lower incidence of bleeding events (25 vs. 55%, $p = 0.212$), and especially decreased need for RBC transfusion (Table 3). These observations showed no statistically significant differences. Rate of survival to hospital discharge (77.5% vs. 60%) or favorable neurological outcome (94.1% vs. 82.4%) and hospital or ICU stay were more favorable in the loading group, but were not statistically different.

Table 3. Outcome of STEMI patients stratified by loading.

	Pre-Clinical Loading N = 40	No Loading N = 20	p-Value *
Patients with bleeding complication, n (%)	10 (25)	11 (55)	0.212
RBC transfusion, n patients	10 (25)	10 (50)	0.053
Mean number of RBC transfusion	2 [±6.1]	4.8 [±8.1]	0.139
Intracranial bleeding, n	0	1	0.429
ICU stay, mean	6.8 [±3.3]	12.2 [±9.8]	0.327
Hospital stay, mean	13.9 [±9.4]	14.9 [±12.7]	0.725
Survival to hospital discharge, %	77.5	60	0.156
Favorable neurological outcome at hospital discharge, % of survivors	94.1	82.4	0.318

Abbreviations: STEMI: ST-segment elevation myocardial infarction; RBC: red blood cell; ICU: intensive care unit. * Chi-square test/Fisher's exact test in categorical variables and *t*-test in metric variables.

4. Discussion

To our knowledge, this is the first systematic evaluation of pre-hospital loading with aspirin and heparin in OHCA. These are the main and novel findings:

In highly selected patients with mainly cardiac origin,

- loading was associated with increased survival to hospital discharge and a more favorable neurological outcome,
- the rates for RBC transfusion and intracranial bleeding were not affected by pre-clinical loading,
- a considerable number of STEMI patients (33%) were not loaded on scene,
- 54% of patients in the loading group had OHCA from non-ischemic cause and had no expected benefit from pretreatment, retrospectively.

Patients in the loading group had an advantageous survival and neurological outcome. Given the non-randomized, uncontrolled registry design, these observations need to be interpreted with caution. The study group represents a highly selected cohort. Rates of witnessed cardiac arrest, bystander CPR and shockable rhythm were high compared to an all-comer cohort [1,3,23]. The majority of patients were male. EMS was activated and CPR was started in each patient. All patients were transported to a hospital, and ROSC could be achieved in a considerable number of patients. Moreover, patients were young and the cohort had a high prevalence of ACS. These are all well-known favorable prognostic factors in OHCA [1,5–7,24], and might have contributed to observed favorable survival and neurological outcome rates in both groups. The groups were not balanced in these important characteristics. Hence, advantageous outcome of the loading group is attributable to the increased rate of witnessed arrest, high percentage of bystander CPR and higher prevalence of ACS than to loading itself.

4.1. Bleeding

Bleeding rates were similar between the groups. Notably, the registry design underestimates the true prevalence of bleeding complications by assessing only RBC transfusion and intracranial bleeding. In the literature, intracranial bleeding has a prevalence of 3.5 to 11.5% in OHCA patients [25–27], and intracranial hemorrhage itself can be the cause of OHCA [25,28]. Overall bleeding complications in OHCA range from 15–20%, and increase to 31–32% in patients treated with eCPR or MCS [29–32]. Mechanical CPR and MCS themselves are associated with increased bleeding risk, and in MCS, access-site bleeding is a frequent complication [33,34]. Current registry data are in line with prior publications, but one should bear in mind that RBC transfusion is an unspecific bleeding event and OHCA patients are at increased bleeding risk even in the absence of antithrombotic/anticoagulatory pretreatment. Future evaluation of loading harm should ideally address all entities of bleeding.

4.2. Undertreatment of STEMI

One-third of STEMI patients were not treated with ASA or UFH in the current registry, even though current guidelines recommend immediate loading at the time of diagnosis [13]. In STEMI patients—in whom coronary artery occlusion is likely—pre-hospital administration of heparin did not affect clinical outcomes in prior analyses. Heparin use led to fewer coronary artery occlusions, but major adverse cardiac events or 30 day survival were not affected [35–37]. In accordance, the current analysis did not reveal clinically significant differences between loaded and non-pretreated STEMI group. At the patient level, the reasoning for withholding ASA and UFH in STEMI remains unclear, but some factors could be involved. First, simple misdiagnosis of ST-segment elevation in pre-hospital settings is a possible explanation. Notably, even extracardiac pathologies like intracranial hemorrhage can mimic transient ischemic ECG patterns like ST-segment elevation and might be misleading [38]. Misjudgment of STEMI equivalents (e.g., posterior infarction) or misinterpretation of bundle branch blockade or paced rhythms are also potential factors. Electrolyte imbalances, conduction disturbances or use of antiarrhythmic drugs might have contributed to bizarre ECG presentations. Of note, Baldi et al. demonstrated that immediate ECG following ROSC can be misleading, showing both false negative or false positive STEMI results [39]. Consequently, these authors recommend delayed ECG acquisition for eight minutes following ROSC to minimize systematic diagnostic errors [39].

4.3. Overtreatment of Non-STEMI OHCA

More than 50% of patients in the loading group had a non-ischemic cause of OHCA. One might assume that loading was not beneficial in these patients, even though the current study was not designed to demonstrate such difference.

In subjects with preclinically unknown intracavitary bleeding or aortic dissection, the administration of antiplatelets or anticoagulants might cause severe harm. Patient selection for pre-treatment is of utmost interest. Current guidelines on NSTE-ACS or resuscitation do not explicitly address pre-hospital loading. To date, only position papers are available. A position paper from the Acute Cardiovascular Care Association of the European Society of Cardiology recommends pre-hospital loading with aspirin and heparin in STEMI and NSTE-ACS with immediate invasive strategy (coronary angiography < 2 h) [40]. The authors point out that there is no scientific evidence for pre-hospital loading in NSTE-ACS patients, overall. Specific recommendations for OHCA are also missing.

Given this vacuum, STEMI and NSTE-ACS guidelines should be considered in OHCA with presumed cardiac cause [13,14]. The European guideline on NSTE-ACS recommends the use of aspirin, and the administration of UFH at the time of diagnosis [14,41]. Troponin measurement is a cornerstone in NSTE-ACS diagnosis [14], but it is not routinely used on scene in daily practice [17,18]. As a consequence, NSTE-ACS remains solely a suspected diagnosis in OHCA patients on scene, but this judgment affects upcoming treatment steps in the chain of survival. The paradigm shift from immediate to delayed coronary angiography in hemodynamic stable NSTE-ACS-OHCA patients currently translates to daily routine [8–10]. Identification and discrimination of patients with total coronary artery occlusion is challenging but crucial. One might speculate that these patients still require immediate coronary angiography including percutaneous coronary intervention. Guidelines recommend immediate angiography in patients with infarct-related cardiogenic shock with hemodynamic instability, ongoing chest pain, life threatening arrhythmias or mechanical infarct complication, but diagnostic modalities are limited in pre-hospital settings [14]. EPs need to assess the individuals' probability of ischemia on clinical criteria. Spirito et al. recently showed that hemodynamic instability does not automatically indicate vessel occlusion [11]. Instead, shockable rhythm and presence of chest pain demonstrated a predictive value for coronary artery occlusion [11]. However, chest pain is not reliably assessable in comatose patients, especially in patients with non-witnessed collapse. In all-comer chest pain cohorts, non-ischemic and even non-cardiac are the most prevalent causes [15,16]. The retrospective data from Spirito and colleagues must be weighed against this non-specific character of chest pain. Diagnostic error remains the Achilles heel of optimized OHCA patient management, and medical history and evidence of chest pain might contribute to decision making, but prospectively validated criteria are missing.

We observed heterogeneity in loading of OHCA patients with both under- and overtreatment. Nescience and uncertainty of EPs are potential mechanisms. In the absence of reliable randomized controlled data, use of pre-hospital antithrombotic and anticoagulatory pretreatment without ischemic cardiac cause of OHCA remains debatable. Future studies should address clinically measurable factors to overcome these gaps in the evidence. These could possibly change the current strategy from unselected to individualized, selected loading strategies in OHCA patients with considerable risk for coronary artery occlusion.

4.4. Limitations

The current analysis followed a non-controlled design in a relatively small cohort. Hence, selection and performance bias are inherent limitations and restrict generalizability. As previously mentioned, the current cohort had a high prevalence of favorable prognostic factors and the majority of patients suffered from ACS. The performance bias was mainly based on loading decision. Administration of ASA and UFH was solely at the treating EP's discretion. Especially in STEMI patients without loading, individual reasoning remains uncertain, but might reflect uncertainty of the EP. As our registry does not regularly include all entities of bleeding events, we decided to only report the routinely measured data (RBC transfusion, intracranial hemorrhage). In doing so, we numerically underestimated bleeding rates of missing events like gastrointestinal, parenchymatous, intrathoracic, abdominal or access-site bleeding. The relatively small sample size restricts statistical power.

5. Conclusions

In this non-traumatic OHCA registry including mainly patients with cardiac cause pre-clinical loading was neither associated with increased intracranial bleeding, nor resulted in higher requirement of red blood cell transfusion. Overtreatment with aspirin and heparin could be documented in 54% of patients presenting with OHCA of non-ischemic origin. One-third of STEMI-OHCA were not loaded, but this undertreatment did not translate to worse survival. The administration of anticoagulatory and antithrombotic pretreatment in OHCA without definite diagnosis of sustained ischemia is debatable in the absence of reliable randomized controlled data. Future prospective studies should address the loading dilemma and evaluate benefit and harm of pre-hospital loading in comatose patients.

Author Contributions: Conceptualization, S.M.-M., S.B. (Simon Braumann) and C.A.; Methodology, S.M.-M. and C.A.; Formal Analysis, S.M.-M. and M.M.M.; Data Curation, S.F.N.; Writing—Original Draft Preparation, S.M.-M. and C.A.; Writing—Review & Editing, S.M.-M., S.H., M.M.M., S.B. (Simon Braumann), S.B. (Stephan Baldus), S.F.N., S.L. and C.A.; Visualization, S.M.-M.; Supervision, S.L. and C.A.; Project Administration, S.B. (Stephan Baldus) and C.A. All authors have read and agreed to the published version of the manuscript.

Funding: This research received no external funding.

Institutional Review Board Statement: Ethical approval was not necessary in this retrospective, non-interventional analysis of the local OHCA registry.

Informed Consent Statement: Patient consent was waived due to retrospective, non-interventional analysis of the local OHCA registry.

Data Availability Statement: The data presented in this study are available on request from the corresponding author. The data are not publicly available due to data protection of patients included.

Acknowledgments: We thank Greta Sommer for her valuable support in data extraction.

Conflicts of Interest: The authors declare no conflict of interest.

References

1. Gräsner, J.-T.; Wnent, J.; Herlitz, J.; Perkins, G.D.; Lefering, R.; Tjelmeland, I.; Koster, R.W.; Masterson, S.; Rossell-Ortiz, F.; Maurer, H.; et al. Survival after out-of-hospital cardiac arrest in Europe—Results of the EuReCa TWO study. *Resuscitation* **2020**, *148*, 218–226. [CrossRef]
2. Gräsner, J.T.; Lefering, R.; Koster, R.W.; Masterson, S.; Böttiger, B.W.; Herlitz, J.; Wnent, J.; Tjelmeland, I.B.; Ortiz, F.R.; Maurer, H.; et al. EuReCa ONE-27 Nations, ONE Europe, ONE Registry: A prospective one month analysis of out-of-hospital cardiac arrest outcomes in 27 countries in Europe. *Resuscitation* **2016**, *105*, 188–195. [CrossRef] [PubMed]
3. Gräsner, J.-T.; Herlitz, J.; Tjelmeland, I.B.; Wnent, J.; Masterson, S.; Lilja, G.; Bein, B.; Böttiger, B.W.; Rosell-Ortiz, F.; Nolan, J.P.; et al. European Resuscitation Council Guidelines 2021: Epidemiology of cardiac arrest in Europe. *Resuscitation* **2021**, *161*, 61–79. [CrossRef]
4. Kiguchi, T.; Okubo, M.; Nishiyama, C.; Maconochie, I.; Ong, M.E.H.; Kern, K.B.; Wyckoff, M.H.; McNally, B.; Christensen, E.F.; Tjelmeland, I.; et al. Out-of-hospital cardiac arrest across the World: First report from the International Liaison Committee on Resuscitation (ILCOR). *Resuscitation* **2020**, *152*, 39–49. [CrossRef] [PubMed]
5. Yan, S.; Gan, Y.; Jiang, N.; Wang, R.; Chen, Y.; Luo, Z.; Zong, Q.; Chen, S.; Lv, C. The global survival rate among adult out-of-hospital cardiac arrest patients who received cardiopulmonary resuscitation: A systematic review and meta-analysis. *Crit. Care* **2020**, *24*, 61. [CrossRef]
6. Reynolds, J.C.; Grunau, B.E.; Rittenberger, J.C.; Sawyer, K.N.; Kurz, M.C.; Callaway, C.W. Association Between Duration of Resuscitation and Favorable Outcome After Out-of-Hospital Cardiac Arrest: Implications for Prolonging or Terminating Resuscitation. *Circulation* **2016**, *134*, 2084–2094. [CrossRef]
7. Kandala, J.; Oommen, C.; Kern, K.B. Sudden cardiac death. *Br. Med. Bull.* **2017**, *122*, 5–15. [CrossRef] [PubMed]
8. Desch, S.; Freund, A.; Akin, I.; Behnes, M.; Preusch, M.R.; Zelniker, T.A.; Skurk, C.; Landmesser, U.; Graf, T.; Eitel, I.; et al. Angiography after Out-of-Hospital Cardiac Arrest without ST-Segment Elevation. *N. Engl. J. Med.* **2021**, *385*, 2544–2553. [CrossRef]
9. Heyne, S.; Macherey, S.; Meertens, M.M.; Braumann, S.; Nießen, F.S.; Tichelbäcker, T.; Baldus, S.; Adler, C.; Lee, S. Coronary angiography after cardiac arrest without ST-elevation myocardial infarction: A network meta-analysis. *Eur. Heart J.* **2023**, *44*, 1040–1054. [CrossRef]

10. Lemkes, J.S.; Janssens, G.N.; van der Hoeven, N.W.; Jewbali, L.S.; Dubois, E.A.; Meuwissen, M.; Rijpstra, T.A.; Bosker, H.A.; Blans, M.J.; Bleeker, G.B.; et al. Coronary Angiography after Cardiac Arrest without ST-Segment Elevation. *N. Engl. J. Med.* **2019**, *380*, 1397–1407. [CrossRef]
11. Spirito, A.; Vaisnora, L.; Papadis, A.; Iacovelli, F.; Sardu, C.; Selberg, A.; Bär, S.; Kavaliauskaite, R.; Temperli, F.; Asatryan, B.; et al. Acute Coronary Occlusion in Patients with Non-ST-Segment Elevation Out-of-Hospital Cardiac Arrest. *J. Am. Coll. Cardiol.* **2023**, *81*, 446–456. [CrossRef]
12. Lott, C.; Truhlář, A.; Alfonzo, A.; Barelli, A.; González-Salvado, V.; Hinkelbein, J.; Nolan, J.P.; Paal, P.; Perkins, G.D.; Thies, K.-C.; et al. European Resuscitation Council Guidelines 2021: Cardiac arrest in special circumstances. *Resuscitation* **2021**, *161*, 152–219. [CrossRef]
13. Ibanez, B.; James, S.; Agewall, S.; Antunes, M.J.; Bucciarelli-Ducci, C.; Bueno, H.; Caforio, A.L.; Crea, F.; Goudevenos, J.A.; Halvorsen, S.; et al. 2017 ESC Guidelines for the management of acute myocardial infarction in patients presenting with ST-segment elevation: The Task Force for the management of acute myocardial infarction in patients presenting with ST-segment elevation of the European Society of Cardiology (ESC). *Eur. Heart J.* **2018**, *39*, 119–177. [PubMed]
14. Collet, J.P.; Thiele, H.; Barbato, E.; Barthélémy, O.; Bauersachs, J.; Bhatt, D.L.; Dendale, P.; Dorobantu, M.; Edvardsen, T.; Folliguet, T.; et al. 2020 ESC Guidelines for the management of acute coronary syndromes in patients presenting without persistent ST-segment elevation. *Eur. Heart J.* **2021**, *42*, 1289–1367. [CrossRef] [PubMed]
15. Pitts, S.; Niska, R.; Xu, J.; Burt, C. National Hospital Ambulatory Medical Care Survey: 2006 emergency department summary. *Natl. Health Stat. Rep.* **2008**, *6*, 1–38.
16. Gulati, M.; Levy, P.D.; Mukherjee, D.; Amsterdam, E.; Bhatt, D.L.; Birtcher, K.K.; Blankstein, R.; Boyd, J.; Bullock-Palmer, R.P.; Conejo, T. 2021 AHA/ACC/ASE/CHEST/SAEM/SCCT/SCMR Guideline for the Evaluation and Diagnosis of Chest Pain: Executive Summary: A Report of the American College of Cardiology/American Heart Association Joint Committee on Clinical Practice Guidelines. *Circulation* **2021**, *144*, e368–e454. [CrossRef]
17. Camaro, C.; Aarts, G.W.; Adang, E.M.M.; van Hout, R.; Brok, G.; Hoare, A.; Rodwell, L.; de Pooter, F.; de Wit, W.; Cramer, G.; et al. Rule-out of non-ST-segment elevation acute coronary syndrome by a single, pre-hospital troponin measurement: A randomized trial. *Eur. Heart J.* **2023**, *44*, 1705–1714. [CrossRef]
18. Stengaard, C.; Sørensen, J.T.; Ladefoged, S.A.; Christensen, E.F.; Lassen, J.F.; Bøtker, H.E.; Terkelsen, C.J.; Thygesen, K. Quantitative point-of-care troponin T measurement for diagnosis and prognosis in patients with a suspected acute myocardial infarction. *Am. J. Cardiol.* **2013**, *112*, 1361–1366. [CrossRef]
19. Braumann, S.; Faber-Zameitat, C.; Macherey-Meyer, S.; Tichelbäcker, T.; Meertens, M.; Heyne, S.; Nießen, F.; Nies, R.J.; Nettersheim, F.; Reuter, H.; et al. Acute Chest Pain—Diagnostic Accuracy and Pre-hospital Use of Anticoagulants and Platelet Aggregation Inhibitors. *Dtsch. Arztebl. Int.* **2023**. [CrossRef]
20. Eckle, V.S.; Lehmann, S.; Drexler, B. Prehospital management of patients with suspected acute coronary syndrome: Real world experience reflecting current guidelines. *Med. Klin. Intensivmed. Notfmed.* **2021**, *116*, 694–697. [CrossRef] [PubMed]
21. Macherey-Meyer, S.; Braumann, S.; Meertens, M.; Heyne, S.; Nießen, S.F.; Tichelbäcker, T.; Baldus, S.; Lee, S.; Adler, C. The PRELOAD Study—Pre-clinical loading in patients with acute chest pain and suspected or definite acute coronary syndrome: An interim analysis. *Clin. Res. Cardiol.* **2023**, V451. [CrossRef]
22. Adler, C.; Paul, C.; Michels, G.; Pfister, R.; Sabashnikov, A.; Hinkelbein, J.; Braumann, S.; Djordjevic, L.; Blomeyer, R.; Krings, A.; et al. One year experience with fast track algorithm in patients with refractory out-of-hospital cardiac arrest. *Resuscitation* **2019**, *144*, 157–165. [CrossRef] [PubMed]
23. Seewald, S.; Ristau, P.; Fischer, M.; Gräsner, J.T.; Brenner, S.; Wnent, J.; Bein, B. Öffentlicher Jahresbericht 2021 des Deutschen Reanimationsregisters: Cardiac Arrest Center. *Anästh. Intensivmed.* **2021**, *62*, V128–V130.
24. Blom, M.T.; Oving, I.; Berdowski, J.; van Valkengoed, I.G.M.; Bardai, A.; Tan, H.L. Women have lower chances than men to be resuscitated and survive out-of-hospital cardiac arrest. *Eur. Heart J.* **2019**, *40*, 3824–3834. [CrossRef]
25. Shin, J.; Kim, K.; Lim, Y.S.; Lee, H.J.; Lee, S.J.; Jung, E.; Kim, J.; Yang, H.J.; Kim, J.J.; Hwang, S.Y. Incidence and clinical features of intracranial hemorrhage causing out-of-hospital cardiac arrest: A multicenter retrospective study. *Am. J. Emerg. Med.* **2016**, *34*, 2326–2330. [CrossRef]
26. Cocchi, M.N.; Lucas, J.M.; Salciccioli, J.; Carney, E.; Herman, S.; Zimetbaum, P.; Donnino, M.W. The role of cranial computed tomography in the immediate post-cardiac arrest period. *Intern. Emerg. Med.* **2010**, *5*, 533–538. [CrossRef]
27. Gelber, J.; Montgomery, M.E.; Singh, A. A prospective study of the incidence of intracranial hemorrhage in survivors of out of hospital cardiac arrest. *Am. J. Emerg. Med.* **2021**, *41*, 70–72. [CrossRef]
28. Agrawal, A.; Cardinale, M.; Frenia, D.; Mukherjee, A. Cerebellar Haemorrhage Leading to Sudden Cardiac Arrest. *J. Crit. Care Med.* **2020**, *6*, 71–73. [CrossRef]
29. Nguyen, M.-L.; Gause, E.; Mills, B.; Tonna, J.E.; Alvey, H.; Saczkowski, R.; Grunau, B.; Becker, L.B.; Gaieski, D.F.; Youngquist, S.; et al. Traumatic and hemorrhagic complications after extracorporeal cardiopulmonary resuscitation for out-of-hospital cardiac arrest. *Resuscitation* **2020**, *157*, 225–229. [CrossRef]
30. García, J.; Jiménez-Brítez, G.; Flores-Umanzor, E.; Mendieta, G.; Freixa, X.; Sabaté, M. Thrombotic and Bleeding Events after Percutaneous Coronary Intervention in Out-of-Hospital Cardiac Arrest with and without Therapeutic Hypothermia. *Rev. Esp. Cardiol. (Engl. Ed.)* **2019**, *72*, 433–435. [CrossRef]

1. Yannopoulos, D.; Bartos, J.; Raveendran, G.; Walser, E.; Connett, J.; Murray, T.A.; Collins, G.; Zhang, L.; Kalra, R.; Kosmopoulos, M.; et al. Advanced reperfusion strategies for patients with out-of-hospital cardiac arrest and refractory ventricular fibrillation (ARREST): A phase 2, single centre, open-label, randomised controlled trial. *Lancet* **2020**, *396*, 1807–1816. [CrossRef] [PubMed]
2. Belohlavek, J.; Smalcova, J.; Rob, D.; Franek, O.; Smid, O.; Pokorna, M.; Horák, J.; Mrazek, V.; Kovarnik, T.; Zemanek, D.; et al. Effect of Intra-arrest Transport, Extracorporeal Cardiopulmonary Resuscitation, and Immediate Invasive Assessment and Treatment on Functional Neurologic Outcome in Refractory Out-of-Hospital Cardiac Arrest: A Randomized Clinical Trial. *JAMA* **2022**, *327*, 737–747. [CrossRef] [PubMed]
3. Gall, E.; Lafont, A.; Varenne, O.; Dumas, F.; Cariou, A.; Picard, F. Balancing thrombosis and bleeding after out-of-hospital cardiac arrest related to acute coronary syndrome: A literature review. *Arch. Cardiovasc. Dis.* **2021**, *114*, 667–679. [CrossRef]
4. Bisdas, T.; Beutel, G.; Warnecke, G.; Hoeper, M.M.; Kuehn, C.; Haverich, A.; Teebken, O.E. Vascular complications in patients undergoing femoral cannulation for extracorporeal membrane oxygenation support. *Ann. Thorac. Surg.* **2011**, *92*, 626–631. [CrossRef] [PubMed]
5. Bloom, J.E.; Andrew, E.; Nehme, Z.; Dinh, D.T.; Fernando, H.; Shi, W.Y.; Vriesendorp, P.; Nanayakarra, S.; Dawson, L.P.; Brennan, A.; et al. Pre-hospital heparin use for ST-elevation myocardial infarction is safe and improves angiographic outcomes. *Eur. Heart J. Acute Cardiovasc. Care* **2021**, *10*, 1140–1147. [CrossRef]
6. Zijlstra, F.; Ernst, N.; de Boer, M.-J.; Nibbering, E.; Suryapranata, H.; Hoorntje, J.C.; Dambrink, J.-H.; Hof, A.W.V.; Verheugt, F.W. Influence of prehospital administration of aspirin and heparin on initial patency of the infarct-related artery in patients with acute ST elevation myocardial infarction. *J. Am. Coll. Cardiol.* **2002**, *39*, 1733–1737. [CrossRef]
7. Emilsson, O.E.; Bergman, S.; Mohammad, M.M.; Olivecrona, G.O.; Götberg, M.; Erlinge, D.; Koul, S. Pretreatment with heparin in patients with ST-segment elevation myocardial infarction: A report from the Swedish Coronary Angiography and Angioplasty Registry (SCAAR). *EuroIntervention* **2022**, *18*, 709–718. [CrossRef]
8. Arnaout, M.; Mongardon, N.; Deye, N.; Legriel, S.; Dumas, F.; Sauneuf, B.; Malissin, I.; Charpentier, J.; Pène, F.; Baud, F.; et al. Out-of-hospital cardiac arrest from brain cause: Epidemiology, clinical features, and outcome in a multicenter cohort. *Crit. Care Med.* **2015**, *43*, 453–460. [CrossRef]
9. Baldi, E.; Schnaubelt, S.; Caputo, M.L.; Klersy, C.; Clodi, C.; Bruno, J.; Compagnoni, S.; Benvenuti, C.; Domanovits, H.; Burkart, R.; et al. Association of Timing of Electrocardiogram Acquisition after Return of Spontaneous Circulation with Coronary Angiography Findings in Patients with Out-of-Hospital Cardiac Arrest. *JAMA Netw. Open* **2021**, *4*, e2032875. [CrossRef]
10. Beygui, F.; Castren, M.; Brunetti, N.D.; Rosell-Ortiz, F.; Christ, M.; Zeymer, U.; Huber, K.; Folke, F.; Svensson, L.; Bueno, H.; et al. Pre-hospital management of patients with chest pain and/or dyspnoea of cardiac origin. A position paper of the Acute Cardiovascular Care Association (ACCA) of the ESC. *Eur. Heart J. Acute Cardiovasc. Care* **2020**, *9* (Suppl. 1), 59–81. [CrossRef]
11. Thiele, H.; Bauersachs, J.; Mehilli, J.; Möllmann, H.; Landmesser, U.; Jobs, A. Kommentar zu den 2020er Leitlinien der Europäischen Gesellschaft für Kardiologie (ESC) zum Management des akuten Koronarsyndroms bei Patienten ohne persistierende ST-Strecken-Hebung. *Der Kardiol.* **2021**, *15*, 19–31. [CrossRef]

Disclaimer/Publisher's Note: The statements, opinions and data contained in all publications are solely those of the individual author(s) and contributor(s) and not of MDPI and/or the editor(s). MDPI and/or the editor(s) disclaim responsibility for any injury to people or property resulting from any ideas, methods, instructions or products referred to in the content.

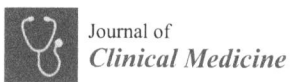

Article

Early Prediction of Mortality after Birth Asphyxia with the nSOFA

Anne-Kathrin Dathe [1,2,3], Anja Stein [1,2], Nora Bruns [1,2], Elena-Diana Craciun [1,2], Laura Tuda [1,2], Johanna Bialas [1,2], Maire Brasseler [1,2], Ursula Felderhoff-Mueser [1,2] and Britta M. Huening [1,2,*]

[1] Neonatology, Paediatric Intensive Care and Paediatric Neurology, Department of Paediatrics I, University Hospital Essen, University of Duisburg-Essen, 45122 Essen, Germany; anne-kathrin.dathe@eah-jena.de (A.-K.D.)
[2] Centre for Translational Neuro- and Behavioural Sciences, C-TNBS, Faculty of Medicine, University of Duisburg-Essen, 45122 Essen, Germany
[3] Department of Health and Nursing, Occupational Therapy, Ernst-Abbe-University of Applied Sciences, 07745 Jena, Germany
* Correspondence: britta.huening@uk-essen.de; Tel.: +49-(0)-201-723-85021

Abstract: (1) Birth asphyxia is a major cause of delivery room resuscitation. Subsequent organ failure and hypoxic–ischemic encephalopathy (HIE) account for 25% of all early postnatal deaths. The neonatal sequential organ failure assessment (nSOFA) considers platelet count and respiratory and cardiovascular dysfunction in neonates with sepsis. To evaluate whether nSOFA is also a useful predictor for in-hospital mortality in neonates ($\geq$36 + 0 weeks of gestation (GA)) following asphyxia with HIE and therapeutic hypothermia (TH), (2) nSOFA was documented at $\leq$6 h of life. (3) A total of 65 infants fulfilled inclusion criteria for TH. All but one infant received cardiopulmonary resuscitation and/or respiratory support at birth. nSOFA was lower in survivors (median 0 [IQR 0–2]; $n = 56$, median GA 39 + 3, female $n = 28$ (50%)) than in non-survivors (median 10 [4–12], $p < 0.001$; $n = 9$, median GA 38 + 6, $n = 4$ (44.4%)). This was also observed for the respiratory ($p < 0.001$), cardiovascular ($p < 0.001$), and hematologic sub-scores ($p = 0.003$). The odds ratio for mortality was 1.6 [95% CI = 1.2–2.1] per one-point increase in nSOFA. The optimal cut-off value of nSOFA to predict mortality was 3.5 (sensitivity 100.0%, specificity 83.9%). (4) Since early accurate prognosis following asphyxia with HIE and TH is essential to guide decision making, nSOFA ($\leq$6 h of life) offers the possibility of identifying infants at risk of mortality.

Keywords: birth asphyxia; nSOFA; outcome prediction; neonate; hypoxic–ischemic encephalopathy (HIE); therapeutic hypothermia; resuscitation; organ dysfunction; critical illness assessment; mortality

1. Introduction

The essential component to neonatal adaptation after birth is the initiation of adequate respiratory effort. Approximately 10–15% of newborns require support for respiratory transition at birth, 3% require positive pressure ventilation by mask, 2% intubation, and only <1% cardiopulmonary resuscitation with chest compressions or epinephrine to establish cardiorespiratory function [1,2]. The major cause for delivery room cardiopulmonary resuscitation is birth asphyxia, a condition of insufficient oxygen supply to vital organs that results in hypoxia, hypercarbia, and metabolic acidosis and, if prolonged, may progress to multiorgan failure, including the developing brain, which is then referred to as hypoxic–ischemic encephalopathy [3,4]. Asphyxia may originate from prenatal, perinatal or postnatal pathology. Prenatal maternal pathologies that increase the risk for birth asphyxia include diabetes mellitus or gestational diabetes, arterial hypertension, placental insufficiency, pregnancy toxemia, eclamptic seizure, infections, or drugs. Perinatal risk factors are, e.g., placental abruption, fetomaternal hemorrhage, amniotic fluid embolism, umbilical cord compression (knot or prolapse), insertio velamentosa of the umbilical cord, placenta previa, or shoulder dystocia. Postnatal causes of birth asphyxia are fetal anemia due to twin-to-twin transfusion in monochoriotic twins or fetal isoimmunization, airway anomalies, neurologic disorders, severe cardiopulmonary disease, infections, congenital malformations, intrauterine growth retardation, or medication effects.

Hypoxic–ischemic encephalopathy is a form of brain dysfunction (i.e., following brain injury) that occurs due to insufficient blood flow to the brain and/or insufficient oxygenation. The pattern of damage in hypoxic–ischemic encephalopathy depends on the severity, duration, and reoccurrence of hypoxia–ischemia and may result in involvement of the deep gray matter (basal ganglia and thalami), brainstem, and/or brain white matter in various combinations [5]. Hypoxic–ischemic encephalopathy is classified into three severity grades, according to Sarnat et al., based on clinical symptoms. For the diagnosis of moderate or severe hypoxic–ischemic encephalopathy (grade II and III), at least three of the six categories (e.g., vigilance, activity, reflexes, muscle tone, or apnea), i.e., a Sarnat Score ≥ 5, must be met [6]. While the Sarnat score is broadly used today, other scores, e.g., the Thompson score, with comparable clinical signs, exist.

Birth asphyxia accounts for 900,000 neonatal deaths worldwide annually and hypoxic–ischemic encephalopathy is estimated to cause up to a quarter of all postnatal deaths [7–9]. In developed countries, birth asphyxia occurs in 1.5–2.5 per 1000 live births and is one of the major causes for the development of cerebral palsy [10].

Therapeutic hypothermia is the only evidence-based neuroprotective therapeutic intervention currently available and is the standard of care in high income countries for moderate and severe hypoxic–ischemic encephalopathy (grade II and III) [11].

Therapeutic hypothermia improved the prognosis significantly: lower incidences of death and less severe cerebral palsy and epilepsy were reported in major randomized controlled trials on hypothermia [12–15]. However, mortality rates and the prevalence of severe disability are still high at 28% and 16–30%, respectively [11,16,17].

In severe hypoxic–ischemic encephalopathy, early prognosis is essential for parental counseling and treatment decisions, such as withdrawal of care. Currently available biomarkers and clinical parameters have in common that they require high personnel and technical resources. Furthermore, applicability and validity are limited in the first hours of life [18]. In a situation of a life-threatening illness, as severe hypoxic–ischemic encephalopathy, accurate and reliable determination of organ dysfunction and mortality risk is urgently needed.

The sepsis-related organ failure assessment (SOFA) score was designed to quantify organ dysfunction and mortality risk in adult intensive care patients with sepsis [19–21]. In recent years, its use is no longer limited to sepsis and the acronym is sometimes translated into sequential organ failure assessment, reflecting the broad dissemination of the SOFA score.

The neonatal modification of the SOFA (nSOFA) was proposed to address the need for a consensus definition of neonatal sepsis in 2020 [22]. nSOFA uses three objective and broadly available clinical parameters to quantify organ dysfunction: respiratory, cardiovascular, and hematological scores (total scores range from 0 to 15).

It was previously used for predicting mortality and severe morbidity in preterm infants [23], preterm infants with late onset sepsis [24], respiratory distress syndrome (RDS) [25], and neonates with proven sepsis [22,26]. Thus, the score was already shown to be predictive independent of the cause of organ dysfunction in the first 24 and 72 h.

The aim of the present study was to evaluate the accuracy of the nSOFA for predicting in-hospital mortality (sensitivity, specificity) following hypoxic–ischemic encephalopathy and therapeutic hypothermia.

2. Materials and Methods

2.1. Participants

For this retrospective study, the charts of all neonates with a gestational age of $\geq 36 + 0$ weeks were reviewed who had received therapeutic hypothermia for hypoxic–ischemic encephalopathy following birth asphyxia at the level III NICU of the University Hospital Essen, Germany, between 1st December 2007 and 31st January 2023.

Therapeutic hypothermia was initiated based on clinical and laboratory criteria derived from large, randomized trials [12–15]. Therapeutic hypothermia after birth asphyxia was officially recommended by the American Heart Association in 2010, followed by the German Guidelines in 2013.

The eligibility criteria for therapeutic hypothermia at our institution did not change substantially in the evaluated time period and were as follows:

Birth asphyxia defined by at least one of the following criteria (block 1):

(a) documented severe acidosis with a pH ≤ 7.00;
(b) base excess of ≤ -16 mmol/l (blood from umbilical cord or neonate within the first 60 min of life);
(c) Apgar score ≤ 5 at 10 min of life;
(d) prolonged cardiorespiratory support (at least 10 min), consisting of chest compressions, epinephrine, intubation, bag and mask ventilation, or continuous positive airway pressure (CPAP).

In addition to moderate to severe hypoxic–ischemic encephalopathy defined by at least one of the following (block 2):

(a) encephalopathy (lethargy, stupor, coma) plus at least one of the following signs: (a1) muscular hypotonia, (a2) abnormal reflexes, or (a3) clinical seizures;
(b) post-2020 modified Sarnat score ≥ 5 (hypoxic–ischemic encephalopathy grade II and III);
(c) clinical seizures;
(d) pathologic amplitude integrates electroencephalogram (aEEG, discontinuous normal voltage, low voltage, burst-suppression, flat trace, or electroencephalographic seizures).

For inclusion in this retrospective study, a reconstruction of the Sarnat score was possible: five points for moderate encephalopathy was already present with invasive ventilation and a clinical neurological sign, such as muscular hypotonia.

Contraindications for therapeutic hypothermia were life-threatening congenital malformation (e.g., diaphragmatic hernia, cerebral malformation), suspected metabolic disease, coagulopathy with active bleeding, cerebral hemorrhage, cerebral venous thrombosis, hemorrhagic infarction, small for gestational age with birth weight < 1800 g, or severe pulmonary hypertension.

2.2. Therapeutic Hypothermia

Therapeutic hypothermia was delivered following a standardized protocol. Whole body hypothermia was initiated as early postnatally as possible but within 6 h after birth (TECOtherm® tcmatt Neo, Tec Com Medizintechnik GmbH, Kabelsketal, Germany). A target temperature of 33.5 to 34.5 °C was monitored via a continuous rectal probe. It was sustained for 72 h followed by a rewarming phase. The temperature was increased 0.5 °C per hour until 37.0 °C was reached. Until 2015, this was performed manually; however, post-2015, a servo-controlled cooling mattress has been used.

2.3. Calculation of nSOFA

The nSOFA is calculated from 3 subcategories for respiratory, cardiovascular, and hematological status (Table 1). The respiratory category takes the status of mechanical ventilation, oxygen saturation (SpO$_2$), and a fraction of inspired oxygen (FiO$_2$) into account (score range 0–8). Cardiovascular status analyses the number of vasoactive drugs necessary to maintain normal blood pressure, including the use of corticosteroids (score range 0–4). The hematologic score is based on the presence and severity of thrombocytopenia (score range 0–3). The total score can therefore range from 0 (best) to 15 (worst) [22]. Data to calculate nSOFA in our cohort were derived from the patient charts, choosing the worst score value from the first 6 h of life, both values from the delivery room and after admission were included. Monitoring included continuous amplitude-integrated electroencephalogram (aEEG), a Thompson score (not standardized in time), and 1–2 hourly vital signs, including changes in ventilator settings. A complete blood count was included in the initial blood work on admission.

Table 1. Neonatal sequential organ failure assessment (nSOFA) [22].

Component	nSOFA Scores				
	0	2	4	6	8
Respiratory score	Not intubated or intubated SpO_2/FiO_2 ratio ≥ 300	Intubated SpO_2/FiO_2 ratio < 300	Intubated SpO_2/FiO_2 ratio < 200	Intubated SpO_2/FiO_2 ratio < 150	Intubated SpO_2/FiO_2 ratio < 100
	0	1	2	3	4
Cardiovascular score	No systemic corticosteroids and no inotropes	Systemic corticosteroid treatment but no inotropes	1 inotrope and no systemic corticosteroids	≥ 2 inotropes or 1 inotrope and systemic corticosteroids	≥ 2 inotropes and systemic corticosteroids
	0	1	2	3	
Hematologic score	Platelet count $\geq 150/nL$	Platelet count 100–149/nL	Platelet count <100/nL	Platelet count <50/nL	

Notes: FiO_2 = fraction of inspired oxygen; SpO_2 = oxygen saturation as measured by pulse oximetry. Medications considered as inotropes (or vasoactive) = dopamine, dobutamine, epinephrine, norepinephrine, vasopressin, and milrinone.

2.4. Endpoint: Death

The endpoint of the study was death. The timepoint of death and causes of death were taken from the medical records and/or death certificates. The decision to withdraw or limit care was based on a combination of clinical considerations—mainly the lack of respiratory effort in ventilated infants, severe CNS injury identified via Magnetic resonance imaging (MRI) or sonography, and severe organ dysfunction. If infants did not show respiratory effort after the cessation of mechanical ventilation, they were not reintubated and palliative care was initiated in the form of adequate analgesia, sedation, and/or weaning of cardiovascular support while maintaining enteral nutrition and warming for comfort.

2.5. Statistical Analysis

Analyses were performed using SPSS 29 (IBM Corp., New York, NY, USA). Patient demographics, clinical characteristics, and nSOFA scores are presented as medians and ranges or interquartile ranges for continuous variables and for categorical variables as counts and category percentages. Mann–Whitney U-tests and Fisher's exact test were used to compare continuous and non-continuous data, respectively. Two-sided p-values < 0.05 were considered statistically significant. The Kaplan–Meier curve was used to visualize time to death and discharge.

Logistic regression was performed to calculate the odds ratio for in-hospital mortality with the nSOFA score as regressor. A receiver operating characteristics curve (ROC) was generated to plot true positive rate (sensitivity) against false positive rate (1—specificity) across varying threshold settings and areas under the receiver operating characteristic curves (AUCs) were calculated. An optimal cut-off value for odds of in-hospital mortality by nSOFA was determined using the Youden index and closest top-left methods. Positive and negative predictive values were calculated.

3. Results

Out of the 6016 infants screened, 79 infants received therapeutic hypothermia due to hypoxic–ischemic encephalopathy (Figure 1). One infant, at 37 + 0 weeks of gestation, was included although the birth weight was 1745 g (contrary to recommendations of the American Heart Association) based on an individual treatment decision. We excluded four infants from the analysis because of a baseline condition with influences on organ function or mortality other than hypoxic–ischemic encephalopathy: two infants with blood culture-proven early onset sepsis, one infant with congenital malformation, and one infant with chromosomal abnormality. Two infants had life-threatening congenital malformations, so they were excluded. Two infants were excluded, since they did not suffer from birth asphyxia but required resuscitation later than in the delivery room. A total of 45 of 79 infants were inborn. Outborn infants were transferred to our institution and therapeutic hypothermia was begun within the first 6 h of life. Of these, Three infants were born outside of a hospital, which led to missing data in one case. Seven additional cases of outborn infants had to be excluded, because data to calculate nSOFA were not sufficient. This led to a final cohort of 65 infants with 21 outborn infants (survival cohort n = 16; non-survival cohort n = 5) (Figure 1).

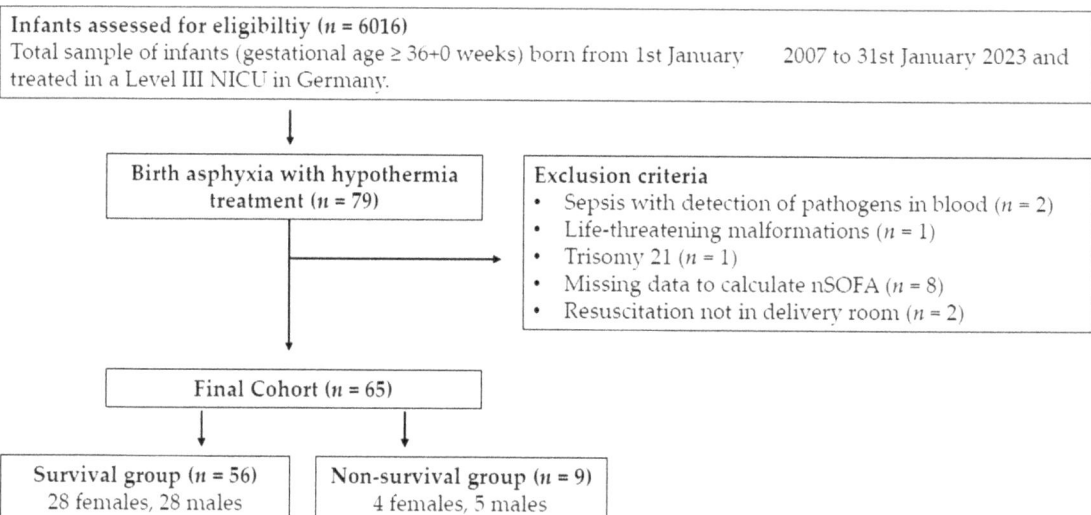

Figure 1. Inclusion and exclusion criteria. Notes: NICU = neonatal intensive care unit.

All neonates fulfilled at least one of the criteria for birth asphyxia (block 1), 26.2% of infants presented with two criteria, and 64.6% with more than two criteria (Table 2).

All infants had at least moderate hypoxic–ischemic encephalopathy as indication for therapeutic hypothermia (block 2). A total of 47.7% infants presented with two criteria and 38.8% with more than two criteria. Clinical signs of hypoxic–ischemic encephalopathy according to criteria (a) were fulfilled by 60 infants; in 13 infants, the Sarnat score was available; and in 21 cases, the Sarnat score was reconstructed (invasive ventilation plus muscular hypotonia). Clinical seizures or pathological aEEG were valid for three and forty infants, respectively.

3.1. Clinical Characteristics

Survivors (n = 56) and non-survivors (n = 9) were similar with respect to gestational age, birth weight, small for gestational age, head circumference, child sex, umbilical cord pH, umbilical base excess (BE), and seizures before and during hypothermia treatment (Table 3). Maternal platelets in blood sample closest to birth showed no group differences (survivor group median 223 [119–385]/nL, non-survivor group median 197 [137–302]/nL). The platelets were less than 160/nL in three cases of each group. There was no platelet count of less than 100/nL. Neither pregnancy-associated nor immunological diseases were present in these mothers. In one case, an amniotic infection syndrome was present.

Table 2. Eligibility criteria for therapeutic hypothermia (number (%)).

	Infants (n = 65)
Block 1	
Birth asphyxia criteria	
(a) Severe acidosis, pH $\leq$ 7.00 [a]	56 (91.8) [c]
(b) Base excess $\leq$ −16 mmol/L [a]	42 (68.9) [c]
(c) Apgar 10 min $\leq$ 5	22 (34.4) [d]
(d) Prolonged delivery room resuscitation [b]	59 (96.7) [c]
Number of criteria block 1:	
One	6
Two	17
>two	42
Block 2	
Hypoxic–ischemic encephalopathy criteria	
(a) Encephalopathy (lethargy, stupor, coma) plus	60 (92.3)
(a1) Muscular hypotonia	51 (78.5)
(a2) Abnormal reflexes	58 (89.2)
(a3) Clinical seizures	3 (4.6)
(b) Sarnat score $\geq$ 5	34 (52.3)
(c) Clinical seizures	3 (4.6)
(d) Pathologic aEEG	40 (70.0) [e]
Number of criteria block 2:	
One	15
Two	31
>two	20

Notes: [a] pH und base excess: Infant's first blood sample was obtained arterial, venous, or capillary and derived either from cord blood or was drawn at admission to the NICU within the first hour of life. [b] Cardiopulmonary resuscitation of at least 10 min includes respiratory support, chest compressions, and Epinephrine. Descriptive statistics are based on [c] n = 61, [d] n = 64, and [e] n = 58, otherwise n = 65 infants.

Non-survivors had lower pH and BE in the infant blood gas analysis during the first hour of life and lower Apgar scores at 1, 5, and 10 min. Non-survivors were more often born via c-section or emergency c-section (Table 3). A comparison of complete Sarnat scores was not possible due to the small number of cases. One surviving infant was born as a twin, but there were no multiple births in the non-survival cohort. All but one infant received cardiopulmonary resuscitation (chest compression and/or epinephrine) and/or respiratory support during transition after birth. Non-survivors were more likely to have received delivery room resuscitation and epinephrine during postnatal care. There was the need for respiratory support in both groups. However, there were more intubations in the non-surviving group while temporary mask ventilation via T-piece was sufficient for stabilization in the group of survivors (Table 3). Death occurred within the first 24 h in five neonates and before 48 h of life in another two neonates. Two infants died later on days 6 and 8 (Figure 2, Table 3). Causes of death were lack of respiratory effort in four cases, multi-organ dysfunction in four cases, and circulatory failure in one case. Four of the non-surviving infants received MRI. In survivors, the median length of hospital stay was 11.3 days with a wide range (Figure 2, Table 3).

3.2. nSOFA Scores in Survivors and Non-Survivors

nSOFA sum scores were lower in survivors than in non-survivors (Mann–Whitney U-test, $p < 0.001$) (Figure 3, Table 4). This also held true for respiratory ($p < 0.001$), cardiovascular ($p < 0.001$), and hematologic sub-scores ($p = 0.003$), respectively (Figure 3, Table 4).

Table 3. Clinical characteristics of survivors and non-survivors.

	Survivors (n = 56)	Non-Survivors (n = 9)
Gestational age, weeks	39 + 3 [36 + 0–41 + 4]	38 + 6 [37 + 2–41 + 2]
Weight at birth, grams	3170 [1745–4400]	3380 [2600–4400]
SGA, n (%)	12 (21.4)	1 (11.1)
Height at birth, cm	50.0 [42.0–58.0]	52.5 [50.0–56.0] [f]
Head circumference at birth, cm	34.0 [30.0–38.0] [g]	34.8 [31.5–38.0] [f]
Female, n (%)	28 (50.0)	4 (44.4)
Multiple birth, n (%)	1 (1.8)	0 (0)
C-section, n (%)	28 (50)	8 (88.9)
Perinatal sentinel event [a], n (%)	22 (39.3)	7 (77.8)
Umbilical cord pH (SD)	6.98 [6.61–7.28] [h]	7.05 [6.59–7.29] [i]
First pH from infant [b]	6.93 [6.75–7.19] [j]	6.74 [6.41–7.23]
Umbilical cord base excess	−15.25 [−33.90–−4.20] [k]	−16.70 [−23.00–−5.00] [l]
First base excess from infant [b]	−17.90 [−28.00–−9.10] [m]	−25.15 [−31.70–−8.70] [f]
Apgar 1 min	2 [0–6] [g]	0 [0–1]
Apgar 5 min	5 [0–8] [g]	0 [0–4]
Apgar 10 min	7 [1–10] [g]	0 [0–4]
Delivery room resuscitation [c], n (%)	13 (23.2)	7 (77.7)
Respiratory support [d], n (%)	55 (98.2)	9 (100)
Intubation, n (%)	23 (41.0)	9 (100)
Mask ventilation via T-piece, n (%)	28 (50.0)	0 (0)
CPAP, n (%)	3 (5.4)	0 (0)
Chest compressions, n (%)	3 (5.3)	0 (0)
Epinephrine, n (%)	4 (7.3) [g]	6 (66.7)
Sarnat score [e]	11 [5–15] [n]	20.5 [18–23] [o]
Sarnat score ≥ 5 (reconstructed) [e], n (%)	25 (45.5) [g]	9 (100)
Seizure activity in aEEG, n (%)		
Before TH, n (%)	2 (3.6) [g]	0 (0)
During TH, n (%)	16 (29.1) [g]	5 (62.5) [f]
Time to death or discharge, days	11.29 [5.43–54.66]	0.97 [0.42–8.50]

Notes: Data are presented as median [range] if not indicated otherwise. SGA = small for gestational age with weight of birth < 10th percentile; cm = centimeter; CPAP = continuous positive airway pressure; TH = therapeutic hypothermia; C-section = caesarean section. [a] Perinatal sentinel events include: placental abruption, uterine rupture, umbilical cord trauma (either cord prolapse, knot, tear, rupture, or compression), shoulder dystocia, severe internal bleeding, trauma, cardiorespiratory arrest, or seizures immediately before birth, [b] pH und base excess: infant's first blood sample was applied arterial, venous, or capillary and derived either from cord blood or was drawn at admission to the NICU within the first hour of life, [c] Delivery room resuscitation includes prolonged chest compression and/or respiratory support for at least 10 minutes postnatally. [d] Respiratory support applied in the delivery room, [e] Sarnat scores displayed here were obtained within the first 6 h of life. A Sarnat score of ≥ 5 was reconstructed if invasive ventilation and clinical neurological signs, such as muscular hypotonias were present. Descriptive statistics are based on [f] n = 8, [g] n = 55, [h] n = 52, [i] n = 7, [j] n = 47, [k] n = 44, [l] n = 4, [m] n = 45, [n] n = 11, and [o] n = 2, otherwise n = 56 in the survival group and n = 9 in the non-survival group.

3.3. Prediction of In-Hospital Mortality by nSOFA

A significant relationship of nSOFA and mortality was confirmed with an odds ratio for mortality of 1.61 [95% CI = 1.24–2.08] per one-point increase in nSOFA score (X^2 (1) = 25.98, $p < 0.001$, Nagelkerkes R^2 = 0.53). The ROC curve for risk of death by nSOFA (Figure 4) had an area under the curve (AUC) of 0.94 (95% CI = 0.88–1.00). The optimal cut-off value of the nSOFA score, according to the Youden index and the closest top-left method was 3.5 (sensitivity 100.0%, specificity 83.9%). Using a cut-off of 3.5 points on the nSOFA score, the positive and negative predictive values were 50.0% and 100.0%, respectively (cross-tabulation in Table 5).

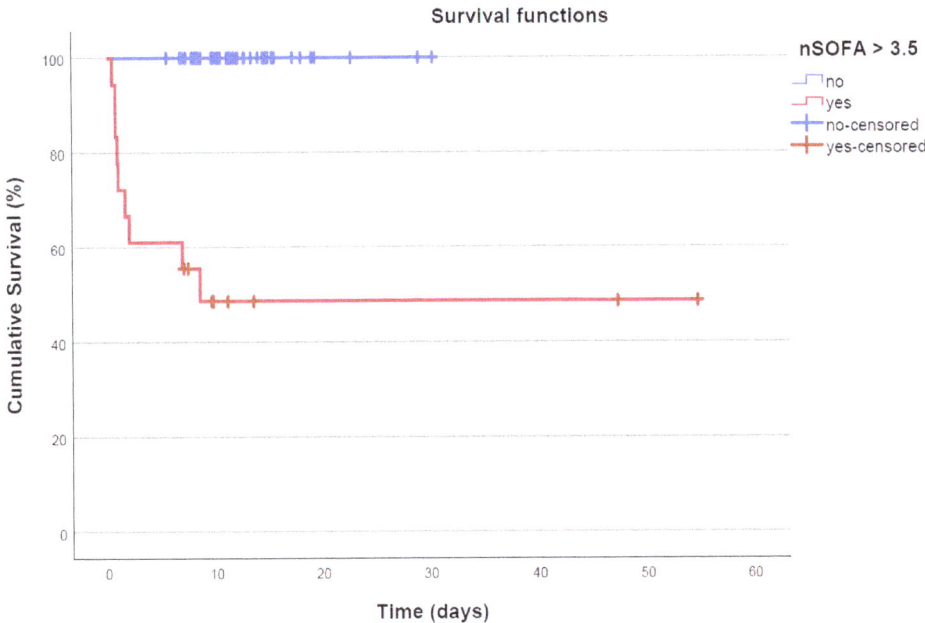

Figure 2. Kaplan–Meier curve of time to mortality or discharge (censor) using an nSOFA cut-off level (as reported later) of 3.5. Notes: The length of hospital stay did not differ between groups with an nSOFA value above 3.5 ($n = 9$, median 9.7 [range 7.0–54.7] days) and below 3.5 ($n = 47$, median 11.4 [5.4 to 30.2] days).

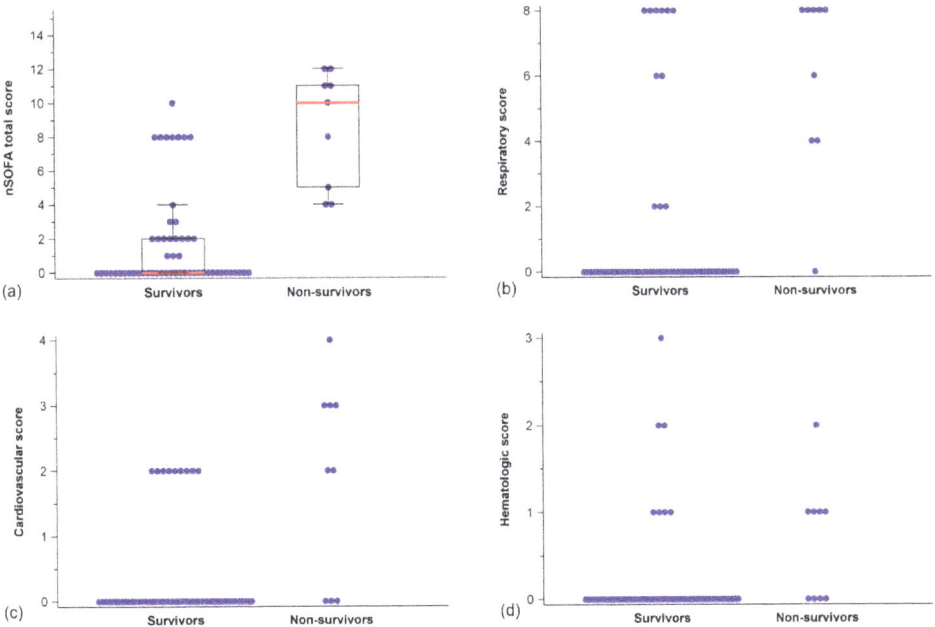

Figure 3. Distribution (scatter plot) of (**a**) nSOFA total scores with box plot (median, IQR), (**b**) respiratory scores, (**c**) cardiovascular scores, and (**d**) hematologic scores in survivors and non-survivors. Notes: The area above the nSOFA cut-off value of 3.5 is colored gray. nSOFA = neonatal sequential organ failure assessment; IQR = interquartile range.

Table 4. Descriptive characteristics of nSOFA total score and sub-scores in survivors and non-survivors.

	Survivors (n = 56)	Non-Survivors (n = 9)	p-Value
nSOFA total score	0 [0–2]	10 [4.5–11.5]	<0.001
Respiratory score	0 [0–0]	8 [4–8]	<0.001
Intubation, n (%)	23 (41.1%)	9 (100.0%)	<0.001
SpO_2/FiO_2 ratio	447.6 [246.9–461.9] [a]	79.0 [55.0–178.3]	<0.001
Cardiovascular score	0 [0–0]	2 [2,3]	<0.001
One inotrope, n (%)	9 (16.1%)	2 (22.2%)	0.642
Two or more inotropes, n (%)	0 (0%)	4 (44.4%)	<0.001
Systemic steroids, n (%)	0 (0%)	1 (11.1%)	0.138
Hematologic score	0 [0–0]	1 [1]	0.003
Platelets/nL	237 [180–279]	132 [110–242]	0.077

Notes: Data are presented as median [interquartile range] if not indicated otherwise. Mann–Whitney U-test and Fisher's exact test were used for continuous and non-continuous data, respectively. [a] n = 52.

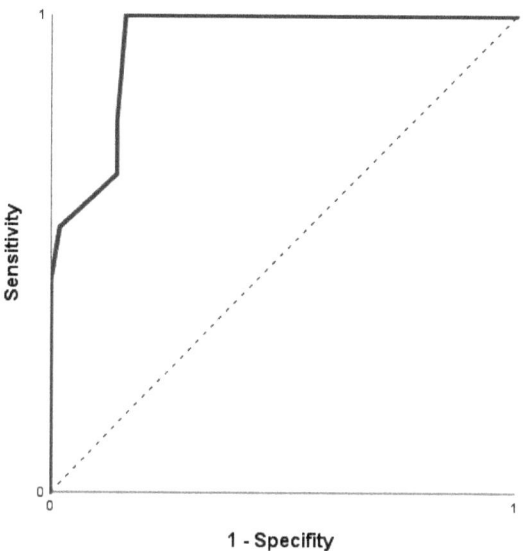

Figure 4. Receiver operating characteristics curve for nSOFA to predict non-survival.

Table 5. Cross-tabulation of nSOFA cut-off value of 3.5 in survivors (n = 56) and non-survivors (n = 9).

		Survivors	Non-Survivors	Total
nSOFA at least 3.5	no	47	0	47
	yes	9	9	18
		56	9	65

Notes: Data are presented as n.

4. Discussion

4.1. Prediction of In-Hospital Mortality

The nSOFA, as a critical illness assessment, proved useful for predicting in-hospital mortality in neonates with hypoxic–ischemic encephalopathy during therapeutic hypothermia. Non-survivors showed significantly higher sum scores, as well as respiratory, cardiovascular, and hematologic sub-scores. A one-point increase in nSOFA increased the odds for in-hospital mortality by 1.6. None of the infants with a nSOFA score < 3.5 died in this cohort (negative predictive value: 100%). Thus, the nSOFA serves well as an operational definition of organ dysfunction identifying neonates at risk for death following hypoxic–ischemic encephalopathy.

Despite the excellent negative predictive value of nSOFA scores of < 3.5, several survivors had nSOFA scores of 8, limiting the positive predictive value of the cut-off value. This is likely due to the fact that the respiratory sub-score has the highest weight in the nSOFA sum score, with mechanical ventilation contributing to 8 points of the possible total of 15. All non-survivors and 41% of survivors were intubated and received mechanical ventilation within the first 6 h of life, which resulted in respiratory sub-scores of 2 to 8 points. The notable effect of respiratory management on the nSOFA was also present in other studies within the first 72 h of life in very preterm infants, as well as in late onset sepsis regardless of gestational age [23,26].

4.2. Respiratory and Cardiovascular Sub-Scores

Factors contributing to the need for mechanical ventilation in hypoxic–ischemic encephalopathy and therapeutic hypothermia are manifold: Hypoxia at birth may prevent the onset of spontaneous breathing, lead to apnea and bradycardia, and prevent physiologic transition of circulation to extrauterine life, resulting in pulmonary hypertension and persistent fetal circulation [3]. Therapeutic hypothermia exerts direct effects on respiration by increasing pulmonary vascular resistance and reducing oxygen consumption and release (hemoglobin dissociation) [27]. Neuroactive medication, injury to the respiratory control center in the brain stem, and status epilepticus affect respiratory drive, potentially exacerbating hypoxia and disturbed CO_2 elimination [28]. In a previous study, it was shown that the need for mechanical ventilation was significantly higher in the group with severe asphyxia and unfavorable outcomes (death and severe brain injury on MRI) compared to infants with better short-term outcomes [29]. However, in this cohort, the need for mechanical ventilation without another sign of organ dysfunction was not inextricably associated with death, calling for caution when interpreting nSOFA scores in neonates on mechanical ventilation who are otherwise stable.

Because the establishment of sufficient oxygenation and ventilation is the most important aspect of delivery room resuscitation, the fact that few neonates require chest compressions and/or the administration of epinephrine should not be misinterpreted. A neonate who experiences birth asphyxia may still develop multi-organ failure and become life-threateningly ill due to the redistribution of cardiac output to vital organs such as the brain, myocardium, and adrenal gland. Reduced perfusion to the other organs may cause local hypoxia/ischemia and may result in organ failure [30]. If birth asphyxia is prolonged, cardiovascular deterioration occurs that eventually causes myocardial dysfunction. The fact that the cardiovascular sub-score showed fewer differences between survivors and non-survivors in this study may indicate that this cohort was less affected, or that cardiovascular impairment in asphyxia is less common than in sepsis, for which the nSOFA was originally developed for.

4.3. Hematologic Sub-Score

Thombocytopenia may result from both asphyxia and therapeutic hypothermia. There is a reduced release of platelets from the bone marrow and an increased destruction of circulating platelets in birth asphyxia, and platelet dysfunction during therapeutic hypothermia. The nadir of platelet count is on the 3rd day of life following asphyxia and 5th day of life during therapeutic hypothermia, suggesting an additive effect of therapeutic hypothermia [31–33]. The influence of therapeutic hypothermia on the early nSOFA score is therefore unlikely. It is reasonable to assume that cardiovascular and hematological sub-scores of the nSOFA increase during the acute phase of post-resuscitation treatment before dropping again. Therefore, these sub-scores may well be important in the sequential use of the nSOFA. Maternal diseases may influence the fetal platelet count as well but the statistical power of this study was not sufficient to investigate these potential confounders.

4.4. Decision Making

However, the early determination of organ dysfunction and the risk of mortality is desirable. All infants in this study had hypoxic–ischemic encephalopathy and therapeutic hypothermia as an expression of moderate to severe brain injury. In such a serious situation, objective and easily accessible prognostic markers can help in parental counseling and decision making.

nSOFA scores > 3.5 were associated with early neonatal death. Five of the nine non-survivors in this study died within the first 24 h of life, and two further neonates died in the first 48 h. In this cohort, neonates who survived this initial critical period were no longer at increased risk thereafter, despite an initial nSOFA score of >3.5. All these early deaths were caused by lack of respiratory effort, circulatory failure, or multi-organ dysfunction. The fact that only four of the non-surviving infants in this study received an MRI (day 5–7) highlights that they presented with such severe symptomatology that the extent of cerebral damage was either not necessary for decision making to discontinue therapy or the infants died despite full therapy. This observation is in accordance with other reports on early neonatal deaths (<72 h), in the phase of clinical instability and critical illness [34,35].

Because this is the first application of the nSOFA score in HIE, it is too early to recommend clinical application at this point. Rather, these data generate the hypothesis that the nSOFA may be useful for classifying mortality risk in the decision-making process in infants with hypoxic–ischemic encephalopathy during therapeutic hypothermia if the results can be reproduced and validated in a larger, prospective multi-center study.

4.5. Available Biomarkers and Clinical Assessments

First-hour clinical parameters, such as umbilical cord pH and Apgar scores have limited reliability in predicting individual mortality. In addition, the Apgar includes subjective components with high inter-observer variability. Currently available biomarkers, physical examination, chemical, electrophysiological, and imaging studies all have specific limitations. Clinical examinations require experience and may be influenced by treatment/medication. Chemical biomarkers, e.g., plasma biomarkers, proteomics, and metabolomics, require specific lab resources and may have a delayed response to the injury [18]. Electrophysiology has a good predictive marker for abnormal brain activity, but it necessitates equipment, resources, and expertise [36]. MRI examinations also involves a large amount of time and effort, the risk of transporting a critically ill infant and limited accuracy of early scans compared to those obtained at the end of the first week of life [37]. Existing neonatal critical illness scores are either designed for very preterm infants (clinical risk index for babies—CRIB I and II; Berlin Score) are too complex and inconvenient for use and/or variables are collected over a longer period of time—up to 24 h after birth (score for neonatal acute physiology (perinatal extension)—SNAP I/II and SNAP-PE I/II; (extended) sick neonatal score—(E)SNS) [38,39]. Scores like Sarnat and Thompson may aid in decision making regarding hypothermia treatment or decision making. However, the results depend on the timing of scoring, as symptoms may evolve over time, and on the expertise of the examiner and may be less predictive of mortality, as our results show [40]. It is therefore desirable to have a very early and at the same time accurate assessment of prognosis, which can easily be performed without technical effort or special expertise.

4.6. Strengths and Limitations

The strength of our study lies in the fact that we were able to show for the first time that the nSOFA offers the potential to identify infants at risk of mortality following hypoxic–ischemic encephalopathy and therapeutic hypothermia within the first 6 h of life. The nSOFA is easy to apply, does not require a large number of human resources or anys technical equipment. It is based on variables that can be objectified and measured even in low-resource settings. The nSOFA may serve as a valuable tool in the process of decision making after severe birth asphyxia with hypoxic–ischemic encephalopathy and therapeutic hypothermia.

The nSOFA has already proven its suitability as a predictor for unfavorable outcomes in neonates diagnosed with sepsis. Therefore, neonates with sepsis, which must be considered a potential confounder, were excluded from our study. From clinical experience, an infant suffering from hypoxic–ischemic encephalopathy may also have sepsis. However, our study had a small sample size, which limits the statistical power to allow for subgroup analysis.

Other limitations of this study need to be recognized. This single-center study was performed retrospectively over a long period. This is due to the fact that the center, although providing the highest level of care, tends to care for a small annual number of infants with hypoxic–ischemic encephalopathy, compared to international standards, with many of them referrals. The German system of care is highly decentralized and special centers for asphyxia treatment do not exist.

Although inclusion criteria and major therapeutic regimes did not substantially change, it cannot be excluded that neonatal intensive care of infants has changed slightly over time.

5. Future Aspects and Conclusions

Therefore, the results of this study should be prospectively replicated in multiple centers and larger samples to investigate influencing factors such as maternal diseases, delivery mode, socio-economic status, and fetal factors, e.g., child sex, small for gestational age, and sepsis. In addition, it may be of interest to explore the extent to which the nSOFA is helpful in future decision making and in counseling with parents. The nSOFA is easy to apply, measurable even in low-resource settings, and might be used to identify infants at risk of in-hospital mortality due to hypoxic–ischemic encephalopathy and therapeutic hypothermia. Early accurate prognosis in hypoxic–ischemic encephalopathy during therapeutic hypothermia is essential for decision making.

Author Contributions: Conceptualization, A.-K.D., A.S., N.B. and B.M.H.; formal analysis, A.-K.D. and N.B.; investigation, E.-D.C., L.T., J.B. and M.B.; methodology, A.S.; validation, A.-K.D., A.S., J.B. and M.B.; writing—original draft, A.-K.D., A.S. and B.M.H.; writing—review and editing, N.B., M.B. and U.F.-M. All authors have read and agreed to the published version of the manuscript.

Funding: This research received no external funding.

Institutional Review Board Statement: The study was conducted in accordance with the Declaration of Helsinki and approved by the Ethics Committee of the University Duisburg-Essen (protocol code 18-8191-BO and 7 June 2018).

Informed Consent Statement: Patient consent was waived due to the retrospective analysis of charts on clinical routine data.

Data Availability Statement: The dataset used and/or analyzed for the study is available from the corresponding author upon reasonable request.

Acknowledgments: We thank Lena Hüning for creating the graphical abstract.

Conflicts of Interest: The authors declare no conflict of interest.

References

1. Perlman, J.M.; Risser, R. Cardiopulmonary resuscitation in the delivery room. Associated clinical events. *Arch. Pediatr. Adolesc. Med.* **1995**, *149*, 20–25. [CrossRef] [PubMed]
2. Madar, J.; Roehr, C.C.; Ainsworth, S.; Ersdal, H.; Morley, C.; Rudiger, M.; Skare, C.; Szczapa, T.; Te Pas, A.; Trevisanuto, D.; et al. European Resuscitation Council Guidelines 2021: Newborn resuscitation and support of transition of infants at birth. *Resuscitation* **2021**, *161*, 291–326. [CrossRef] [PubMed]
3. Rainaldi, M.A.; Perlman, J.M. Pathophysiology of Birth Asphyxia. *Clin. Perinatol.* **2016**, *43*, 409–422. [CrossRef]
4. Aziz, K.; Chadwick, M.; Baker, M.; Andrews, W. Ante- and intra-partum factors that predict increased need for neonatal resuscitation. *Resuscitation* **2008**, *79*, 444–452. [CrossRef] [PubMed]
5. Volpe, J.J. Neonatal encephalopathy: An inadequate term for hypoxic-ischemic encephalopathy. *Ann. Neurol.* **2012**, *72*, 156–166. [CrossRef]
6. Sarnat, H.B.; Sarnat, M.S. Neonatal encephalopathy following fetal distress. A clinical and electroencephalographic study. *Arch. Neurol.* **1976**, *33*, 696–705. [CrossRef]

7. World Health Organization. Perinatal Asphyxia. Available online: https://www.who.int/teams/maternal-newborn-child-adolescent-health-and-ageing/newborn-health/perinatal-asphyxia (accessed on 26 January 2023).
8. Liu, L.; Oza, S.; Hogan, D.; Chu, Y.; Perin, J.; Zhu, J.; Lawn, J.E.; Cousens, S.; Mathers, C.; Black, R.E. Global, regional, and national causes of under-5 mortality in 2000-15: An updated systematic analysis with implications for the Sustainable Development Goals. *Lancet* **2016**, *388*, 3027–3035. [CrossRef]
9. McIntyre, S.; Nelson, K.B.; Mulkey, S.B.; Lechpammer, M.; Molloy, E.; Badawi, N.; Newborn Brain Society Guidelines and Publications Committee. Neonatal encephalopathy: Focus on epidemiology and underexplored aspects of etiology. *Semin. Fetal Neonatal Med.* **2021**, *26*, 101265. [CrossRef]
10. Kurinczuk, J.J.; White-Koning, M.; Badawi, N. Epidemiology of neonatal encephalopathy and hypoxic-ischaemic encephalopathy. *Early Hum. Dev.* **2010**, *86*, 329–338. [CrossRef]
11. Tagin, M.A.; Woolcott, C.G.; Vincer, M.J.; Whyte, R.K.; Stinson, D.A. Hypothermia for neonatal hypoxic ischemic encephalopathy: An updated systematic review and meta-analysis. *Arch. Pediatr. Adolesc. Med.* **2012**, *166*, 558–566. [CrossRef]
12. Simbruner, G.; Mittal, R.A.; Rohlmann, F.; Muche, R.; neo.nEURO.network Trial Participants. Systemic hypothermia after neonatal encephalopathy: Outcomes of neo.nEURO.network RCT. *Pediatrics* **2010**, *126*, e771–e778. [CrossRef] [PubMed]
13. Azzopardi, D.V.; Strohm, B.; Edwards, A.D.; Dyet, L.; Halliday, H.L.; Juszczak, E.; Kapellou, O.; Levene, M.; Marlow, N.; Porter, E.; et al. Moderate hypothermia to treat perinatal asphyxial encephalopathy. *N. Engl. J. Med.* **2009**, *361*, 1349–1358. [CrossRef]
14. Shankaran, S.; Laptook, A.R.; Ehrenkranz, R.A.; Tyson, J.E.; McDonald, S.A.; Donovan, E.F.; Fanaroff, A.A.; Poole, W.K.; Wright, L.L.; Higgins, R.D.; et al. Whole-body hypothermia for neonates with hypoxic-ischemic encephalopathy. *N. Engl. J. Med.* **2005**, *353*, 1574–1584. [CrossRef] [PubMed]
15. Jacobs, S.E.; Morley, C.J.; Inder, T.E.; Stewart, M.J.; Smith, K.R.; McNamara, P.J.; Wright, I.M.; Kirpalani, H.M.; Darlow, B.A.; Doyle, L.W.; et al. Whole-body hypothermia for term and near-term newborns with hypoxic-ischemic encephalopathy: A randomized controlled trial. *Arch. Pediatr. Adolesc. Med.* **2011**, *165*, 692–700. [CrossRef] [PubMed]
16. Liu, X.; Jary, S.; Cowan, F.; Thoresen, M. Reduced infancy and childhood epilepsy following hypothermia-treated neonatal encephalopathy. *Epilepsia* **2017**, *58*, 1902–1911. [CrossRef] [PubMed]
17. Perez, A.; Ritter, S.; Brotschi, B.; Werner, H.; Caflisch, J.; Martin, E.; Latal, B. Long-term neurodevelopmental outcome with hypoxic-ischemic encephalopathy. *J. Pediatr.* **2013**, *163*, 454–459. [CrossRef]
18. Ahearne, C.E.; Boylan, G.B.; Murray, D.M. Short and long term prognosis in perinatal asphyxia: An update. *World J. Clin. Pediatr.* **2016**, *5*, 67–74. [CrossRef] [PubMed]
19. Seymour, C.W.; Liu, V.X.; Iwashyna, T.J.; Brunkhorst, F.M.; Rea, T.D.; Scherag, A.; Rubenfeld, G.; Kahn, J.M.; Shankar-Hari, M.; Singer, M.; et al. Assessment of Clinical Criteria for Sepsis: For the Third International Consensus Definitions for Sepsis and Septic Shock (Sepsis-3). *JAMA* **2016**, *315*, 762–774. [CrossRef]
20. Shankar-Hari, M.; Phillips, G.S.; Levy, M.L.; Seymour, C.W.; Liu, V.X.; Deutschman, C.S.; Angus, D.C.; Rubenfeld, G.D.; Singer, M.; Sepsis Definitions Task Force. Developing a New Definition and Assessing New Clinical Criteria for Septic Shock: For the Third International Consensus Definitions for Sepsis and Septic Shock (Sepsis-3). *JAMA* **2016**, *315*, 775–787. [CrossRef]
21. Singer, M.; Deutschman, C.S.; Seymour, C.W.; Shankar-Hari, M.; Annane, D.; Bauer, M.; Bellomo, R.; Bernard, G.R.; Chiche, J.D.; Coopersmith, C.M.; et al. The Third International Consensus Definitions for Sepsis and Septic Shock (Sepsis-3). *JAMA* **2016**, *315*, 801–810. [CrossRef]
22. Wynn, J.L.; Polin, R.A. A neonatal sequential organ failure assessment score predicts mortality to late-onset sepsis in preterm very low birth weight infants. *Pediatr. Res.* **2020**, *88*, 85–90. [CrossRef]
23. Berka, I.; Korcek, P.; Janota, J.; Stranak, Z. Neonatal Sequential Organ Failure Assessment (nSOFA) Score within 72 Hours after Birth Reliably Predicts Mortality and Serious Morbidity in Very Preterm Infants. *Diagnostics* **2022**, *12*, 1342. [CrossRef]
24. Fleiss, N.; Coggins, S.A.; Lewis, A.N.; Zeigler, A.; Cooksey, K.E.; Walker, L.A.; Husain, A.N.; de Jong, B.S.; Wallman-Stokes, A.; Alrifai, M.W.; et al. Evaluation of the Neonatal Sequential Organ Failure Assessment and Mortality Risk in Preterm Infants with Late-Onset Infection. *JAMA Netw. Open* **2021**, *4*, e2036518. [CrossRef]
25. Shi, S.; Guo, J.; Fu, M.; Liao, L.; Tu, J.; Xiong, J.; Liao, Q.; Chen, W.; Chen, K.; Liao, Y. Evaluation of the neonatal sequential organ failure assessment and mortality risk in neonates with respiratory distress syndrome: A retrospective cohort study. *Front. Pediatr.* **2022**, *10*, 911444. [CrossRef] [PubMed]
26. Srikanth, M.; Kumar, N. Utility of Neonatal Sequential Organ Failure Assessment (nSOFA) Score for Neonatal Mortality prediction. *J. Neonatol.* **2022**, *36*, 189–193. [CrossRef]
27. Polderman, K.H. Mechanisms of action, physiological effects, and complications of hypothermia. *Crit. Care Med.* **2009**, *37*, S186–S202. [CrossRef]
28. Szakmar, E.; Jermendy, A.; El-Dib, M. Correction: Respiratory management during therapeutic hypothermia for hypoxic-ischemic encephalopathy. *J. Perinatol.* **2019**, *39*, 891. [CrossRef]
29. Giannakis, S.; Ruhfus, M.; Markus, M.; Stein, A.; Hoehn, T.; Felderhoff-Mueser, U.; Sabir, H. Mechanical Ventilation, Partial Pressure of Carbon Dioxide, Increased Fraction of Inspired Oxygen and the Increased Risk for Adverse Short-Term Outcomes in Cooled Asphyxiated Newborns. *Children* **2021**, *8*, 430. [CrossRef] [PubMed]
30. Jensen, A.; Garnier, Y.; Berger, R. Dynamics of fetal circulatory responses to hypoxia and asphyxia. *Eur. J. Obstet. Gynecol. Reprod. Biol.* **1999**, *84*, 155–172. [CrossRef] [PubMed]

31. Christensen, R.D.; Baer, V.L.; Yaish, H.M. Thrombocytopenia in late preterm and term neonates after perinatal asphyxia. *Transfusion* **2015**, *55*, 187–196. [CrossRef]
32. Boutaybi, N.; Razenberg, F.; Smits-Wintjens, V.E.; van Zwet, E.W.; Rijken, M.; Steggerda, S.J.; Lopriore, E. Neonatal thrombocytopenia after perinatal asphyxia treated with hypothermia: A retrospective case control study. *Int. J. Pediatr.* **2014**, *2014*, 760654. [CrossRef] [PubMed]
33. Valeri, C.R.; Feingold, H.; Cassidy, G.; Ragno, G.; Khuri, S.; Altschule, M.D. Hypothermia-induced reversible platelet dysfunction. *Ann. Surg.* **1987**, *205*, 175–181. [CrossRef] [PubMed]
34. Sarkar, S.; Barks, J.D.; Bhagat, I.; Donn, S.M. Effects of therapeutic hypothermia on multiorgan dysfunction in asphyxiated newborns: Whole-body cooling versus selective head cooling. *J. Perinatol.* **2009**, *29*, 558–563. [CrossRef] [PubMed]
35. Al Amrani, F.; Racine, E.; Shevell, M.; Wintermark, P. Death after Birth Asphyxia in the Cooling Era. *J. Pediatr.* **2020**, *226*, 289–293. [CrossRef]
36. Murray, D.M.; Boylan, G.B.; Ryan, C.A.; Connolly, S. Early EEG findings in hypoxic-ischemic encephalopathy predict outcomes at 2 years. *Pediatrics* **2009**, *124*, e459–e467. [CrossRef]
37. Thayyil, S.; Chandrasekaran, M.; Taylor, A.; Bainbridge, A.; Cady, E.B.; Chong, W.K.; Murad, S.; Omar, R.Z.; Robertson, N.J. Cerebral magnetic resonance biomarkers in neonatal encephalopathy: A meta-analysis. *Pediatrics* **2010**, *125*, e382–e395. [CrossRef]
38. Dorling, J.S.; Field, D.J.; Manktelow, B. Neonatal disease severity scoring systems. *Arch. Dis. Childhood Fetal Neonatal Ed.* **2005**, *90*, F11–F16. [CrossRef]
39. Garg, B.; Sharma, D.; Farahbakhsh, N. Assessment of sickness severity of illness in neonates: Review of various neonatal illness scoring systems. *J. Matern. Fetal Neonatal Med.* **2018**, *31*, 1373–1380. [CrossRef]
40. Mrelashvili, A.; Russ, J.B.; Ferriero, D.M.; Wusthoff, C.J. The Sarnat score for neonatal encephalopathy: Looking back and moving forward. *Pediatr. Res.* **2020**, *88*, 824–825. [CrossRef]

Disclaimer/Publisher's Note: The statements, opinions and data contained in all publications are solely those of the individual author(s) and contributor(s) and not of MDPI and/or the editor(s). MDPI and/or the editor(s) disclaim responsibility for any injury to people or property resulting from any ideas, methods, instructions or products referred to in the content.

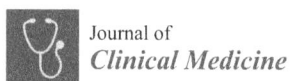

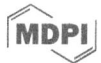

Article

The Impact of Head Position on Neurological and Histopathological Outcome Following Controlled Automated Reperfusion of the Whole Body (CARL) in a Pig Model

Domagoj Damjanovic [1,*], Jan-Steffen Pooth [2], Yechi Liu [1], Fabienne Frensch [1], Martin Wolkewitz [3], Joerg Haberstroh [4], Soroush Doostkam [5], Heidi Ramona Cristina Schmitz [4], Katharina Foerster [6], Itumeleng Taunyane [1], Tabea Neubert [1], Christian Scherer [1], Patric Diel [1], Christoph Benk [1], Friedhelm Beyersdorf [1] and Georg Trummer [1]

[1] Department of Cardiovascular Surgery, University Medical Center Freiburg, Faculty of Medicine, University of Freiburg, Hugstetter Str. 55, D-79106 Freiburg, Germany
[2] Department of Emergency Medicine, University Medical Center Freiburg, Faculty of Medicine, University of Freiburg, D-79106 Freiburg, Germany
[3] Institute of Medical Biometry and Statistics, Division Methods in Clinical Epidemiology, Faculty of Medicine and Medical Center, University of Freiburg, D-79104 Freiburg, Germany
[4] Experimental Surgery, Center for Experimental Models and Transgenic Service, University Medical Center Freiburg, Faculty of Medicine, University of Freiburg, Breisacher Str. 66, D-79106 Freiburg, Germany
[5] Institute of Neuropathology, University Medical Center Freiburg, Faculty of Medicine, University of Freiburg, Breisacherstr. 64, D-79106 Freiburg, Germany
[6] Center for Experimental Models and Transgenic Service, University Medical Center Freiburg, Faculty of Medicine, University of Freiburg, Stefan-Meier-Str. 17, D-79104 Freiburg, Germany
* Correspondence: domagoj.damjanovic@uniklinik-freiburg.de; Tel.: +49-761-270-24010

Abstract: **Introduction:** Based on extracorporeal circulation, targeted reperfusion strategies have been developed to improve survival and neurologic recovery in refractory cardiac arrest: Controlled Automated Reperfusion of the whoLe Body (CARL). Furthermore, animal and human cadaver studies have shown beneficial effects on cerebral pressure due to head elevation during conventional cardiopulmonary resuscitation. Our aim was to evaluate the impact of head elevation on survival, neurologic recovery and histopathologic outcome in addition to CARL in an animal model. **Methods:** After 20 min of ventricular fibrillation, 46 domestic pigs underwent CARL, including high, pulsatile extracorporeal blood flow, pH–stat acid–base management, priming with a colloid, mannitol and citrate, targeted oxygen, carbon dioxide and blood pressure management, rapid cooling and slow rewarming. N = 25 were head-up (HUP) during CARL, and N = 21 were supine (SUP). After weaning from ECC, the pigs were extubated and followed up in the animal care facility for up to seven days. Neuronal density was evaluated in neurohistopathology. **Results:** More animals in the HUP group survived and achieved a favorable neurological recovery, 21/25 (84%) versus 6/21 (29%) in the SUP group. Head positioning was an independent factor in neurologically favorable survival ($p < 0.00012$). Neurohistopathology showed no significant structural differences between HUP and SUP. Distinct, partly transient clinical neurologic deficits were blindness and ataxia. **Conclusions:** Head elevation during CARL after 20 min of cardiac arrest independently improved survival and neurologic outcome in pigs. Clinical follow-up revealed transient neurologic deficits potentially attributable to functions localized in the posterior perfusion area, whereas histopathologic findings did not show corresponding differences between the groups. A possible explanation of our findings may be venous congestion and edema as modifiable contributing factors of neurologic injury following prolonged cardiac arrest.

Keywords: ischemia-reperfusion; extracorporeal life support; venous return; porcine cardiac arrest model; bundle of care; targeted CPR; eCPR; VA-ECMO; pathophysiology of cardiac arrest

Citation: Damjanovic, D.; Pooth, J.-S.; Liu, Y.; Frensch, F.; Wolkewitz, M.; Haberstroh, J.; Doostkam, S.; Cristina Schmitz, H.R.; Foerster, K.; Taunyane, I.; et al. The Impact of Head Position on Neurological and Histopathological Outcome Following Controlled Automated Reperfusion of the Whole Body (CARL) in a Pig Model. *J. Clin. Med.* **2023**, *12*, 7054. https://doi.org/10.3390/jcm12227054

Academic Editors: Stephan Marsch and Timur Sellmann

Received: 25 July 2023
Revised: 27 October 2023
Accepted: 7 November 2023
Published: 13 November 2023

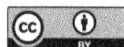

Copyright: © 2023 by the authors. Licensee MDPI, Basel, Switzerland. This article is an open access article distributed under the terms and conditions of the Creative Commons Attribution (CC BY) license (https://creativecommons.org/licenses/by/4.0/).

1. Introduction

Neurologically favorable survival in cardiac arrest (CA) is dramatically low despite advanced life support and high quality cardiopulmonary resuscitation (CPR) [1–4]. Therapy bundles and a system-based approach rather than stand-alone interventions might improve these outcomes [5–10].

On the *tissue and cellular level*, one of the main therapeutic objectives in such bundles is in the mitigation of ischemia-reperfusion injury (IRI). Controlled Automated Reperfusion of the whoLe body (CARL) is an individualized therapy bundle based on extracorporeal circulation that is designed to reduce IRI. With CARL, favorable neurologic recovery has been be achieved in a porcine cardiac arrest model, even after 20 min of normothermic cardiac arrest [11,12].

From a *macro-hemodynamic perspective*, traditionally, the restoration of arterial perfusion of organs and tissues has been considered the primary aim during cardiac arrest. More recent resuscitation research, however, suggests that cerebral venous drainage and venous return to the central circulation are equally as important. The assumption that venous congestion during cardiac arrest adds to neuronal damage has led to the development and marketing of devices designed to increase venous return during CPR, thereby improving survival and neurologic outcome.

Elevated positioning of the head is another simple intervention to enhance cerebral venous drainage. In neuro-critical care, as well as post-resuscitation care, it is an established measure for prophylaxis and therapy of increased intracranial pressure (ICP) [13]. Following the concept of *intra-arrest* venous congestion as an important pathophysiologic contributor to bad neurologic outcome, head elevation has been applied *during* conventional CPR and was shown to reduce ICP in an animal model [14,15].

It has been combined with other methods for enhancing venous return in further studies [16]. However, to our best knowledge, it has not yet been studied in conjunction with extracorporeal circulation.

The aim of our study was, therefore, to evaluate the impact of head elevation on survival, neurologic recovery and neuronal loss in combination with CARL therapy.

2. Methods

Animal experiments were approved by the local ethics committee (Freiburg, Germany, approval number G-15/148) and performed in accordance with the rules and regulations of the German animal protection law and the animal care guidelines of the European Community (2010/63/EU). The ARRIVE Checklist is added as Supplement S1.

The basic protocol of this chronic porcine cardiac arrest model has already been published in detail [11]. Figure 1 depicts the timeline of the experiment. This study was conducted as a pooled analysis. Experiments were carried out in an open-label parallel-group design. The group allocation was non-randomized, block-wise.

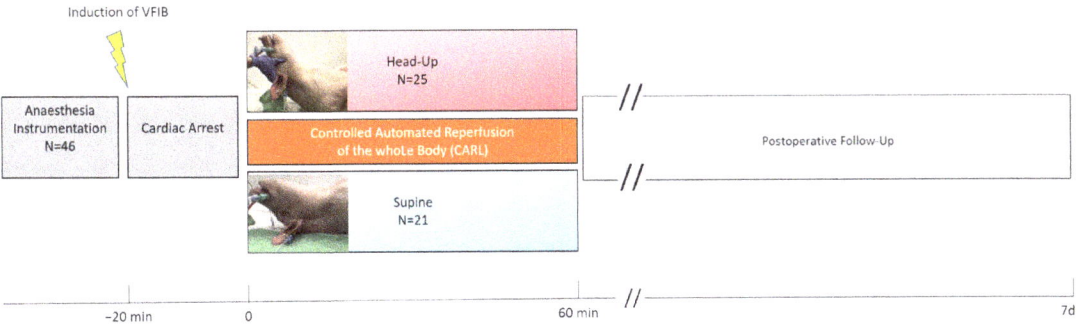

Figure 1. Timeline of the experiment. VFIB: ventricular fibrillation.

Twenty-eight juvenile domestic pigs were anesthetized, and ventricular fibrillation was induced. Before anesthesia, they were fasted overnight with free access to water. After 20 min of normothermic CA, CARL was started. It comprises a targeted reperfusion therapy bundle based on arteriovenous extracorporeal membrane oxygenation. This, in brief, consists of high, pulsatile extracorporeal blood flow, pH–stat acid–base management, priming with a colloid (20% human albumin (Albiomin 200 g/L, Biotest Pharma GmbH, Dreieich, Germany; 200 g/L, Baxalta Deutschland GmbH, Unterschleissheim, Germany; or 200 g/L, Octapharma GmbH, Langenfeld, Germany, respectively, depending on availability)) or Gelatin-Polysuccinate (Gelafundin 40 g/L, B. Braun Melsungen AG, Melsungen, Germany)), mannitol and citrate [17], tight oxygen and carbon dioxide control, rapid cooling and slow rewarming before weaning off the extracorporeal circulation and ECC [11]. Instead of electric defibrillation, ventricular fibrillation was preferably terminated through cardioplegic potassium bolus [18]. The hyperosmolar priming solution has a neuroprotective potential, whereas pharmacologic defibrillation via secondary cardioplegia aims at cardioprotection through avoidance of the harmful impact of serial electric defibrillations on cardiac tissue. A detailed overview of the CARL therapy, including rationales for its single components, as well as images and an explanatory video, can be found in Ref. [19].

Head elevation was conducted using a standardized pillow (towel roll), with additional regular inclinations for up to 90°. This is depicted in Supplement S3/Supplementary Figure S1. An additional 18 animals from historic groups with an otherwise identical intervention protocol were added for pooled analysis regarding head positioning.

Overall, 25/46 pigs underwent CARL with head-up positioning HUP (sixteen current, nine historic sample), and the other 21 were positioned supine (SUP) (twelve current, nine historic sample).

After completion of the reperfusion protocol, animals were weaned off the ECC and the ventilator and subsequently extubated. Follow-up in the CEMT facility was conducted for up to seven days. Postoperative care was conducted following a standard protocol. On postoperative day (POD) 3, interim analysis and scoring were performed in accordance with this protocol. The assessors were trained members of the research group, supervised by a veterinarian, not blinded to the group allocation. The neurologic outcome was characterized using a species-specific neurologic deficit score. A score of 500 denotes brain death, whereas animals with NDS < 50 were able to stand up independently, walk without help and eat on their own. A score < 50 was, therefore, defined as a surrogate of favorable neurologic outcome or significant potential for rehabilitation, respectively. Upon clinical suspicion, distinct neurologic deficits were evaluated separately. Following regulatory requirements, a prespecified set of criteria was applied for early termination of the survival experiment (NDS > 200 after 24 h or >120 after 48 h, suspicion of vegetative state, inhumane suffering, inadequate non-neurologic recovery or poor general health status) [11].

After completion of clinical follow-up and euthanasia, the porcine brains were retrieved for neuro–histopathologic workup, for which hematoxylin–eosin staining was used. For this purpose, a frontal craniotomy was performed. After transecting at the level of the medulla oblongata, brains were extracted as a whole and immediately immersed in formaldehyde 4%. Following one week of immersion, the brains were dissected, and 5 mm samples of the frontal lobe, cerebellar vermis and hippocampus were obtained, respectively. In identifying those areas as our regions of interest, we sought to procure a representation of both the territories of the anterior and occipital cerebral blood supply, respectively. Furthermore, the hippocampal region has been identified as one of the most susceptible regions for cerebral ischemia-reperfusion injury following cardiac arrest [20]. In the next step, the samples were dehydrated and embedded in paraffin. 3μm slices of the samples underwent hematoxylin–eosin staining. Consequently, slides were masked and digitalized, and representative areas were examined in terms of neuron count to determine neuron density. Only neurons with a clearly identifiable nucleus were considered to be viable and have been included in the total count.

Statistical Methods

Continuous baseline characteristics were compared between the groups (HUP and SUP) using the Kruskal–Wallis rank sum test. Kaplan–Meier survival curves were calculated to compare survival up to 7 days between the groups. Regarding NDS, linear mixed models (see Brown and Prescott, 1999) have been fitted with a random intercept (subject = pig). The continuous response variable "NDS" is modeled as a linear function of time (continuous) and group (HUP or SUP), including an interaction term. We further included all baseline characteristics if they showed significant variations between the groups. All computations were performed using the statistical software R system (version 4.3.0). They are added as Supplement S2.

3. Results

Baseline characteristics of the animals are shown in Table 1.

Table 1. Baseline characteristics. HUP: head-up, SUP: supine.

	HUP (n = 25)	SUP (n = 21)	
Male:Female	21:4	19:2	ns
Mean Body Weight (kg)	52.12 ± 3.71	54.40 ± 6.09	ns

- Intra-operative course

After starting reperfusion, electric defibrillation was inevitable to terminate VF in three pigs. In all other animals, secondary cardioplegia through a potassium bolus was sufficient for rhythm conversion. Intraoperative monitoring revealed no systematic differences between the animals with good or bad neurologic outcome. Table 2 shows mean arterial blood pressure values during the experiment, i.e., at baseline and during controlled reperfusion. Blood flow rates achieved were high, as targeted; mean cardiac index during the first 15 min of reperfusion was ≥ 5.0 L/min/m^2 in all but two animals (4.87 and 4.95 L/min/m^2).

Table 2. MAP and NSE. Mean arterial blood pressure (MAP) values in mmHg at baseline and after 15, 30, 45 and 60 min of controlled reperfusion. Neuron Specific Enolase (NSE) values in µg/L found at baseline, end of surgery, on postoperative day 1 and at the end of the experiment on day 7, immediately before euthanasia. HUP: head-up, SUP: supine. ns: not significant. Results are shown as mean +/− SD.

	HUP (n = 25)	SUP (n = 21)	
MAP (mmHg)			
Baseline	77.16 ± 13.60	81.30 ± 10.83	ns
15 min	110.11 ± 14.02	109.21 ± 15.56	ns
30 min	105.01 ± 16.92	104.19 ± 13.95	ns
45 min	107.08 ± 14.14	109.97 ± 8.60	ns
60 min	101.80 ± 17.38	109.85 ± 18.85	ns
Baseline	0.78 ± 0.22	0.53 ± 0.17	ns
End of surgery	0.59 ± 0.17	0.46 ± 0.12	ns
Day 1	10.79 ± 2.33	6.73 ± 1.41	ns
Day 7	9.99 ± 8.20	10.81 ± 9.69	ns

- Survival, neurologic outcome and clinical status

Forty-five out of forty-six pigs were successfully weaned off ECC after 1 h of CARL. One animal could not be weaned off ECC due to refractory hemodynamic failure, and was excluded from further analysis. In all others, extubation was possible after 3 h from the start of the intervention. In Table 2, the time course of neuron-specific enolase as a surrogate marker of neurologic injury can be appreciated. No significant differences were found between the HUP and the SUP group. NSE did, however, predict worse outcomes in the NDS score, i.e., animals that did not achieve the predefined threshold of NDS = 50 for good neurologic outcome on day 1 and day 7, respectively ($p = 0.04787$ and $p = 0.003094$). Figure 2 shows a higher survival probability in the head-up group compared to the supine group over the follow-up period of one week, displayed as a Kaplan–Meier survival curve. Figure 3 depicts the development of the NDS values over time, with a threshold of 50 points considered to be a good recovery. Starting with scores between 100 and 150 on the first day after the intervention, more animals in the head-up group achieved neurological recovery compared to supine positioning: 21/25 (84%) vs. 6/20 (30%). During clinical follow-up, predominant clinical problems were transient blindness and ataxia in otherwise alert animals, most of whom started eating and drinking early on in the postoperative course. After adjusting for different confounders, such as plasma hemoglobin, priming composition (gelatin or albumin, see Table 3), priming osmolality or sodium concentration, head positioning remained an independent factor in neurologically favorable survival ($p < 0.00012$).

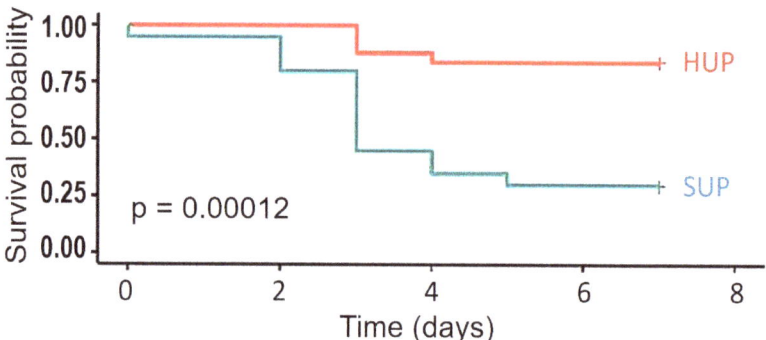

Figure 2. Survival probability following the experiments, in correlation to head positioning. HUP: head-up, SUP, supine.

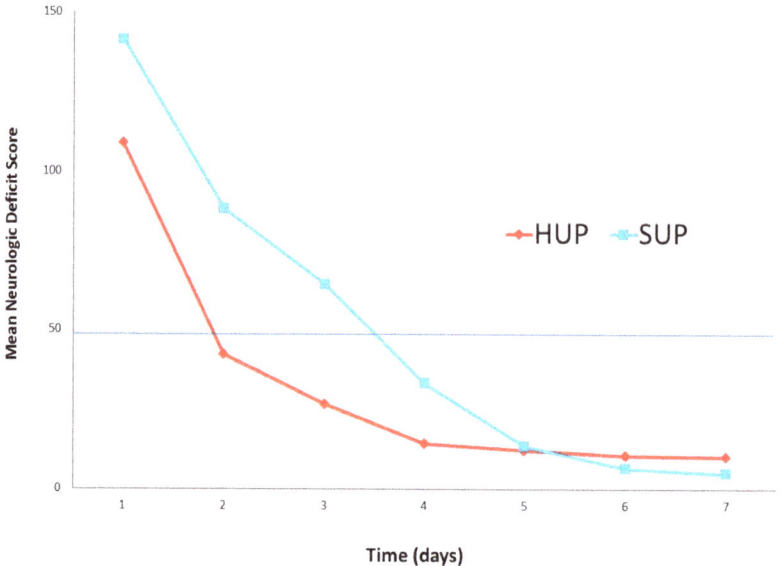

Figure 3. Mean neurologic deficit score during the postoperative course. HUP: Head-up, SUP, supine.

Table 3. Hemoglobin, priming composition, neurologic recovery and survival. Data are presented as mean ± standard deviation. [a] $p = 0.9077$, [b] $p = 0.001069$, [c] $p = 0.002414$. HUP: head-up, SUP: supine. NDS [1–7]: neurologic deficit score [Days 1–7]. Favorable neurologic survival was defined as NDS < 50.

	HUP (n = 25)	SUP (n = 20)
Hemoglobin (g/dL)	9.28 ± 0.79	9.35 ± 0.89 [a]
Sodium Priming (mmol/L)	146.24 ± 10.45	144.59 ± 9.61 [b]
Osmolality of Priming (mosm/kg)	549.40 ± 20.06	524.39 ± 28.93 [c]
Survival (days)	6.06 ± 1.64	4.10 ± 2.12
NDS1	108.96 ± 52.52	141.37 ± 61.79
NDS2	42.40 ± 31.66	88.29 ± 42.10
NDS3	26.80 ± 33.16	64.53 ± 43.54
NDS4	14.48 ± 17.80	33.33 ± 40.55
NDS5	12.38 ± 15.17	13.57 ± 21.99
NDS6	10.71 ± 13.30	6.67 ± 11.06
NDS7	10.24 ± 13.14	5.00 ± 11.18
Favourable Neurologic Survival	21	6

Neurohistopathology

Figure 4 shows a neurohistopathologic evaluation of neuron density in the cerebellum, frontal cortex and hippocampus in correlation to the head position. Samples were available for workup in $n = 24$ in the HUP and $n = 12$ in the SUP group. Four sham animals did not undergo ischemia, CPR or extracorporeal circulation. A significantly lower neuron count was found in the hippocampus of head-up animals compared to controls, while all other differences were not statistically significant.

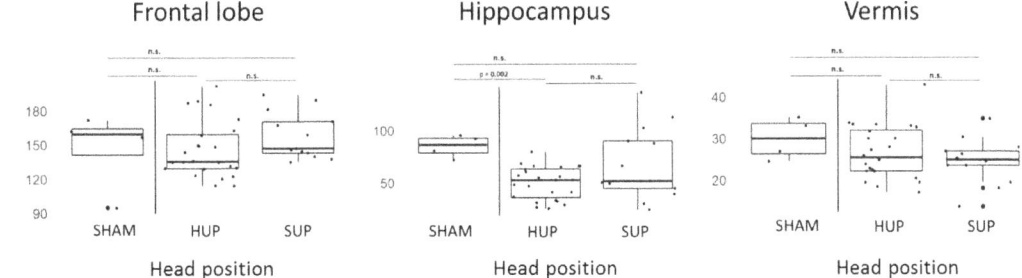

Figure 4. Neurohistopathologic analysis of total number of neurons per square millimeter in frontal lobe, hippocampus and vermis. Boxplots (median, interquartile range) are shown in correlation to head position. SHAM: sham animals. HUP: head-Up; SUP: supine. ns: not significant. Samples were available for workup in N = 24 in the HUP and N = 12 in the SUP group. Sham animal controls did not undergo ischemia, CPR or extracorporeal circulation. Head-up animals had significantly lower neuron counts in the hippocampus when compared to controls. All other differences were not statistically significant.

4. Discussion

In this experimental large animal cardiac arrest study, we showed that (1) in conjunction with the CARL therapy bundle, elevation and repeated inclination of the head after 20 min of normothermic cardiac arrest improved survival and neurologic recovery compared to supine positioning, but (2) without corresponding damage patterns in histopathology. To our best knowledge, this is the first translational study to combine elevation of the head with extracorporeal reperfusion following prolonged cardiac arrest. Furthermore, post-interventional follow-up for several days allowed for clinical assessment, characterization of neurologic deficits and dynamics of recovery. The majority of translational resuscitation studies are conducted as physiology-centered terminal experiments, without awakening the animals after the intervention, and hence without the opportunity for neurologic scoring and follow-up. Instead, data on trajectories of decreased intracranial pressure, improved cerebral perfusion or metabolism, respectively, have been reported in several studies on head elevation during CPR [14,15,21–24]. Two systematic reviews and meta-analyses provide a further synopsis [25,26]. The results of studies using a postoperative follow-up are conflicting: One randomized study by Park et al. found lower ROSC-rates and 24 h survival in pigs undergoing CPR after 15 min of untreated cardiac arrest, with the whole body tilted 30 degrees head-up. Neurologic outcomes were not reported [27]. More recently, Moore et al. showed an improved neurologic survival with HUP in one study with Yorkshire pigs in a 24 h follow-up period after 10 min of untreated cardiac arrest, followed by 9 min of CPR [16]. Therefore, the results of our study may complement the predominantly physiologic data at least to some extent, providing information on the most robust and most desired target outcome of CPR, the neurologically favorable outcome.

The neurologic deficit score we used for that purpose is a standardized instrument that supports comparability with other translational studies in resuscitation research. Regarding the severity of functional impairment, mean deficit scores under 150 are considerably low already after 24–48 h, given the major insult of 20 min no-flow-time. The score comprises different neuro-functional aspects. However, the clinical constellations we observed, i.e., ataxia and transient blindness, were not fully covered. This is further discussed in the Section 4.2.

The enhancement of venous drainage from the brain to the thorax, which has been reported with conventional CPR, might be a possible explanation for this observation in our study as well, although it was not directly measured.

4.1. Structural Correlation of Damage Patterns

Traditional veterinary anatomical studies, as well as recent functional magnetic resonance imaging studies, show structural representation of visual functions and posturing in the posterior cerebral and cerebellar areas. Lesions herein are consistent with visual impairment and postural problems seen in the postoperative course in many of the animals. In the supine position, intravascular *stasis* during arrest is likely to predominate in the posterior areas. An impaired *venous* drainage through the prominent prevertebral venous plexus and *venous* congestion in the sinus sigmoideus, transversus and the pronounced confluens sinuum will gradually affect adjacent areas, that is, the abovementioned posterior parts again. Stasis and congestion will result in tissue edema. This might explain the transient nature of visual loss, with regression of the edema leading to the regaining of sight. An MRI study on a Yucatan pig by Habib et al. further illustrates the relation between porcine cerebral venous vasculature and possible ways of drainage [28].

The structural damage patterns (loss of neurons) actually seen in the histopathologic workup of our sample do not match the clinical findings. These were (1) obvious neurologic damage in all animals immediately after profound ischemia-reperfusion injury and (2) significantly better functional recovery in the head-up group, despite its increased loss of hippocampal neurons, when compared to the sham and supine groups. In the literature, the hippocampus; basal ganglia; frontal, parietal, temporal and occipital cortices; as well as the cerebellar cortex, were found to be most susceptible to ischemia and hypoxia, respectively [18]. Methodological limitations in recovery and workup of brain tissue specimens may have contributed to these conflicting findings (see Section 4.2.). Another possible explanation is that neurologic damage was not only transient from a clinical perspective, but also in terms of reversible tissue edema. This edema cannot be detected by the histopathological methods used herein, and might have been more pronounced and less regredient in the supine group. The increased hippocampal neuron loss observed in the tissue of HUP animals obviously had less of a clinically relevant impact on the neuro-functional status and recovery than other histopathologically inapparent changes. Furthermore, neuron-specific enolase (NSE) concentrations did not differ between the groups; they did, however, predict worse neurologic outcome. As a serum marker of neuronal injury, NSE was only moderately elevated. Notably, the molecule is also contained in erythrocytes and hence can be elevated due to hemolysis, e.g., when extracorporeal circulation is applied. Due to the mechanism of experimental injury itself and the extracorporeal reperfusion with a dual blood pump configuration, respectively, higher NSE-values could have been expected. In humans, the prognostic utility of NSE in predicting poor outcomes after cardiac arrest has been studied extensively. Reported cut-off values range between 33 and 120 µg/L [28]. Following extracorporeal cardiopulmonary resuscitation, Haertel et al. found NSE serum levels of >55.9 µg/L after 48 h post-arrest to be predictive of worse neurologic outcomes [29]. In pigs, Vammen et al. described mean NSE values below 10 µg/L up to 48 h following 11 min of untreated cardiac arrest, with markedly higher levels in more severely affected animals [30]. NSE values are time-dependent and prone to confounding [31]. Therefore, current international guidelines for post-resuscitation care suggest that NSE should only be used in conjunction with other prognostic tests because "no single test has sufficient specificity to eliminate false positives" [28]. In previously published work from our group by Foerster et al., even after 20 min of untreated cardiac arrest, low levels of 4.6 and 1.5 µg/L in a hypothermic group versus 5.6 µg/L and 4.3 µg/L in a normothermic group were found on day 1 and day 7 of the follow-up period, respectively [12]. According to Taunyane et al., an up to twenty-fold increase to 7.95 µg/L at the end of the experiment compared to the baseline was only seen in an uncontrolled reperfusion group with 15 min of cardiac arrest, 10 min conventional CPR and 60 min of normothermic reperfusion [11].

The clinical course in our study might support the veno-congestive edema hypothesis, as would the benefit of head elevation ex juvantibus. In summary, intraoperative physiology, structural changes, serum markers and clinical outcomes can differ significantly. In isolation, the acute setting obviously has limited predictive value, which underlines the need for clinical correlation and long-term neurologic follow-up in translational resuscitation research.

4.2. Limitations

Due to the complexity of the experimental model and the therapy bundle applied, it is possible that not all confounders were known or controlled for, respectively. Furthermore, we did not directly measure cerebral tissue perfusion or intracranial pressure in real time to prove the congestion hypothesis. Anticoagulation was necessary during extracorporeal circulation. The concurrent intracranial bleeding risk following invasive ICP measurement was deemed unacceptably high in this experimental setting. In the histopathologic workup, there is an increased dropout-rate of specimens in the supine group, which is in part due to the retrospective nature of the analysis. As mentioned above, a historic sample of the study population, which underwent the same experimental procedure, has been added for pooled analysis. This included the post hoc consideration of historic histopathologic samples, some of which were no longer available. From an ethical standpoint in translational animal research, we decided to use all available information and, hence, the biggest possible number of samples instead of eliminating samples from the HUP group to achieve a 1:1 ratio.

The only moderately increased NSE levels we observed are consistent with previous findings in this research model by Foerster et al. [12] and Taunyane et al. [11]. The best test performance of NSE has been described at 48 and 72 h post-cardiac arrest, with "only limited evidence" for the period after 72 h [28]. Following our protocol, blood sampling was only possible on day 1 and day 7 or at end of the experiment, respectively. Hence, we might have missed the relevant time window and true peak levels.

The NDS score used to formalize clinical observations cannot account for specific constellations, as found in our study. It is an inherent limitation of the score and our mode; due to the interdependence between the visual system and the equilibrium sense, visual impairment directly affects postural control, even if there is no further damage to the vestibular or cerebellar apparatus itself. Thus, transient blindness and gait disturbance may lead to an overestimation of neurologic damage in otherwise alert and physiologically interacting animals. This overestimation could have prevented some of these animals with significant recovery potential from crossing the pre-defined 72 h cut-off point, therefore being sacrificed early. On the other hand, the NDS does not cover aspects of general well-being or non-neurological injury, which might induce suffering and trigger premature sacrifice in translational survival experiments. We did not use formal scoring systems for general well-being; however, we are not aware of major non-neurological impairments in this study sample.

4.3. Transferability

The transferability of these translational research results to resuscitation in humans might be limited by the different vascular anatomy, especially regarding venous drainage of the brain. However, recent experimental data suggest a potentially beneficial role in human patients. A first clinical study involving a bundled head-up/torso-up approach by Pepe et al. showed a doubling of resuscitation rates, i.e., return of spontaneous circulation on hospital arrival after introducing the bundle [32]. Rates of neurologic recovery remained proportional, however, and the bundle also included other adjustments of the CPR-management, i.e., using the Impedance Threshold Device (ITD) and Active Compression-Decompression Device (ACD), as well as performing pit crew CPR. A more recent observational study by Moore et al. displayed no difference in primary or secondary endpoints among 860 patients with Out-of-Hospital Cardiac Arrest (OHCA) undergoing conventional CPR versus 222 propensity-score-matched OHCA patients with automated sequential elevation of the head and torso using an automated device (ITD or ACD) [33]. The group did find, however, a higher likelihood of survival and neurological recovery when device therapy was initiated early [34].

5. Conclusions

Our study suggests an improved neurologic recovery with head elevation during extracorporeal circulation within the CARL therapy bundle following twenty minutes of untreated ventricular fibrillation in pigs. Within this complex translational research model, clinical follow-up revealed neurologic deficit patterns, which were not directly supported by histopathologic findings. Our results may serve as a basis to reconsidering traditional pathomechanisms and recovery potential in prolonged cardiac arrest.

Supplementary Materials: The following supporting information can be downloaded at: https://www.mdpi.com/article/10.3390/jcm12227054/s1, Supplement S1: ARRIVE checklist, Animal Research: Reporting In Vivo Experiments; Supplement S2: 2023_07_25_Heads-up-CARL; Supplement S3: Figure S1, Head positioning in the pig during the experiment.

Author Contributions: Conceptualization, C.B., F.B. and G.T.; methodology, S.D., K.F., I.T. and G.T.; validation, G.T.; formal analysis, J.-S.P., M.W. and I.T.; investigation, D.D., J.-S.P., Y.L., F.F., J.H., S.D., H.R.C.S., I.T., C.S. and G.T.; resources, P.D., C.B. and G.T.; data curation, J.-S.P., I.T., T.N., C.S. and P.D.; writing—original draft preparation, D.D.; writing—review and editing, J.-S.P., T.N., C.S. and C.B. visu-alization, J.-S.P.; supervision, S.D., C.B., F.B. and G.T.; project administration, I.T., C.B., F.B. and G.T. All authors have read and agreed to the published version of the manuscript.

Funding: The animal research was funded by Resuscitec GmbH, Freiburg, Germany.

Institutional Review Board Statement: The animal study protocol was approved by the local animal welfare committee of the city of Freiburg, Germany, Regierungspräsidium Freiburg (G-15/148 and date of approval: 21 January 2016).

Informed Consent Statement: Not applicable.

Data Availability Statement: Preliminary data to this publication have been presented at the European Resuscitation Council annual conference 2018 in Bologna, Italy. "Beneficial effects of head-elevation during Controlled Automated Reperfusion of the WhoLe Body (CARL) in the pig model", Damjanovic, Domagoj et al., Resuscitation, Volume 130, e35 [35]. The data presented in this study are available on reasonable request from the corresponding author.

Acknowledgments: We would like to cordially thank all CEMT staff, animal keepers, laboratory staff and neurohistopathology staff for their dedicated support.

Conflicts of Interest: Friedhelm Beyersdorf, Christoph Benk and Georg Trummer are shareholders of Resuscitec GmbH. Jan-Steffen Pooth, Christian Scherer, Christoph Benk and Georg Trummer receive salaries for part-time employment at Resuscitec GmbH. Domagoj Damjanovic had been a part-time employee at Resuscitec GmbH until 6/2022, and was a speaker at an online symposium by Getinge. All other authors declare no conflict of interest.

References

1. Reynolds, J.C.; Grunau, B.E.; Elmer, J.; Rittenberger, J.C.; Sawyer, K.N.; Kurz, M.C.; Singer, B.; Proudfoot, A.; Callaway, C.W. Prevalence, natural history, and time-dependent outcomes of a multi-center North American cohort of out-of-hospital cardiac arrest extracorporeal CPR candidates. *Resuscitation* **2017**, *117*, 24–31. [CrossRef] [PubMed]
2. Yukawa, T.; Kashiura, M.; Sugiyama, K.; Tanabe, T.; Hamabe, Y. Neurological outcomes and duration from cardiac arrest to the initiation of extracorporeal membrane oxygenation in patients with out-of-hospital cardiac arrest: A retrospective study. *Scand. J. Trauma Resusc. Emerg. Med.* **2017**, *25*, 95. [CrossRef] [PubMed]
3. Reynolds, J.C.; Frisch, A.; Rittenberger, J.C.; Callaway, C.W. Duration of resuscitation efforts and functional outcome after out-of-hospital cardiac arrest: When should we change to novel therapies? *Circulation* **2013**, *128*, 2488–2494. [CrossRef]
4. Grunau, B.; Scheuermeyer, F.X.; Stub, D.; Boone, R.H.; Finkler, J.; Pennington, S.; Carriere, S.A.; Cheung, A.; MacRedmond, R.; Bashir, J.; et al. Potential Candidates for a Structured Canadian ECPR Program for Out-of-Hospital Cardiac Arrest. *CJEM* **2016**, *18*, 453–460. [CrossRef] [PubMed]
5. Yannopoulos, D.; Bartos, J.A.; Martin, C.; Raveendran, G.; Missov, E.; Conterato, M.; Frascone, R.J.; Trembley, A.; Sipprell, K.; John, R.; et al. Minnesota Resuscitation Consortium's Advanced Perfusion and Reperfusion Cardiac Life Support Strategy for Out-of-Hospital Refractory Ventricular Fibrillation. *J. Am. Heart Assoc.* **2016**, *5*, e003732. [CrossRef] [PubMed]
6. Adabag, S.; Hodgson, L.; Garcia, S.; Anand, V.; Frascone, R.; Conterato, M.; Lick, C.; Wesley, K.; Mahoney, B.; Yannopoulos, D. Outcomes of sudden cardiac arrest in a state-wide integrated resuscitation program: Results from the Minnesota Resuscitation Consortium. *Resuscitation* **2017**, *110*, 95–100. [CrossRef] [PubMed]
7. Okubo, M.; Atkinson, E.J.; Hess, E.P.; White, R.D. Improving trend in ventricular fibrillation/pulseless ventricular tachycardia out-of-hospital cardiac arrest in Rochester, Minnesota: A 26-year observational study from 1991 to 2016. *Resuscitation* **2017**, *120*, 31–37. [CrossRef]
8. Stub, D.; Bernard, S.; Pellegrino, V.; Smith, K.; Walker, T.; Sheldrake, J. Refractory cardiac arrest treated with mechanical CPR, hypothermia, ECMO and early reperfusion (the CHEER trial). *Resuscitation* **2015**, *86*, 88–94. [CrossRef]
9. Belohlavek, J.; Kucera, K.; Jarkovsky, J.; Franek, O.; Pokorna, M.; Danda, J.; Skripsky, R.; Kandrnal, V.; Balik, M.; Kunstyr, J.; et al. Hyperinvasive approach to out-of hospital cardiac arrest using mechanical chest compression device, prehospital intraarrest cooling, extracorporeal life support and early invasive assessment compared to standard of care. A randomized parallel groups comparative study proposal. *Prague OHCA Study J. Transl. Med.* **2012**, *10*, 163. [CrossRef]
10. Belohlavek, J.; Smalcova, J.; Rob, D.; Franek, O.; Smid, O.; Pokorna, M.; Horák, J.; Mrazek, V.; Kovarnik, T.; Zemanek, D.; et al. Effect of Intra-arrest Transport, Extracorporeal Cardiopulmonary Resuscitation, and Immediate Invasive Assessment and Treatment on Functional Neurologic Outcome in Refractory Out-of-Hospital Cardiac Arrest: A Randomized Clinical Trial. *JAMA* **2022**, *327*, 737–747. [CrossRef]
11. Taunyane, I.C.; Benk, C.; Beyersdorf, F.; Foerster, K.; Cristina Schmitz, H.; Wittmann, K.; Mader, I.; Doostkam, S.; Heilmann, C.; Trummer, G. Preserved brain morphology after controlled automated reperfusion of the whole body following normothermic circulatory arrest time of up to 20 minutes. *Eur. J. Cardio-Thorac. Surg. Off. J. Eur. Assoc. Cardio-Thorac. Surg.* **2016**, *50*, 1025–1034. [CrossRef] [PubMed]
12. Foerster, K.; Benk, C.; Beyersdorf, F.; Cristina Schmitz, H.; Wittmann, K.; Taunyane, I.; Heilmann, C.; Trummer, G. Twenty minutes of normothermic cardiac arrest in a pig model: The role of short-term hypothermia for neurological outcome. *Perfusion* **2018**, *33*, 270–277. [CrossRef] [PubMed]
13. Freeman, W.D. Management of Intracranial Pressure. *Contin. Minneap. Minn.* **2015**, *21*, 1299–1323. [CrossRef] [PubMed]
14. Ryu, H.H.; Moore, J.C.; Yannopoulos, D.; Lick, M.; McKnite, S.; Shin, S.D.; Kim, T.Y.; Metzger, A.; Rees, J.; Tsangaris, A.; et al. The Effect of Head Up Cardiopulmonary Resuscitation on Cerebral and Systemic Hemodynamics. *Resuscitation* **2016**, *102*, 29–34. [CrossRef]

15. Moore, J.C.; Holley, J.; Segal, N.; Lick, M.C.; Labarère, J.; Frascone, R.J.; Dodd, K.W.; Robinson, A.E.; Lick, C.; Klein, L.; et al. Consistent head up cardiopulmonary resuscitation haemodynamics are observed across porcine and human cadaver translational models. *Resuscitation* **2018**, *132*, 133–139. [CrossRef]
16. Moore, J.C.; Salverda, B.; Rojas-Salvador, C.; Lick, M.; Debaty, G.; Lurie, K.G. Controlled sequential elevation of the head and thorax combined with active compression decompression cardiopulmonary resuscitation and an impedance threshold device improves neurological survival in a porcine model of cardiac arrest. *Resuscitation* **2021**, *158*, 220–227. [CrossRef]
17. Pooth, J.-S.; Brixius, S.J.; Scherer, C.; Diel, P.; Liu, Y.; Taunyane, I.C.; Damjanovic, D.; Wolkewitz, M.; Haberstroh, J.; Benk, C.; et al. Limiting calcium overload after cardiac arrest: The role of human albumin in controlled automated reperfusion of the whole body. *Perfusion* **2023**, *38*, 622–630. [CrossRef]
18. Brixius, S.J.; Pooth, J.-S.; Haberstroh, J.; Damjanovic, D.; Scherer, C.; Greiner, P.; Benk, C.; Beyersdorf, F.; Trummer, G. Beneficial Effects of Adjusted Perfusion and Defibrillation Strategies on Rhythm Control within Controlled Automated Reperfusion of the Whole Body (CARL) for Refractory Out-of-Hospital Cardiac Arrest. *J. Clin. Med.* **2022**, *11*, 2111. [CrossRef]
19. Beyersdorf, F.; Trummer, G.; Benk, C.; Pooth, J.-S. Application of cardiac surgery techniques to improve the results of cardiopulmonary resuscitation after cardiac arrest: Controlled automated reperfusion of the whole body. *JTCVS Open* **2021**, *8*, 47–52. [CrossRef]
20. Högler, S.; Sterz, F.; Sipos, W.; Schratter, A.; Weihs, W.; Holzer, M.; Janata, A.; Losert, U.; Behringer, W.; Tichy, A.; et al. Distribution of neuropathological lesions in pig brains after different durations of cardiac arrest. *Resuscitation* **2010**, *81*, 1577–1583. [CrossRef]
21. Debaty, G.; Shin, S.D.; Metzger, A.; Kim, T.; Ryu, H.H.; Rees, J.; McKnite, S.; Matsuura, T.; Lick, M.; Yannopoulos, D.; et al. Tilting for perfusion: Head-up position during cardiopulmonary resuscitation improves brain flow in a porcine model of cardiac arrest. *Resuscitation* **2015**, *87*, 38–43. [CrossRef] [PubMed]
22. Kim, T.; Shin, S.D.; Song, K.J.; Park, Y.J.; Ryu, H.H.; Debaty, G.; Lurie, K.; Hong, K.J. The effect of resuscitation position on cerebral and coronary perfusion pressure during mechanical cardiopulmonary resuscitation in porcine cardiac arrest model. *Resuscitation* **2017**, *113*, 101–107. [CrossRef] [PubMed]
23. Putzer, G.; Braun, P.; Martini, J.; Niederstätter, I.; Abram, J.; Lindner, A.K.; Neururer, S.; Mulino, M.; Glodny, B.; Helbok, R.; et al. Effects of head-up vs. supine CPR on cerebral oxygenation and cerebral metabolism—A prospective, randomized porcine study. *Resuscitation* **2018**, *128*, 51–55. [CrossRef] [PubMed]
24. Rojas-Salvador, C.; Moore, J.C.; Salverda, B.; Lick, M.; Debaty, G.; Lurie, K.G. Effect of controlled sequential elevation timing of the head and thorax during cardiopulmonary resuscitation on cerebral perfusion pressures in a porcine model of cardiac arrest. *Resuscitation* **2020**, *149*, 162–169. [CrossRef]
25. Huang, C.-C.; Chen, K.-C.; Lin, Z.-Y.; Chou, Y.-H.; Chen, W.-L.; Lee, T.-H.; Lin, K.-T.; Hsieh, P.-Y.; Chen, C.H.; Chou, C.-C.; et al. The effect of the head-up position on cardiopulmonary resuscitation: A systematic review and meta-analysis. *Crit. Care* **2021**, *25*, 376. [CrossRef] [PubMed]
26. Varney, J.; Motawea, K.R.; Mostafa, M.R.; AbdelQadir, Y.H.; Aboelenein, M.; Kandil, O.A.; Ibrahim, N.; Hashim, H.T.; Murry, K.; Jackson, G.; et al. Efficacy of heads-up CPR compared to supine CPR positions: Systematic review and meta-analysis. *Health Sci. Rep.* **2022**, *5*, e644. [CrossRef]
27. Park, Y.J.; Hong, K.J.; Shin, S.D.; Kim, T.Y.; Ro, Y.S.; Song, K.J.; Ryu, H.H. Worsened survival in the head-up tilt position cardiopulmonary resuscitation in a porcine cardiac arrest model. *Clin. Exp. Emerg. Med.* **2019**, *6*, 250–256. [CrossRef] [PubMed]
28. Nolan, J.P.; Sandroni, C.; Böttiger, B.W.; Cariou, A.; Cronberg, T.; Friberg, H.; Genbrugge, C.; Haywood, K.; Lilja, G.; Moulaert, V.R.M.; et al. European Resuscitation Council and European Society of Intensive Care Medicine guidelines 2021: Post-resuscitation care. *Intensive Care Med* **2021**, *47*, 369–421. [CrossRef]
29. Haertel, F.; Babst, J.; Bruening, C.; Bogoviku, J.; Otto, S.; Fritzenwanger, M.; Gecks, T.; Ebelt, H.; Moebius-Winkler, S.; Schulze, P.C.; et al. Effect of Hemolysis Regarding the Characterization and Prognostic Relevance of Neuron Specific Enolase (NSE) after Cardiopulmonary Resuscitation with Extracorporeal Circulation (eCPR). *J. Clin. Med.* **2023**, *12*, 3015. [CrossRef]
30. Vammen, L.; Munch Johannsen, C.; Magnussen, A.; Povlsen, A.; Riis Petersen, S.; Azizi, A.; Løfgren, B.; Andersen, L.W.; Granfeldt, A. Cardiac Arrest in Pigs with 48 hours of Post-Resuscitation Care Induced by 2 Methods of Myocardial Infarction: A Methodological Description. *J. Am. Heart Assoc.* **2021**, *10*, e022679. [CrossRef]
31. Czimmeck, C.; Kenda, M.; Aalberts, N.; Endisch, C.; Ploner, C.J.; Storm, C.; Nee, J.; Streitberger, K.J.; Leithner, C. Confounders for prognostic accuracy of neuron-specific enolase after cardiac arrest: A retrospective cohort study. *Resuscitation* **2023**, *192*, 109964. [CrossRef] [PubMed]
32. Pepe, P.E.; Scheppke, K.A.; Antevy, P.M.; Crowe, R.P.; Millstone, D.; Coyle, C.; Prusansky, C.; Garay, S.; Ellis, R.; Fowler, R.L.; et al. Confirming the Clinical Safety and Feasibility of a Bundled Methodology to Improve Cardiopulmonary Resuscitation Involving a Head-Up/Torso-Up Chest Compression Technique. *Crit. Care Med.* **2019**, *47*, 449–455. [CrossRef] [PubMed]
33. Moore, J.C.; Pepe, P.E.; Scheppke, K.A.; Lick, C.; Duval, S.; Holley, J.; Salverda, B.; Jacobs, M.; Nystrom, P.; Quinn, R.; et al. Head and thorax elevation during cardiopulmonary resuscitation using circulatory adjuncts is associated with improved survival. *Resuscitation* **2022**, *179*, 9–17. [CrossRef] [PubMed]

34. Moore, J.C.; Duval, S.; Lick, C.; Holley, J.; Scheppke, K.A.; Salverda, B.; Rojas-Salvador, C.; Jacobs, M.; Nystrom, P.; Quinn, R.; et al. Faster time to automated elevation of the head and thorax during cardiopulmonary resuscitation increases the probability of return of spontaneous circulation. *Resuscitation* **2022**, *170*, 63–69. [CrossRef]
35. Damjanovic, D.; Haberstroh, J.; Foerster, K.; Wolkewitz, M.; Taunyane, I.; Liu, Y.; Pooth, J.-S.; Fastenau, R.; Frensch, F.; Neubert, T.; et al. Beneficial effects of head-elevation during Controlled Automated Reperfusion of the WhoLe Body (CARL) in the pig model. *Resuscitation* **2018**, *130*, e35. [CrossRef]

Disclaimer/Publisher's Note: The statements, opinions and data contained in all publications are solely those of the individual author(s) and contributor(s) and not of MDPI and/or the editor(s). MDPI and/or the editor(s) disclaim responsibility for any injury to people or property resulting from any ideas, methods, instructions or products referred to in the content.

MDPI AG
Grosspeteranlage 5
4052 Basel
Switzerland
Tel.: +41 61 683 77 34

Journal of Clinical Medicine Editorial Office
E-mail: jcm@mdpi.com
www.mdpi.com/journal/jcm

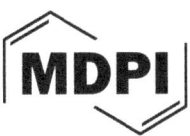

Disclaimer/Publisher's Note: The statements, opinions and data contained in all publications are solely those of the individual author(s) and contributor(s) and not of MDPI and/or the editor(s). MDPI and/or the editor(s) disclaim responsibility for any injury to people or property resulting from any ideas, methods, instructions or products referred to in the content.

www.ingramcontent.com/pod-product-compliance
Lightning Source LLC
LaVergne TN
LVHW070625100526
838202LV00012B/730